An Atlas of
Veterinary Surgery

An Atlas of

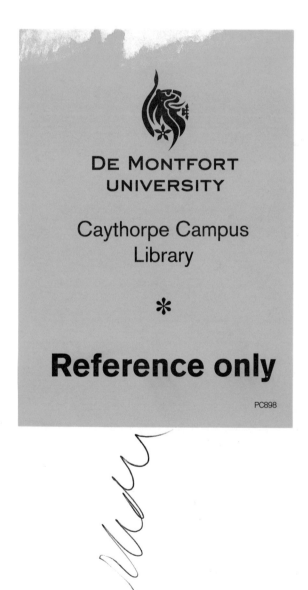

JOHN HICKMAN MA, FRCVS

FORMERLY READER IN ANIMAL SURGERY

DEPARTMENT OF CLINICAL VETERINARY MEDICINE

UNIVERSITY OF CAMBRIDGE

Veterinary Surgery

JOHN E.F. HOULTON

MA, VetMB, DSAO, DVR, MRCVS

UNIVERSITY SURGEON

DEPARTMENT OF CLINICAL VETERINARY MEDICINE

UNIVERSITY OF CAMBRIDGE

BARRIE EDWARDS

BVSc, DVetMed, FRCVS

PROFESSOR OF EQUINE STUDIES

DEPARTMENT OF VETERINARY CLINICAL SCIENCE

UNIVERSITY VETERINARY FIELD STATION

LIVERPOOL

THIRD EDITION

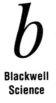

**Blackwell
Science**

© 1973, 1980, 1995 by
Blackwell Science Ltd
Editorial Offices:
Osney Mead, Oxford OX2 OEL
25 John Street, London WC1N 2BL
23 Ainslie Place, Edinburgh EH3 6AJ
238 Main Street, Cambridge
 Massachusetts 02142, USA
54 University Street, Carlton
 Victoria 3053, Australia

Other Editorial Offices:
Arnette Blackwell SA
1, rue de Lille
75007 Paris
France

Blackwell Wissenschafts-Verlag GmbH
Kurfürstendamm 57
10707 Berlin
Germany

Blackwell MZV
Feldgasse 13
A-1238 Wien
Austria

First published 1973
Italian edition 1977
Spanish edition 1977
Second edition 1980
Portuguese edition 1980
ELBS edition 1983
Third edition 1995

Set by Setrite Typesetters, Hong Kong
Printed and bound in Great Britain
at the University Press, Cambridge

DISTRIBUTORS

Marston Book Services Ltd
PO Box 87
Oxford OX2 ODT
(*Orders*: Tel: 01865 791155
 Fax: 01865 791927
 Telex: 837515)

North America
Blackwell Science, Inc.
238 Main Street
Cambridge, MA 02142
(*Orders*: Tel: 800 215-1000
 617 876-7000
 Fax: 617 492-5263)

Australia
Blackwell Science Pty Ltd
54 University Street
Carlton, Victoria 3053
(*Orders*: Tel: 03 347-0300)

A catalogue record for this title
is available from the British Library

ISBN 0−632−03268−5

Library of Congress
Cataloging-in-Publication Data

Hickman, John.
 An atlas of veterinary surgery/
John Hickman, John E.F. Houlton,
Barrie Edwards. — 3rd ed.
 p. cm.
 Includes bibliographical references
(p.) and index.
 ISBN 0−632−03268−5
 1. Veterinary surgery — Atlases.
I. Houlton, John E.F.
II. Edwards, Barrie. III. Title.
SF911.H5 1995
636.089'791 — dc20

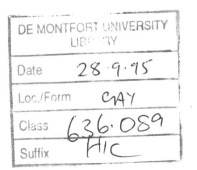

Contents

Preface to Third Edition

Since the publication of the first edition there have been many changes in operative surgery. Fundamental changes have occurred such as the development of synthetic absorbable suture materials and the refinement of anaesthetic techniques. Improved understanding of tissue healing has lead to new suture patterns being adopted and the development of new instruments, such as staple guns and arthroscopes, has changed many procedures, particularly in equine surgery.

It would be impossible to include all of these in one volume and maintain the original concept of the *Atlas*. Thus we have attempted to concentrate on the basic surgical procedures and make no apology for omitting others. A bibliography is provided from which readers can obtain information about those not included here.

The original format is largely unchanged although many new figures have been included and new procedures added. Section 10 has been considerably revised in view of the now widespread application of the AO/ASIF principles of fracture repair. The terminology has been changed to conform with that used in *Anatomica Veterinaria*, although to maintain the style of the first edition some terms in common usage have been retained.

Sadly, Robert Walker is no longer with us although his influence is still very much in evidence. I am pleased, however, to welcome my two new co-authors, happy in the knowledge that they will perpetuate Robert's ideals. These ideals are summed up by the words of Sir Robert Hutchinson who wrote 'from inability to let well alone, from too much zeal for the new and contempt for what is old, from putting knowledge before wisdom, science before art and cleverness before common sense; from treating patients as cases, and making the cure of the disease more grievous than the endurance of the same — Good Lord, deliver us'.

JOHN HICKMAN

Preface to First Edition

The best way of learning to perform an operation is to assist or watch an expert. Therefore any book on operative surgery must emphasize the visual aspects. In this book we have attempted to illustrate by line drawings and diagrams most of the standard surgical procedures employed in veterinary surgery. We have tried to describe each operation stage by stage with drawings, and have only used captions and text for clarification. No two surgeons perform an operation in exactly the same way. In consequence we have concentrated on the standard techniques that have stood the test of time and have illustrated those methods which we, through experience, have come to prefer. No attempt has been made to introduce accepted variations or operations which can only be performed in special centres.

To prevent unnecessary repetition care has been taken not to over-illustrate or to duplicate simple procedures. Some operations are difficult to illustrate satisfactorily with drawings and in these cases diagrams have been introduced. At the same time special attention has been given to the accuracy of anatomical relationships, although only the important blood vessels and nerves have been included.

The book is divided into 12 sections, each of which deals with the surgical procedures either on a regional basis or as a surgical discipline. The illustrations for each operation have been arranged in sequence with accompanying captions and explanatory text interposed.

Although this book deals essentially with the technique of individual operations we considered it would not fulfil its purpose unless the basic surgical principles, not only of each body system, but surgery in general were introduced. This latter has been dealt with in Section 1 and has been reduced to the practical measures we employ and have found adequate.

As far as possible the anatomical terminology of *Anatomy of the Domestic Animals* by Sisson and Grossman and *Anatomy of the Dog* by Miller, Christensen and Evans has been used except where common usage has demanded otherwise. A bibliography has been included at the end of the book which includes standard and more recent works to give readers an introduction into the literature, should they wish to pursue any specific aspects in more detail. Most of the orthopaedic instruments in daily use which have not been illustrated in the text will be found at the end of Section 10 — Orthopaedic Surgery.

Primarily, this book has been written for veterinary students, but it is hoped it will serve as a useful book for those engaged in general practice.

Section 1
General Surgical Principles

The success of operative surgery depends not only on an understanding of the basic principles of dividing tissues, haemostasis and wound closure but also on a well-equipped operating theatre which is maintained by a trained staff who have an organized and established routine for sterilizing instruments and for preparing and assisting at operations.

No operating theatre provides all the ideal requirements but this is no excuse for not attaining the highest possible acceptable standards of asepsis within the theatre facilities and the equipment available.

1 The types of operation vary from those carried out on normal uninfected tissues such as routine ovariohysterectomy and most orthopaedic procedures; operations on the gastro-intestinal tract, during which the intestinal contents may contaminate both instruments and the surgeon's hands;

and finally the exploration of grossly infected tissue such as infected sinuses and fistulae.

Potentially infected cases should always be kept to the end of a surgical list and particular care should be taken to avoid the transfer of infection through instruments, drapes and clothing. To this end, it is normal practice in operations that involve opening portions of the gastro-intestinal tract to make use of an additional, distinctively coloured side-towel. On this towel are placed all the instruments that are used to open and close the bowel so that they may be discarded as potentially contaminated before abdominal closure is undertaken.

2 It should be an established rule that no persons shall be permitted to enter the operating theatre without first changing into appropriate protective clothing, which should include theatre boots, cap, mask and scrub suit.

Operating theatre routine

PREPARING THE INSTRUMENT TROLLEYS

If trolleys are prepared for a series of operations it is impossible to guarantee their sterility even if they have been carefully covered and therefore instrument trolleys should be prepared immediately before the operation (Figs 1.1–1.5).

PREPARATION OF PERSONNEL

After the instrument trolley has been prepared the nurse then gets ready to assist with the operation. This involves scrubbing-up and putting on a sterile gown and gloves.

Scrubbing-up

Care must be taken when scrubbing-up to ensure the hands and forearms are cleansed thoroughly with special attention being paid to the nails and between the fingers. See Figs 1.6–1.11.

Putting on a sterile gown

As it is impossible to render the hands completely sterile by washing and scrubbing they must not come into contact with any part of the outside of the gown. See Figs 1.12–1.14.

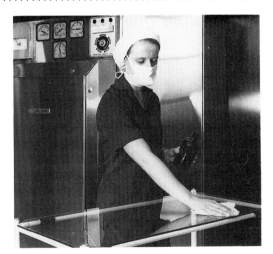

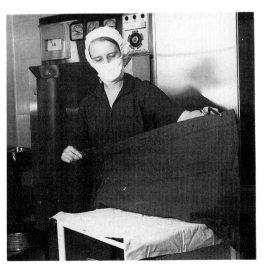

Fig. 1.1. The surface of the trolley is wiped clean with an antiseptic solution (1 per cent cetrimide BP).

Fig. 1.2. Using Cheatle forceps the trolley is first covered with a sterile impervious material and then with a sterile drape.

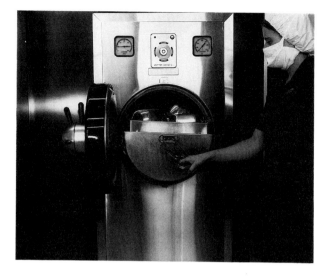

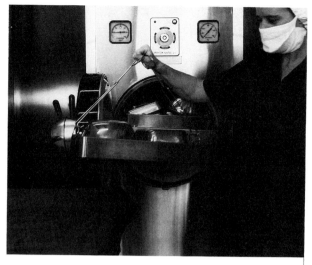

Fig. 1.3. The sterilizer is opened and the autoclave tray withdrawn.

Fig. 1.4. Instrument tray being removed from the sterilizer and placed on the draped instrument trolley.

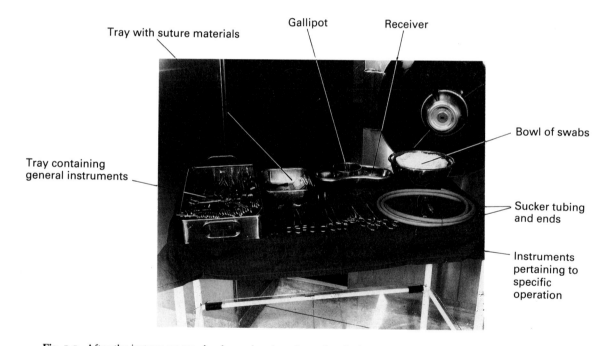

Tray with suture materials

Gallipot

Receiver

Tray containing general instruments

Bowl of swabs

Sucker tubing and ends

Instruments pertaining to specific operation

Fig. 1.5. After the instrument tray has been placed on the trolley the instruments and accessories are laid out using sterile Cheatle forceps. This figure shows a standard general instrument trolley.

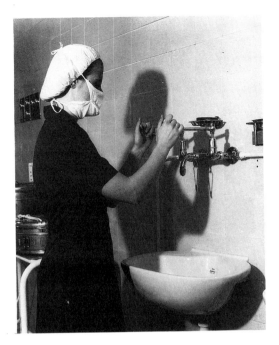

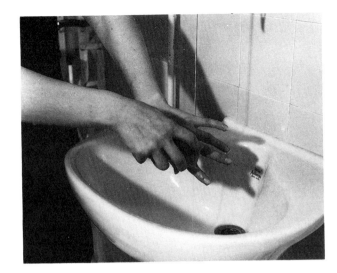

Fig. 1.7. The forearms and hands are scrubbed with a conventional nail brush and soap for not less than 3 minutes with special attention to the nails and between the fingers.

Fig. 1.6. The hot and cold water taps are adjusted to obtain a satisfactory flow of water at an agreeable temperature.

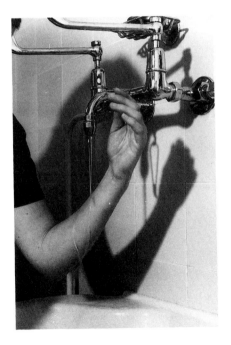

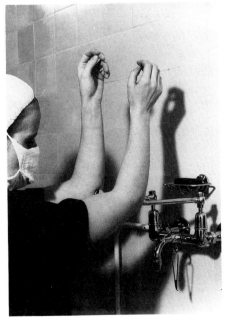

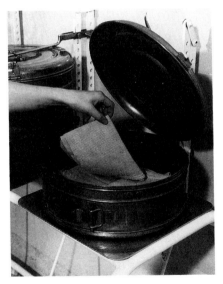

Fig. 1.10. The sterile towel for drying the hands is removed from a drum.

Fig. 1.8. The correct position of the arm when rinsing to ensure that the water flows from the hand to the elbow.

Fig. 1.9. The correct method of using the elbows to turn off the taps.

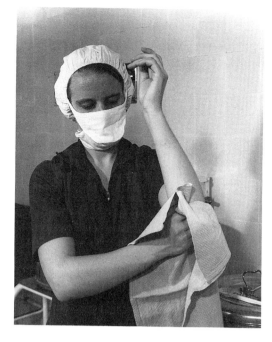

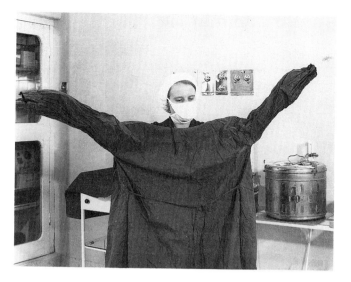

Fig. 1.13. Correct method of putting on a sterile gown: Stage 1. The arms are thrust through the sleeves and then held up to allow the gown to unravel and fall into position.

Fig. 1.11. Correct method of drying the hand and forearm. Note that the elbow is dried last.

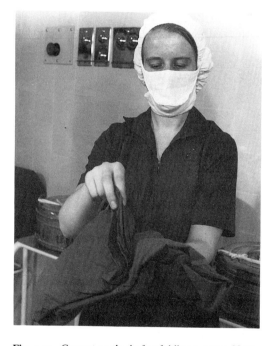

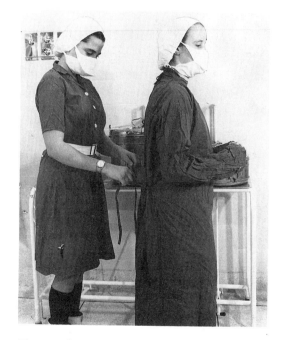

Fig. 1.12. Correct method of unfolding a gown. Note that it has been folded with the inside to the outside to prevent the outside coming into contact with the hands.

Fig. 1.14. Stage 2. Assistant adjusts the gown from behind and ties the tapes.

Putting on sterile gloves

The principle of putting on sterile gloves ensures that at no time does the hand come into contact with the outside of the gloves. The gloves in their paper envelope are lifted out of the drum and placed on a sterile towel. The envelope is then opened so that the packet of powder and each glove can be removed separately.

Open method

For method see Figs 1.15–1.17.

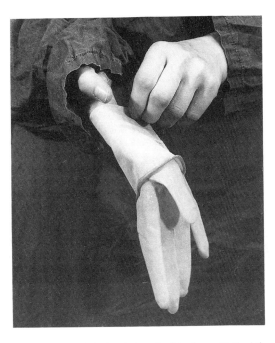

Fig. 1.15. The right-hand glove is picked up with the left hand, holding the inside of the cuff only, and the right hand inserted.

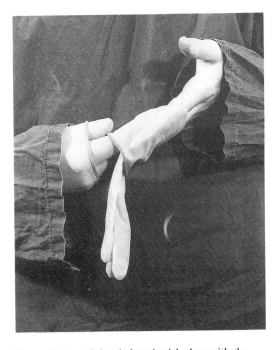

Fig. 1.16. The left-hand glove is picked up with the gloved right hand and held so that it is only in contact with the outside of the glove. The left hand is then inserted.

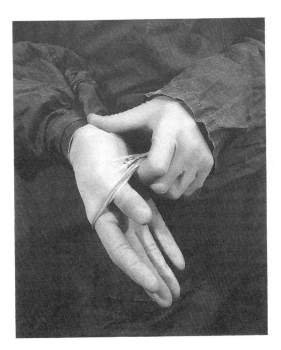

Fig. 1.17. Correct method of turning back the first cuff. The second cuff is turned back in like manner.

Closed method

The closed method (Figs 1.18–1.21) reduces the risk of contamination caused by touching the wrist while pulling the cuff of the glove over the sleeve of the gown.

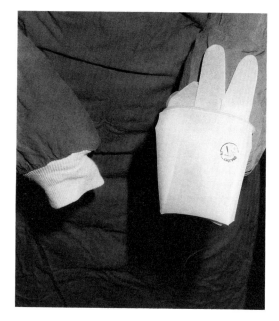

Fig. 1.18. The left hand is kept within the sleeve of the gown so that no part of the hand is exposed. The glove is grasped by the gown-covered right hand and laid along the left wrist.

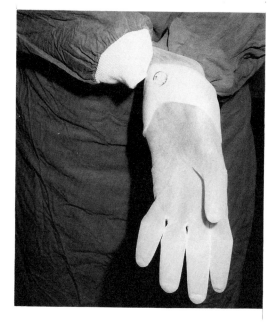

Fig. 1.19. The fingers of the left hand are worked through the end of the gown as the glove and sleeve of the gown are pulled simultaneously over the wrist. The right hand is kept within the sleeve of the gown. The left glove only comes into contact with the right-hand sleeve of the gown.

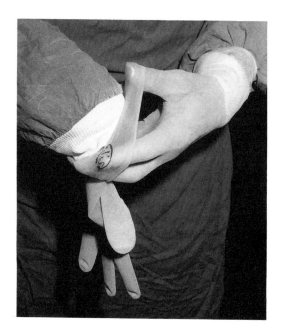

Fig. 1.20. The right-hand glove is put on in similar fashion to Fig. 1.19, keeping the fingers within the sleeve of the gown until the glove is over the wrist. The glove of the left hand only touches the outside of the right-hand glove and the sleeve of the gown.

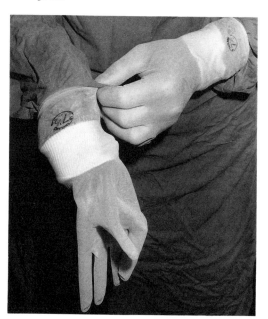

Fig. 1.21. The glove and sleeve are then pulled over the wrist.

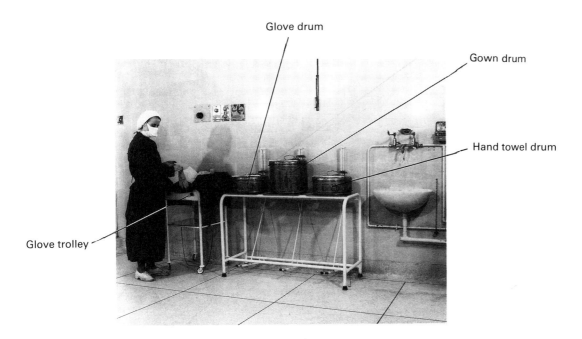

Fig. 1.22. A suitable layout of facilities to enable theatre personnel to proceed from scrubbing-up to putting on sterile gloves in an orderly and methodical manner.

PREPARING FOR THE OPERATION

The theatre nurse having prepared the instrument trolley and put on a sterile gown and gloves has next to arrange the instruments. These have to be placed so that she can most readily assist the surgeon throughout the operation.

In most cases this is best attained by laying up a Mayo table with a set of general instruments and swabs from the instrument trolley (Fig. 1.23). The Mayo table is placed over the foot of the operating table where it is accessible to both surgeon and nurse (Fig. 1.24). The instrument trolley is then left with any special instruments required for a particular operation, reserve instruments and swabs and suture materials for closure.

In addition to instruments there are certain items of operating theatre equipment which are essential if acceptable standards of surgical practice are to be attained. These include a transfusion stand, swab rack, suction machine and diathermy unit (Figs 1.25–1.27).

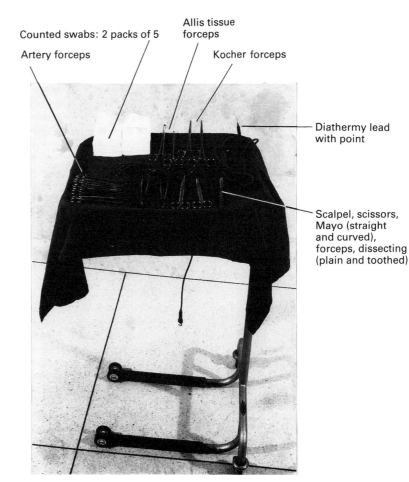

Fig. 1.23. Mayo table with instruments for immediate use.

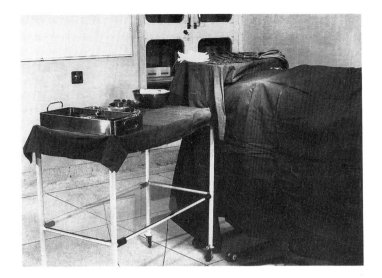

Fig. 1.24. Arrangement of instrument trolley and Mayo table in relation to the patient. The nurse stands with the instrument trolley on her left and facing the surgeon on the opposite side of the table.

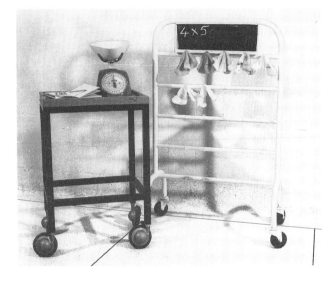

Fig. 1.25. Swab-rack. It is necessary to have a system to check the total number of swabs used during an operation. Swabs should be packed in units of five and the number of packs put out for each operation indicated on the swab-rack. Used swabs are hung upon the rack and are counted at the end of the operation. This figure subtracted from the total put out should give the number of unused swabs. Any discrepancy must be accounted for before the incision is closed.

In addition, blood lost during surgery can be easily estimated by weighing each pack of swabs and each swab used. This information is essential if the blood loss is to be accurately assessed.

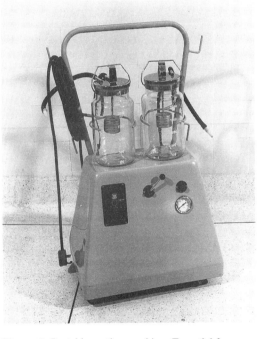

Fig. 1.26. Portable suction machine. Essential for aspirating fluid from the abdominal or thoracic cavities, nasopharynx, trachea and bronchi. It is important to ensure that the tubing is in good condition, without punctures and of adequate bore to prevent blockage or collapse.

These machines have a spark-free switching mechanism and a flame-proof motor. They are all basically of the same design. The pump creates a vacuum in the glass suction bottle into which the aspirated fluid collects. Incorporated into the cap of the suction bottles are internal connections to the pump unit and external connections for the suction tubing. It is advisable to select a unit to which two suction tubes can be connected, one for use by the surgeon and the other for the anaesthetist.

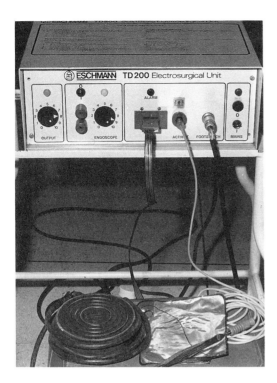

Fig. 1.27. Surgical diathermy unit. A surgical diathermy machine produces a high frequency alternating current ranging between 500 kilocycles and 5 megacycles. When this current is passed through the body from a large neutral or indifferent electrode to a small active electrode there is an intense concentration of current under the small active electrode. This produces a destructive heat effect which results in the coagulation or disruption of the tissues immediately under the active electrode.

The local effect depends on the waveform. An interrupted waveform results in the coagulation of tissues and therefore is used to seal blood vessels and avoids the need to ligate them. A continuous waveform produces a destructive effect on the tissues and is used for cutting.

A variety of active electrodes are available which range from long needles for coagulation to small blades for cutting. These electrodes fit into an insulated handle which has a standard socket to enable electrodes to be easily changed during an operation.

It is necessary to complete the electrical circuit back to the machine after the current has passed through the patient. This is achieved by a second large neutral or indifferent electrode and conductive gel.

When using a surgical diathermy machine care must be taken to prevent burns of the patient. These can occur if the indifferent electrode becomes dry or any exposed part of the patient comes in contact with any metal parts of the operating table or accessories. Also the possibility of explosions exist if anaesthetics such as ether or cyclopropane are being administered.

Preparing the patient

Care must be taken to bring the patient to the operation table in the best possible state to withstand both the anaesthetic and the surgical procedures. To this end attention must be directed to premedication to overcome fear and anxiety, to ensuring that the circulating body fluids are within normal limits and that the operation site has been rendered aseptic.

Prolonged starvation or depriving the patient of fluids is not recommended. In the dog, food need not be withheld for more than 2 or 3 hours prior to surgery even for operations on the gastro-intestinal tract. In the horse a bran mash should be given the evening prior to surgery, after which it must be muzzled but an opportunity to drink to within 3 hours of operation is permissible. In premedicated operations on ruminants water should be withheld for at least 6 hours and green foodstuffs and other easily fermentable food for at least 24 hours before anaesthesia.

PRE-OPERATIVE FLUID THERAPY

Many disease conditions give rise to abnormal losses of fluid and electrolytes from the body. These losses are due either to diarrhoea and vomiting or to interference with the normal circulation of fluid and electrolytes within the body as occurs in cases of intestinal obstruction.

Such losses initially cause a reduction of the extracellular fluid volume and are borne by the interstitial fluid, but if the losses continue they lead to reduction in the circulating blood volume, to impaired renal function, and to changes in the acid–base balance of the body. The body responds to a diminished circulating blood volume in the early stages by selective vaso-constriction. As this is likely to be inhibited by the induction of general anaesthesia it is important to assess fluid and electrolyte deficits so that they may be replaced before surgery is undertaken.

Fluid therapy should always be given by the intravenous route and preferably into the jugular vein. The use of the jugular vein allows the patient to move about with relative freedom without danger of obstructing the drip flow, and also enables measurements to be taken of the central venous pressure. Modern disposable equipment makes intravenous therapy a comparatively simple undertaking, and the use of pliable intravenous cannulae overcomes many of the difficulties that used to be associated with long-term intravenous therapy in animals. The carefully tapered end of all plastic cannulae is easily damaged and splayed, in which state it can inflict serious damage to the endothelium of the vein. In all cases, therefore, a small skin incision must first be made under local anaesthesia at the proposed site of venepuncture so that the needle and plastic cannula (Fig. 1.28) have to penetrate the minimum of tissue before puncturing the vein wall. Jugular venepuncture is greatly simplified if the dog is restrained on its side, and a small sandbag is placed under its neck.

Estimation of fluid loss

The clinical examination of a dehydrated animal will show the characteristic signs of venous engorgement of the conjunctiva, dry mucous membranes and a dry inelastic skin, but various other methods are available which enable the extent of the fluid loss to be more accurately assessed:

1 The haematocrit or packed cell volume will be increased in cases of dehydration.

2 Plasma protein levels will be raised. This estimation tends to be more helpful than the haematocrit which may be misleading in cases of established anaemia.

3 Blood urea levels are raised when haemoconcentration leads to poor renal perfusion, but they are also raised in cases of primary renal dysfunction.

4 Urinary output is naturally reduced when renal perfusion is poor. A measured increase of the urinary output is of value in order to assess the efficacy of rehydration. Repeated catheterization of the bladder is undesirable owing to the risk of introducing infection, and use should be made of an indwelling catheter (Fig. 1.29). Urine may then be continuously collected by attaching a plastic bag to the catheter, or the catheter may be blocked by an obturator, and urine collected at regular intervals. In the male, a polythene catheter is inserted into the bladder, fixed by means of a stitch through the corpus cavernosum of the penis, and then cut off so that 1 cm of catheter protrudes from the end of the penis. The end of the catheter will thus lie within the prepucial orifice and will not be interfered with by the patient.

5 Monitoring the central venous pressure (CVP). Measurement of the CVP is a valuable indication of both the fluid deficit and of the amount of fluid that may safely be given to rectify that deficit. It is thus a dynamic guide to the blood volume in relation to the pumping ability of the heart.

A suitable flexible cannula is inserted into the jugular vein, so that its tip lies adjacent to the right atrium. The cannula is attached by one limb of a

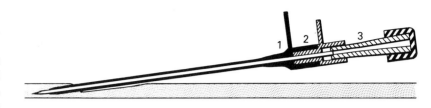

Fig. 1.28. Plastic trochar and cannula for short-term intravenous infusion, consisting of (1) plastic cannula, (2) needle, and (3) obturator with rubber diaphragm. The assembled cannula is inserted into the vein and the needle and obturator are withdrawn. The cannula is fixed in position by means of a skin stitch.

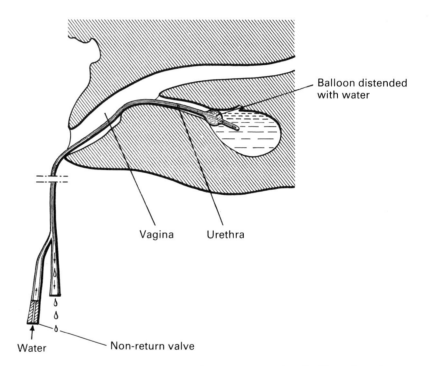

Fig. 1.29. The Foley self-retaining catheter for use in the female. The catheter is inserted and the small balloon inflated by water injected into the non-return valve.

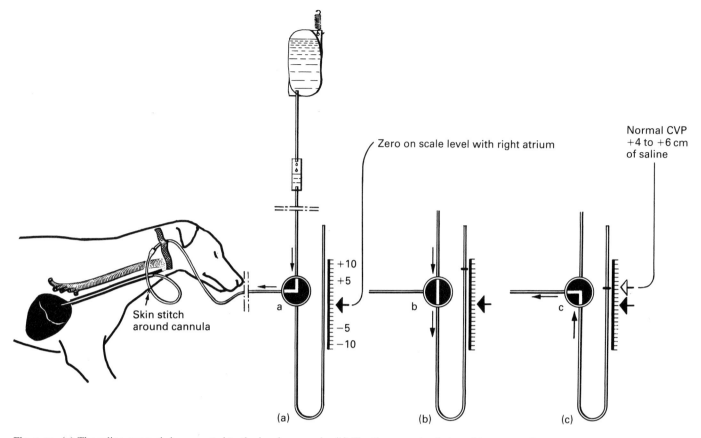

Fig. 1.30. (a) The saline reservoir is connected to the jugular cannula. (b) The three-way tap is turned to connect the saline reservoir to the manometer tubing, which is filled to some 10–12 cm above the zero mark on the scale. (c) The manometer is connected to the jugular cannula. The saline level will drop until it approximates in pressure to the blood in the right atrium, at which level it will oscillate up and down in time with respiration.

Normal CVP in the dog is between +4 and +6 cm of saline. A negative CVP is invariably an indication of severe hypovolaemia. In these circumstances, fluid may be run into the patient until a normal CVP is established. Care must be taken in cases where the CVP is higher than normal, as this is an indication of right-sided heart failure.

three-way tap to a bag of saline, and by the other limb to a piece of open ended, flexible transparent drip tubing of at least 120 cm in length. This must dip well below the level of the patient so that it provides a reservoir of saline sufficient to prevent air being aspirated into the jugular vein. A length of at least 45 cm of this open-ended tubing is strapped to the giving-set stand alongside a centimetre scale, which is adjusted with the zero mark on a level with the patient's right atrium. Once this tubing is filled with saline and is connected to the jugular cannula, it acts as a simple saline manometer, giving a direct reading of the pressure of venous blood in the right atrium (Fig. 1.30).

Control of haemorrhage

It is ideal to perform an operation in a bloodless field. In the majority of cases this is not possible and haemorrhage has to be dealt with as the operation proceeds. Major haemorrhage can be avoided by following lines of cleavage to avoid blood vessels and by isolating and ligating large blood vessels, but the innumerable small blood vessels which are unavoidably severed have to be picked up with artery forceps and either tied off or sealed by diathermy.

A tourniquet can be used to produce a bloodless field for operations on the limbs (Figs 1.31–1.33). Before applying a tourniquet the limb is exsanguinated by means of a rubber bandage applied from the foot to the level of the tourniquet.

A tourniquet correctly applied will compress the vessels sufficiently just to stop the arterial flow. If excessive pressure is used or if a tourniquet is left on an exsanguinated limb for more than 1 hour the ischaemia may result in damage to muscle and nerve fibres.

When a tourniquet is used to produce a bloodless field it is important that, as far as possible, all large

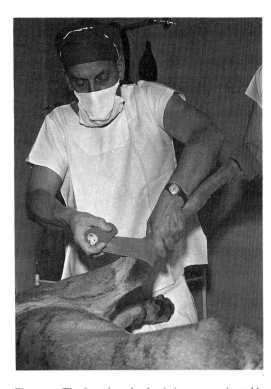

Fig. 1.31. The front leg of a dog being exsanguinated by applying a rubber bandage from the extremity.

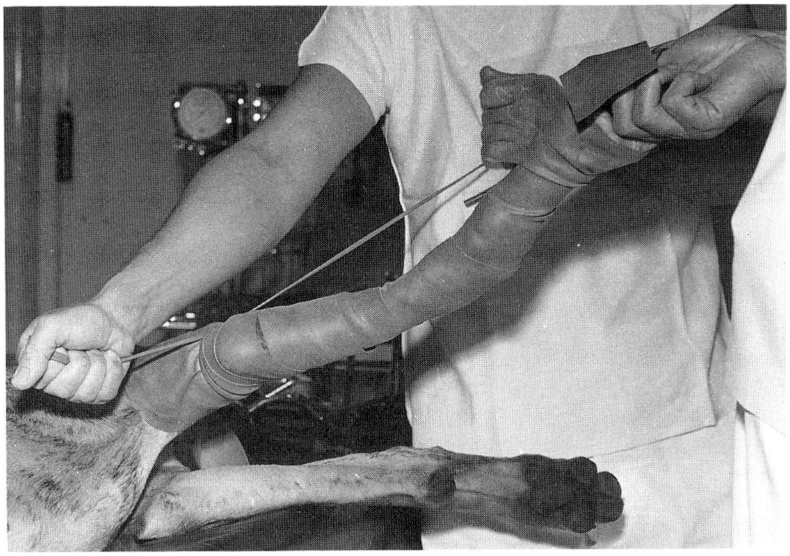

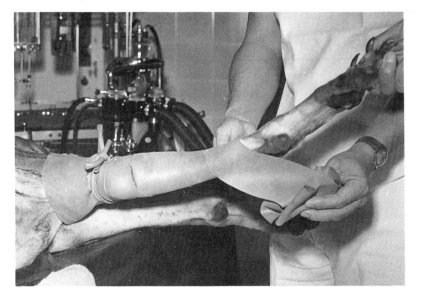

Fig. 1.32. A length of rubber tubing is used as a tourniquet and tied above the elbow. In the hind leg it is tied above the stifle joint.

blood vessels are conserved, but if severed they must be ligated. Many small vessels will be severed and when the tourniquet is released considerable haemorrhage will occur. This haemorrhage may be prevented either by releasing the tourniquet and picking up the blood vessels before closure or controlled by applying a pad and pressure bandage before releasing the tourniquet. The latter method saves time and although inevitably there is some haemorrhage it is of little consequence.

PREPARING THE OPERATION AREA

The principle of aseptic surgery aims at preventing bacteria from contaminating the operation area. Theoretically it is possible to operate in a sterile atmosphere, with sterile instruments and the site surrounded by sterile drapes, but the skin itself is impossible to sterilize completely.

Normal healthy skin produces enzymes which destroy most pathogenic organisms on its surface and the organisms present in the hair follicles, sebaceous and sweat glands are generally non-pathogenic. Unfortunately the pathogens are destroyed but slowly and many are located in hairy, dirty and greasy areas which are inaccessible to the enzymes. Therefore the skin preparation is based

Fig. 1.33. The rubber bandage is unravelled from the extremity to expose the operation site.

on removing the hair and dirt which protects the bacteria from the enzymes and then sterilizing the skin by the application of an antiseptic.

In elective procedures the first pre-surgical skin preparation is performed in the kennel or loose-box and consists of clipping the hair and washing the site clean with a cationic detergent and bacteri-cide such as 1 per cent chlorhexidine (Fig. 1.34). If an open or contaminated wound is present it must be thoroughly cleaned under anaesthesia before

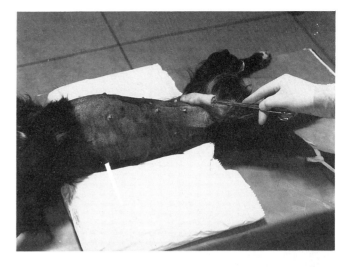

Fig. 1.34. (*Right*) Dog positioned for a laparotomy. The clipped operation area is painted with an antibacterial agent (2 per cent iodine or 1 per cent chlorhexidine gluconate in spirit) using a swab held in sponge-holding forceps. The area painted must be much larger than that required for the purpose of the operation. The application should commence at the site of the incision and continue in ever widening squares until the area is covered. After the first application has dried a second application is made using a fresh swab.

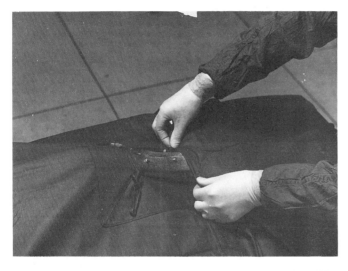

Fig. 1.35. A laparotomy sheet with a rectangular window in the middle is draped over the patient. The window is positioned over the site of incision and the proximal edge held in position with towel clips. The distal edge is folded over to reduce the area of skin exposed to the minimum required.

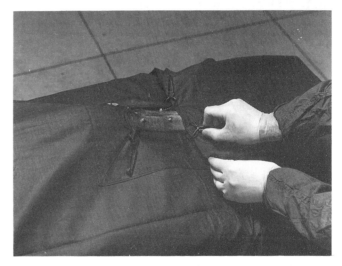

Fig. 1.36. The edge of the window is folded over and retained in position with towel clips.

the patient is brought into the operating theatre. Sterile isotonic saline or lactated Ringer's solution are good wound irrigants.

It is no longer considered necessary to cover the area with sterile material and make the incision through it or to clip drapes to the edge of the skin incision. Satisfactory asepsis is obtained by protecting the area with sterile drapes but obviously leaving the minimum of skin exposed (Figs 1.35–1.36).

Surgical approach

INCISION

An incision is fundamental to all surgical procedures. Surgical incisions (Figs 1.37–1.38) must be of adequate length. The length of the incision does not bear any relationship to healing time.

DISSECTION

To expose tissue it is necessary to separate anatomical structures by either sharp or blunt dissection (Figs 1.39–1.41). Sharp dissection with a scalpel results in less damage to tissues than so-called

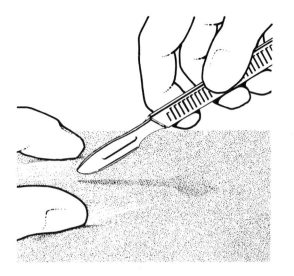

Fig. 1.37. The skin is tensed by the operator using the index finger and thumb of the left hand as stretcher and presser. The scalpel is held with the handle resting in the palm of the hand and with the blade at an angle of about 30° to the skin. The incision is made at right angles to the surface of the skin, which only requires light pressure to divide it.

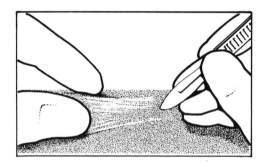

Fig. 1.38. To make a 'stab' or 'puncture' incision, the side of the scalpel blade is held against the middle finger which acts as a stop. The length of blade thus exposed controls the maximum depth of the incision.

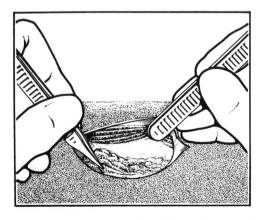

Fig. 1.39. The handle of a scalpel being used to separate tissues by blunt dissection.

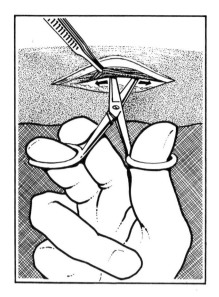

Fig. 1.40. A line of cleavage is found by inserting and then opening the blades of a pair of scissors or artery forceps.

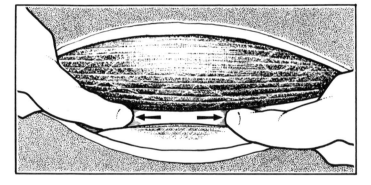

Fig. 1.41. Two large muscles can be separated or their line of cleavage established by placing the index finger of each hand together, thrusting them between the muscles and then drawing them apart.

blunt dissection which is used to separate connective tissue planes and to avoid damage to blood vessels and nerves.

INSTRUMENTS FOR INCISION AND DISSECTION

Scalpels

These are probably the oldest instruments in surgery and are used for incision, dissection and excision (Fig. 1.42). There is a great variety of scalpels, many of which are designed for special purposes, and they include cartilage knives, tenotomy knives, and bistouries which are used for laying open sinuses and fistulae.

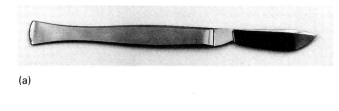

(a)

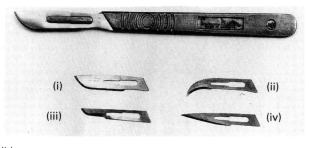

(i) (ii)

(iii) (iv)

(b)

Fig. 1.42. (a) Standard solid or forged scalpel. The dorsal edge of the blade is straight, passing to a point with the cutting edge on the ventral aspect which is rounded or 'bellied' to different degrees. They are manufactured in sizes from 1 to 6, the blade lengths varying from 2.5 to 6.5 cm. (b) Scalpel handle with detachable blade. There are six sizes of scalpel handle and a large selection of blades of different shapes and sizes. They have almost replaced the solid scalpel as the blades are sharp and the minimum of labour is required for their upkeep. (i) Small general purpose blade, (ii) blade for opening abscesses, (iii) blade for fine dissection, and (iv) tenotomy blade.

Scissors

There is a large variety of shapes and sizes of scissors. Scissors may have both points sharp, both blunt or one sharp and one blunt. Scissors can be used as an alternative to a scalpel for cutting and dissection. Often they are safer than a scalpel in deep wounds and for opening the peritoneum. Mayo scissors (Fig. 1.43) are the most useful for general purposes and the curved on flat variety are especially useful for dissecting close to a rounded mass. Metzenbaum scissors are preferred for fine dissection as they have smaller blades.

Dissecting forceps

These forceps, as the name implies, enable the surgeon to grip and hold tissues when dissecting. A number of varieties is available and their suitability depends on the type of tissue to be held (Fig. 1.44).

HAEMOSTASIS

The methods of controlling haemorrhage are either by direct pressure, or by picking up the vessel with forceps and tying it off with fine suture material (Fig. 1.45) or by sealing it by diathermy (Fig. 1.46).

Transfixing ligature

The best method of preventing a ligature from slipping is to pass the material through the tissue and tie it before completing the ligature around the tissue mass (Fig. 1.47). This technique is useful when it is impossible to isolate a large vessel from

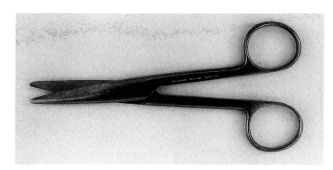

(a)

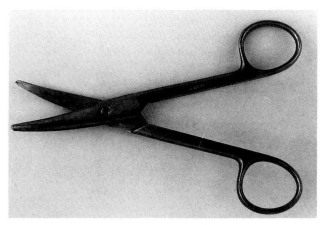

(b)

Fig. 1.43. (a) Mayo's straight scissors, and (b) Mayo's curved on flat scissors.

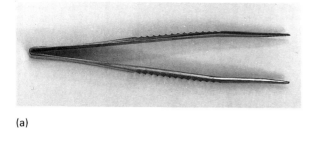

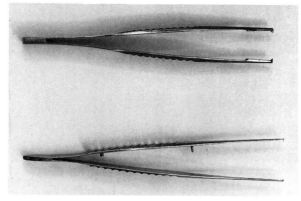

(a)

(b)

Fig. 1.44. (a) Dissecting forceps — serrated jaws used for holding soft tissue, blood vessels and nerves and hollow organs such as stomach, intestine and the bladder. (b) Dissecting forceps — toothed forceps with strong teeth required for holding skin and fascia and for slippery tissue such as fat and glands. Forceps with fine teeth are required for dissecting delicate structures.

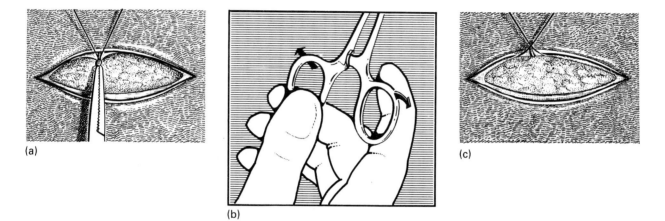

(a)

(b)

(c)

Fig. 1.45. Tying-off a blood vessel. (a) The bleeding point is clamped with artery forceps and 'tied-off' either immediately or at the termination of the operation. The forceps are held almost horizontal to assist the surgeon to tie the first throw of a ligature around the vessel or clamped tissue. (b) One-hand method employed by the assistant to release the artery forceps. (c) As the forceps are released the surgeon maintains tension on the suture and completes a reef knot. The surplus length of suture is cut off a short distance from the ligature.

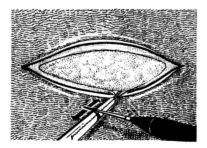

Fig. 1.46. Diathermy. The vessel is picked up with artery forceps which are touched by a diathermy needle, which results in occlusion of the vessel.

its surrounding tissues or when occluding a uterine stump or hernia sac.

Instruments for controlling haemorrhage

Artery forceps are designed for preventing and arresting haemorrhage at operation (Fig. 1.48). Either the vessel alone or the piece of tissue containing the bleeding point is clamped. Their action is to exert pressure on the vessel and compress its walls together.

WOUND CLOSURE

A surgical incision inflicts the minimum of trauma to the wound edges. If these cut edges are held

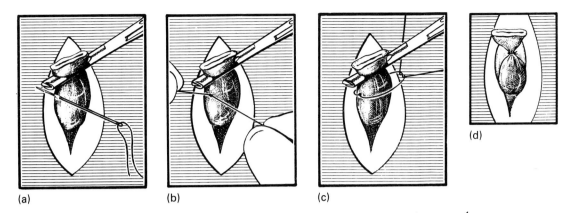

Fig. 1.47. (a) Using a needle the ligature material is passed through the edge of the tissue. (b) The ligature material is tied and held in position with a single knot. (c) Both ends of the ligature material are passed round the tissues and tied opposite the first knot. (d) As the forceps are removed the knot is pulled tight and completed with a second knot so that the ligature lies in the crushed tissues.

securely together with sutures, union will occur in between 7 and 10 days and the end result will be a thin line of scar tissue which will be almost obliterated with the passage of time.

To achieve this result an inert suture material of sufficient strength is used to keep the edges of the wound immobilized and in apposition until healing is established. It has to be attached to the type of needle which is most easily passed through the tissues causing the least damage. The correct material has to be selected in relation to the type of wound, to the tissues being co-apted and to the degree of tissue tension. Finally the suture has to be tied with a secure knot.

SUTURE AND LIGATURE MATERIALS

In the past the selection of surgical sutures was based largely on the physical characteristics of the material itself. In making a rational choice from the ever-widening array of products available today, however, one should also take into consideration the biological interaction of the suture material and the tissue, which can alter the mechanical properties of the suture and the physical properties of the wound.

Based on *in vivo* measurements of material degradation, sutures can be placed into two classifications, absorbable and non-absorbable. Sutures that undergo rapid degradation in tissues and lose tensile strength within 60 days are considered absorbable. Those maintaining tensile strength for longer than 60 days are referred to as non-absorbable.

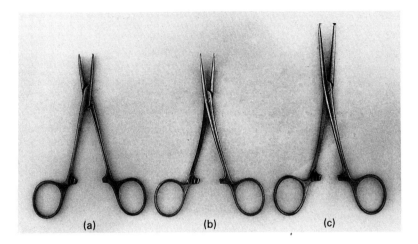

Fig. 1.48. (a) Spencer Wells artery forceps are the standard artery forceps in general use. The jaws are designed with transverse serrations to provide a firm hold and the arms have a double ratchet catch. (b) Dunhill artery forceps. Similar to the Spencer Wells type but curved on flat. (c) Kocher's artery forceps. They have teeth and are especially useful for seizing blood vessels which have retracted into tough fibrous tissue.

Absorbable sutures

Currently five types of absorbable sutures are commercially available.

Surgical gut

Surgical gut is substantially pure collagen and is prepared from the submucous layer of the intestine of lambs. It is available in plain and chromic forms.

Plain catgut evokes a severe sterile pyogenic reaction in tissues and within 3 days rapidly loses its tensile strength. Therefore it should not be used when the tissue layers are under tension. It is seldom used except in plastic surgery and for ligating small blood vessels.

Chromic catgut is produced by hardening strands of plain catgut by immersion in a chromic salt solution thereby decreasing its tissue reactivity, while increasing its resistance to digestion and its tensile strength. It is classified by the duration of its effective tensile strength in tissues. The absorption period is given in days (i.e. 10-day, 20-day, but the most popular for all general purposes is the medium or 15–20-day variety). It is used to ligate blood vessels, co-apt muscle and fascia and for suturing peritoneum, stomach, intestines and bladder. When used for these latter purposes, it is customary for it to be mounted on an atraumatic needle.

Collagen sutures

Collagen sutures, which are derived from the long flexor tendons of steers, are similar to catgut with regard to tissue reaction, tensile strength and histological profile. They are only made in fine sizes.

Synthetic absorbable sutures

Synthetic absorbable sutures were introduced to reduce the variability in absorption and subsequent loss of tensile strength associated with natural products.

Polyglycolic acid and polyglactin 910

The synthetic absorbable sutures polyglycolic acid (Dexon) and polyglactin 910 (Vicryl) have largely replaced catgut. They are made from braided filaments of polymerized glycolic acid (Dexon) or glycolic acid and lactic acid (Vicryl). The materials resemble dry silk in texture and maintain their tensile strength in the presence of both normal and infected body fluids. They are degraded in the body in an orderly manner by hydrolysis. This markedly reduces the inflammatory process compared with that associated with enzymatic absorption of catgut. Because neither of these suture materials contains protein they are non-antigenic. The breaking strength of polyglycolic acid and polyglactin 910 diminishes more or less in a straight line compared with the almost exponential decline of the strength of catgut in tissues. Their more consistent and reliable disappearance pattern gives them a major advantage over catgut.

Inherent disadvantages of these materials are poor knot security and a tendency to drag through tissue and to cut soft organs. It is necessary, therefore, to use a surgeon's knot with multiple throws to overcome the low coefficient of friction and prevent slippage. In order to make the sutures smoother, to decrease pulling, and to improve overall handling the manufacturers have coated them with an absorbable lubricant.

Polydioxanone

Polydioxanone (PDS) is a monofilament, synthetic absorbable suture which retains its strength in tissue twice as long as other synthetic absorbable materials, thereby providing extended wound support. It is absorbed by slow hydrolysis and is completely removed within 6 months. The material is easily handled and has good knot security.

Non-absorbable sutures

The non-absorbable suture materials are characterized by their tensile strength and ease of manipulation. These features enable them to hold tissues together until a stable union is established. In the past it was generally accepted that non-absorbable materials were only used when the sutures were to be removed. This is no longer necessary as many of them are inert in tissues and can be left indefinitely. The sutures constitute only small inert foreign bodies which are zoned off by fibrous tissue.

Silk

Obtainable as either twisted or plaited gossamer strands. It has a high tensile strength, handles easily and knots well. It requires meticulous sterilization as bacteria tend to lodge in the strands. Its chief disadvantages are the tissue reaction it provokes and its tendency to perpetuate any minor wound infection as a foreign body giving rise to a sinus which persists until the stitch is removed. In spite of these disadvantages it is common practice to use silk, serum-proofed in order to reduce capillary attraction, in sizes ranging from 0.7 to 2.0 metric for nerve anastomosis and in vascular and ophthalmic surgery.

Nylon

Monofilament nylon has a high tensile strength, smooth surface, uniform texture and calibre, and is relatively inert and unabsorbable. It is non-capillary and therefore an ideal material for skin sutures. Its chief disadvantage is that it tends to break and knots tied with it tend to slip unless they are double tied and the ends left relatively long. If it is used as a buried suture the sharp ends may irritate the tissues and provoke a tissue reaction.

Braided nylon is made up of a large number of very fine nylon threads spun and braided together. It is of high tensile strength, is flexible, easy to handle and produces a stable knot. It tends to provoke some tissue reaction and therefore should not be left as a buried suture. Its best use is as an alternative to monofilament nylon for skin sutures when the tissues are under tension.

Polypropylene

Polypropylene (Prolene) is available in monofilament form. It has greater knot security than nylon due to its ability to deform and flatten when tied. Nevertheless multiple knots are required to ensure knot security. Polypropylene is one of the most inert and non-reactive suture materials and loses very little strength *in situ* over a 2-year period. It is more suitable for use in infected wounds than the braided synthetic materials.

Polyesters

Uncoated polyester (Mersilene). Polyester fibre suture, which is also a polymer, is available as a braided strand. It has excellent tensile strength and causes minimal tissue reaction. Because of the multifilament nature of the polyester sutures, bacteria and tissue fluids can penetrate their interstices producing a nidus for infection. Consequently, they must only be used under aseptic conditions.

Coated polyester (Ethibond). Coating the suture with polybutylate decreases the capillary action and tissue drag but also results in reduced knot-holding ability.

Multifilament polyamide

Multifilament polyamide polymer encased in a tubular outer sheath (Vetafil, Supramid) has high tensile strength and causes little cellular reaction in tissues. It behaves like a monofilament suture provided the outer sheath is not damaged. It is packaged in plastic dispensers in which it is chemically sterilized. It is suitable for skin closure but should only be buried under strict aseptic conditions.

Metal wire

Suture wire is prepared from either stainless steel or tantalum. It is available in monofilament or twisted (multifilament) forms. The latter is more flexible and is less likely to kink, but both are difficult to handle and have a tendency to cut tissues as well as surgeons' gloves. However, it is the strongest of all suture materials and one of the most unreactive. Unlike the braided synthetics, stainless steel does not harbour bacteria and can be used in the presence of infection.

SUTURE NEEDLES

Suture needles are classified according to their shape and cross-section. They may be straight, curved, half-curved or circular and on cross-section either round or triangular (Fig. 1.49).

The design of the needle selected depends on the site of the operation and the type of tissues to be co-apted. It should be as small in calibre as the suture material will permit and in general a straight needle is preferable to a curved one as it is easier to handle and to anticipate where the point will emerge.

It is customary to thread monofilament nylon twice through the eye of a needle to prevent the end from pulling out. This procedure results in a large knot which damages delicate tissues, but it can be overcome by threading the material only once or by using an eyeless atraumatic needle to which the suture is swaged. Eyeless needles are advisable for all gastro-intestinal, cardiovascular and ophthalmic surgery.

Round-bodied needles

These needles should always be used except where resistance to tissues demands a cutting point for easy penetration. They do not cut tissues and cause only the minimum of trauma. They are used in particular for thin membranes which tear easily such as the peritoneum and for the wall of the gastro-intestinal tract, bladder, mucous membranes and fat.

Cutting needles

The conventional cutting needle is triangular in cross-section and has two opposing cutting edges with the third on the inside curvature of the needle. For particularly tough tissues which are difficult to penetrate a reverse cutting needle is used. This also has two opposing cutting edges but with the

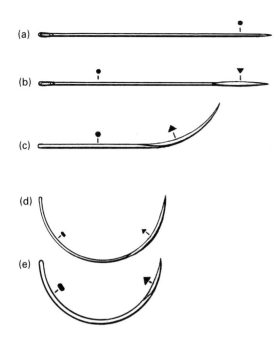

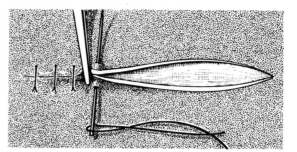

Fig. 1.50. Skin incision being closed with interrupted sutures. To ensure accurate apposition of the skin edges they are held together with dissecting forceps and the straight cutting needle is passed through both edges with a single thrust. Note that the knots have been pulled to one side away from the edge of the incision. Properly inserted interrupted sutures give good apposition and holding power.

Fig. 1.49. Types of suture needles recommended for general surgery, with cross-sections shown above each. (a) Round-bodied straight needle. Used for delicate tissues which easily tear such as the peritoneum, mucous membranes and liver. (b) Cutting needle, straight. Used on strong tissues which are not easily damaged such as skin, fascia and tendon. (c) Cutting needle, half-curved. One half of the needle is straight and the other half is curved, so that the point lies at 45° from the needle eye line. This needle is particularly useful for penetrating thick and tough tissue such as the skin of farm animals. (d) Cutting needle, half-circle. This needle allows the point to cut into tissue at almost 180° from the direction of the eye. Used on all strong tissues in the depth of wounds. The round-bodied half-circle needle is very popular for gastro-intestinal surgery. (e) Mayo needle. A very strong half-circle needle with a cutting point and a large square eye. A most satisfactory needle for penetrating tough tissues and especially when stitching in depth and when excessive leverage is required.

third cutting edge on the outer curvature of the needle. These needles cut a tract through the tissues and leave sharp angles which under tension can easily be converted into a tear.

METHODS OF SUTURING

When tissues are divided they must be held together until normal healing has taken place. There are various and elaborate methods of suturing but it must not be overlooked that the purpose of suturing is to hold the tissues together in the optimum position for healing and this should be achieved by the simplest methods and by using the minimum amount of suture material.

Absence of undue tension is an essential pre-

requisite to perfection in suturing and sutures should only be pulled sufficiently tight to bring the edges of the wound into perfect apposition and to control bleeding. If tension is excessive the sutures may cut through or give rise to areas of ischaemic tissue which contribute to wound breakdown.

Simple or interrupted sutures

The commonest suture in general use (Fig. 1.50). A needle, with suture material attached, is passed through the borders of the tissue. This single loop of suture is then tied. The distance that the needle is inserted from the edge of the tissue and the distance between the sutures is a matter for individual judgement but must be related to the size of the wound and the tension of the tissues. The bite from the cut edge and the space between sutures should not be less than the thickness of the tissue being sutured.

Continuous suture

Formed by passing a needle through the divided tissues, securing the first stitch with a knot and then continually passing and repassing the needle and suture through the whole length of the wound, finally securing the suture with a second knot (Fig. 1.51). This suture saves time but must not be pulled too tight as it results in ischaemia of the tissue's edge and should it break then the whole wound may disrupt.

Mattress suture, horizontal

This is an interrupted suture made by passing a

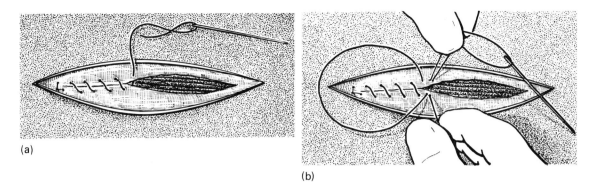

(a)

(b)

Fig. 1.51. (a) Muscle fascia being co-apted with a continuous suture. (b) Method of tying the second knot.

needle through the wound edges as for a simple interrupted suture and then recrossing so as to form a loop at one side and two free ends on the other, which are then tied (Fig. 1.52).

Mattress suture, vertical

This suture is used to close skin incisions. It takes a double bite of the skin, one very near the skin edge and the other some distance away (Fig. 1.53). It combines good apposition and strength when compared with the simple suture.

Inversion suture

This suture is designed to invert the wound edge, and was commonly used in gastro-intestinal surgery. Healing of the apposed peritoneal surfaces is very rapid and prevents leakage from the gastro-intestinal tract. Similar sutures are used to close the uterus following Caesarean section. Inversion sutures may be interrupted or continuous. They must penetrate the submucosa, but preferably should not penetrate the mucous membrane (Fig. 1.54).

Removing sutures

Skin sutures should not be removed for at least 7–9 days after operation by which time a firm union should be established. Any individual sutures that become loose or cut into the tissue causing irritation must be removed forthwith. The common practice of gradually removing sutures over 2 or 3 days commencing on the 7th day has much to commend it.

To remove a suture one end should be picked up with dissecting forceps and tensed, thus allowing one blade of the scissors (Fig. 1.55) to be passed under the loop which is cut close to the skin. This

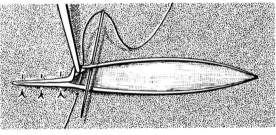

Fig. 1.52. Skin incision being closed with a horizontal mattress suture. This suture tends to evert the skin edges, especially if pulled too tight. It is a good suture for tissues under tension and for friable tissues, such as the liver, as it does not cut through like a simple suture.

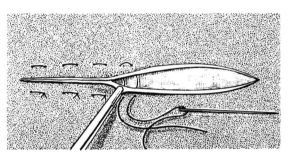

(a)

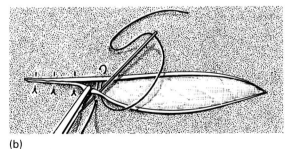

(b)

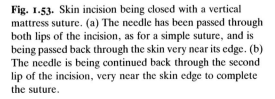

Fig. 1.53. Skin incision being closed with a vertical mattress suture. (a) The needle has been passed through both lips of the incision, as for a simple suture, and is being passed back through the skin very near its edge. (b) The needle is being continued back through the second lip of the incision, very near the skin edge to complete the suture.

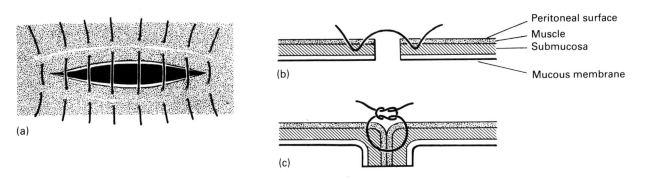

Peritoneal surface
Muscle
Submucosa
Mucous membrane

Fig. 1.54. (a) A series of inversion sutures before tying. (b) The stitch must penetrate into the submucosa. (c) The inverted edges of the wound.

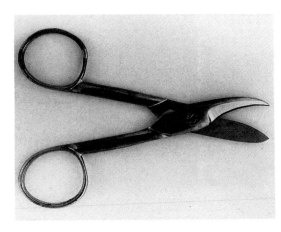

Fig. 1.55. Suture scissors. These scissors, as the name implies, are especially designed for the expeditious removal of sutures. The curved and pointed blade is for easy insertion between the skin and suture material.

ensures that the material which has been lying on the surface, and is probably contaminated, does not pass through the subcutaneous tissues when withdrawn.

TYING KNOTS

The object of a knot is to lock a strand of suture material in position until it has accomplished its purpose. Because knots are invariably subjected to some tension a variety of complicated knots has been advocated but they have no place in surgery. The surgeon's or reef knot, securely and carefully tied meets all requirements. It is important that the first throw is made to lie flat, and if added precautions are to be taken against the knot slipping then either make two throws when tying the first knot or tie a third knot.

Knots are most effectively tied using both hands (Fig. 1.56). The one-handed tie is popular but the first throw does not always lie flat which is essential

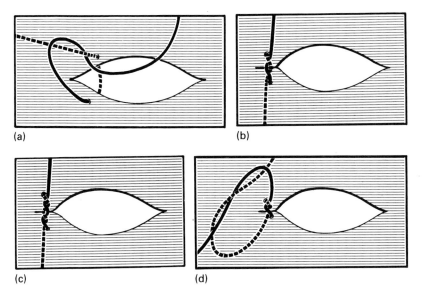

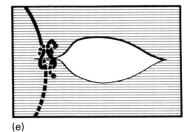

Fig. 1.56. The two-hand tie. (a) The end of the material with the needle attached (dotted line) is held in the left hand and tensed. Using the right hand, the free end of the material is looped over and under the tensed portion. (b) The two ends of the material are pulled to form the throw of the knot which is made to lie flat against the tissue. (c) A second loop has been made as an assurance against slipping. This manoeuvre is especially useful when the tissues are under tension. (d) The free end is reverse looped around the end attached to the needle. (e) Reverse loop being pulled tight to complete the knot. This is called a surgeon's or reef knot.

to obtain a secure knot. All surgeons must learn to tie knots using needle holders or artery forceps (Fig. 1.57) as this technique is useful when the end of the suture material is short, when working in a deep cavity, or when the material is slippery.

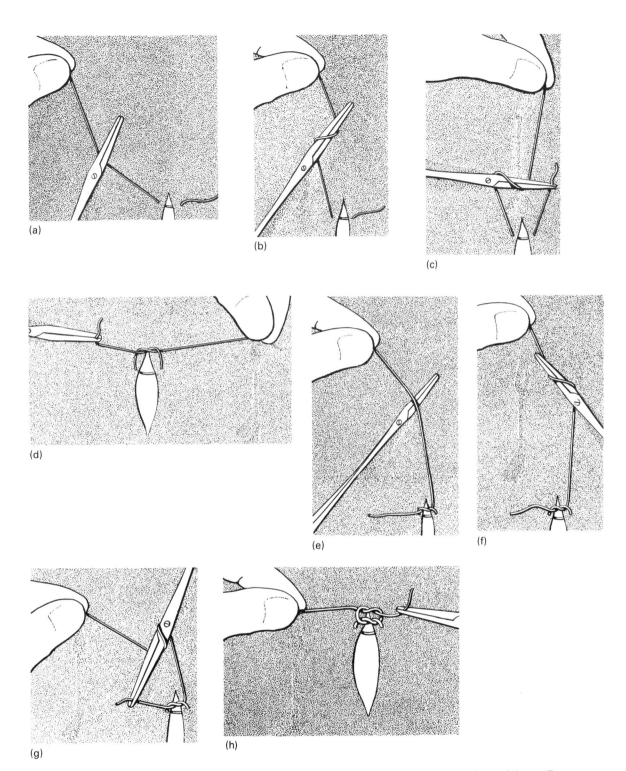

Fig. 1.57. Tying a knot with forceps. (a) The material is pulled through until only a short end remains, and the needle holder placed over the long end. (b) The point of the needle holder is passed under and then over the long end. (c) The short end of the material is picked up. (d) The short end is pulled through the loop formed around the needle holder to complete the first throw. (e) The needle holder is placed under the long end. (f) The point of the needle holder is passed over and then under the long end. (g) The short end of the first throw is picked up. (h) The short end is pulled through the loop formed around the needle holder to complete the knot.

Section 2
Surgery of the Head and Neck

The external ear

HAEMATOMA

A haematoma of the ear is most frequently seen in the dog, cat, and pig, and is caused by violent head shaking. This results in the rupture of blood vessels and the accumulation of blood between the perichondrium of the auricular cartilage and medial integument, the haematoma appearing as a cyst-like swelling of the medial aspect of the ear. Unless it is treated surgically by removing the blood clot (Figs 2.1−2.3), providing drainage and obliterating the cavity, resorption of the haemorrhage is accompanied by extensive cicatricial contraction which results in a crumpled and distorted ear. Before surgery is undertaken the cause of the head shaking must be diagnosed and treated.

Post operation, the ears are strapped together over the top of the head with adhesive tape.

A SPLIT EAR

Cuts extending through all layers of the ear will not unite, unless the skin edges are brought into apposition and infection controlled. In most cases the skin retracts exposing the auricular cartilage which prevents accurate co-aption of the skin edges. This is overcome by freeing the skin and removing a strip of auricular cartilage, which permits the skin edges to be accurately sutured together (Figs 2.4−2.6).

Post operation, the ear should be bandaged over the top of the head between two layers of cotton wool.

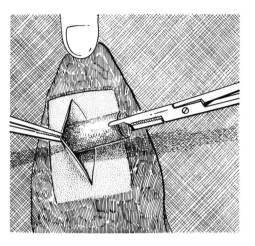

Fig. 2.2. The cavity is evacuated of all blood clots and fibrinous deposits which are carefully removed with a cotton wool tampon or gauze swab.

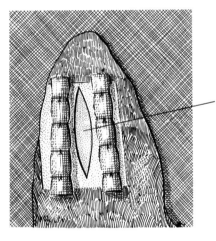

Auricular cartilage

Fig. 2.3. The cavity is occluded by placing a roll of gauze on each side of the incision and retaining it in position with a series of interrupted sutures, using monofilament nylon, which pass through all layers of the ear.

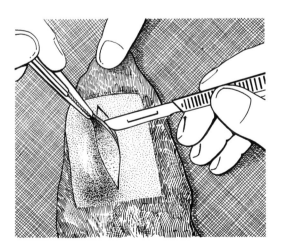

Fig. 2.1. An elliptical section of skin, extending the length of the haematoma and 0.2−0.5 cm in width, is removed with a scalpel.

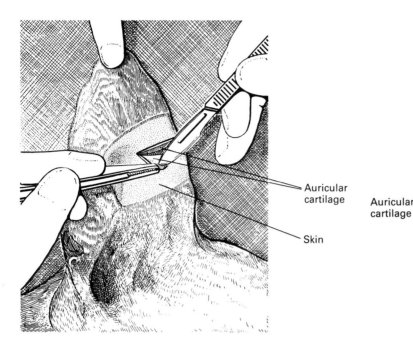

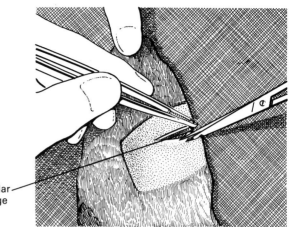

Fig. 2.5. A strip of the exposed auricular cartilage is removed from both edges.

Fig. 2.4. The skin on both surfaces of the cut is carefully freed by dissection from the auricular cartilage.

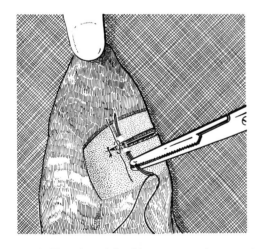

Fig. 2.6. The edges of the skin are accurately co-apted. on both the internal and external surfaces of the ear with interrupted sutures using monofilament nylon.

AURAL RESECTION — DOG

In many cases chronic infections of the external auditory meatus do not respond satisfactorily to conservative methods of treatment because of the absence of drainage, the tendency for ulceration to occur due to local inflammatory swelling and the lack of ventilation. Surgical exposure of the external auditory meatus usually provides the necessary drainage and ventilation.

There are two common forms of aural resection — lateral wall resection and vertical canal ablation. The lateral wall resection facilitates drainage from the horizontal aural canal and improves aeration of the remainder of the ear.

Vertical canal ablation involves removal of the medial wall as well as the lateral wall, leaving the patient with the horizontal canal opening through a stoma in the skin. Vertical canal ablation permits excision of the verrucose proliferations typical of chronic otitis externa.

Lateral wall resection

In the modified Zepp technique adequate drainage is ensured by the creation of a cartilaginous lip which acts as a baffle plate (Figs 2.7–2.12).

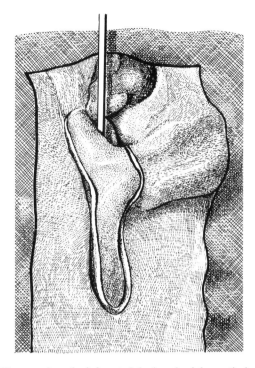

Fig. 2.7. A probe is inserted the length of the vertical part of the external auditory canal. A flap of skin is fashioned by commencing it at the cranial edge of the external opening to the auditory meatus and extending it parallel with and half as far again below the junction of the vertical and horizontal canals. It is then curved round and brought up the caudal edge of the conchal cartilage to terminate at the posterior edge of the tragus.

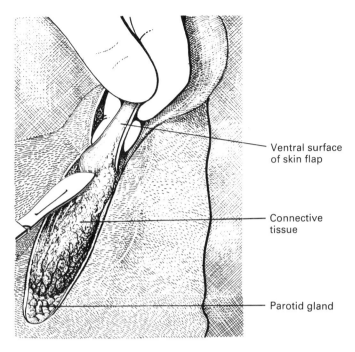

Fig. 2.8. The flap of skin is dissected free and reflected to expose the underlying connective tissue covering the conchal cartilage and the parotid gland.

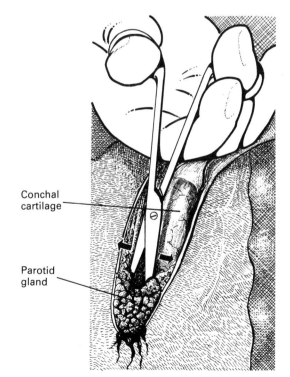

Fig. 2.9. The conchal cartilage is exposed by blunt dissection taking care not to damage the parotid gland.

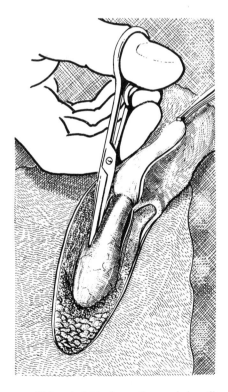

Fig. 2.10. Using straight scissors the conchal cartilage is cut down its cranial and caudal edges. It may be necessary to make slight adjustments to these cuts, in order to ensure that the entrance to the horizontal canal is widely exposed after the cartilage is reflected ventrally.

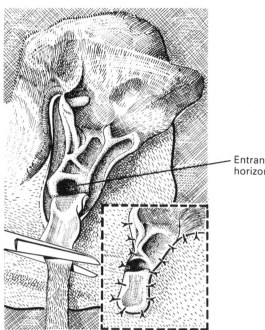

Entrance to
horizontal canal

Fig. 2.11. The central portion of the conchal cartilage together with the skin flap is reflected ventrally. The skin edges are co-apted to the integument of the ear canal with interrupted sutures of monofilament nylon. The reflected cartilage is severed to form a cartilaginous lip which is stitched to the distal edge of the skin incision (inset).

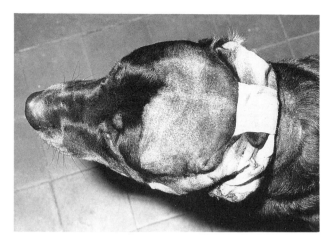

Fig. 2.12. Post operation, the ears are strapped together with adhesive tape over the top of the head. Healing tends to be slower than normal and stitches should be left in for at least 10 days.

Vertical canal ablation

When carrying out this procedure (Figs 2.13–2.17) it is essential to provide an adequate stoma for the horizontal ear canal. Failure to do this may lead to the accumulation of exudates and the development of pressure within the canal, which will eventually destroy the ear drum and the middle ear.

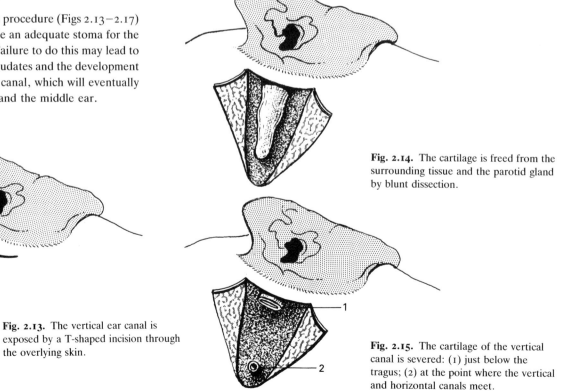

Fig. 2.13. The vertical ear canal is exposed by a T-shaped incision through the overlying skin.

Fig. 2.14. The cartilage is freed from the surrounding tissue and the parotid gland by blunt dissection.

Fig. 2.15. The cartilage of the vertical canal is severed: (1) just below the tragus; (2) at the point where the vertical and horizontal canals meet.

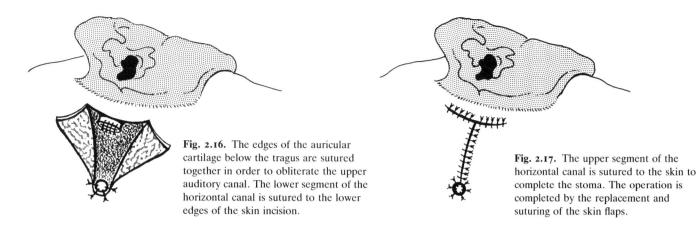

Fig. 2.16. The edges of the auricular cartilage below the tragus are sutured together in order to obliterate the upper auditory canal. The lower segment of the horizontal canal is sutured to the lower edges of the skin incision.

Fig. 2.17. The upper segment of the horizontal canal is sutured to the skin to complete the stoma. The operation is completed by the replacement and suturing of the skin flaps.

The face

OPENING THE FACIAL SINUSES – HORSE

Chronic inflammation of the facial sinuses frequently follows respiratory infections such as influenza or strangles and is also associated with necrosis of the turbinate bones, dental disease, foreign bodies or malignant neoplasms. Pus formed in the frontal sinus gravitates into the superior maxillary sinus and escapes via the nostrils as a purulent and foetid discharge.

In many cases it is necessary to open the sinuses to make a diagnosis and to treat the infection by providing drainage (Figs 2.18–2.19). Although the frontal and superior maxillary sinuses are confluent both must be opened to obtain satisfactory drainage and to enable them to be flushed out. If the septum between the superior and inferior maxillary sinus has been destroyed by necrosis then the latter has to be opened to provide drainage.

The operation of trephining can be performed with the horse standing under sedation and local analgesia but, in the majority of cases, it is advisable to perform the operation with the horse recumbent and under general anaesthesia. There are a number of recognized sites for opening the facial sinuses but the following are those most frequently employed and meet the requirements for drainage and flushing out the cavities (Figs 2.20–2.21).

In cases where the sinuses are opened for exploratory purposes only, a semi-circular skin flap is raised over the area to be trephined. At the completion of the operation this skin flap is sutured in position over the trephine hole, thus preventing the formation of unsightly scar tissue.

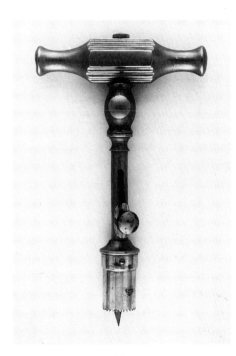

Fig. 2.18. A standard trephine with adjustable trocar. The following sizes are available: 0.6–1.25-cm, 1.9-cm and 2.5-cm diameters.

Frontal sinus

High site

Take a line joining the supraorbital processes, bisect it and trephine in the inferior angle of the intersection, 1.5–2.5 cm below and to one side of this point.

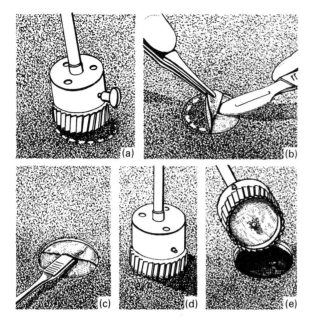

Fig. 2.19. (a) With either a 1.9-cm or 2.5-cm trephine, mark the overlying skin. (b) Incise the skin around the outside of the trephine marks and dissect it off the underlying periosteum. (c) Scrape the periosteum off the exposed bone with either a periosteal elevator or curette. (d) The centre of the exposed area of bone is penetrated with the trocar point of the trephine. (e) The trephine is worked, first with a to-and-fro movement until it bites and then with a continuous rotary movement in one direction until the isolated disc of bone comes away in the trephine.

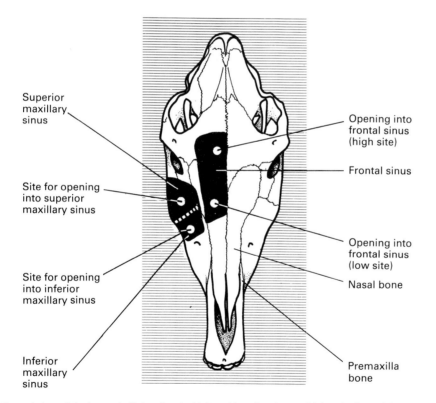

Fig. 2.20. Frontal view of the horse skull showing the high and low sites for trephining the frontal sinus and the sites for trephining the superior and inferior maxillary sinuses. The area of the sinuses is shown in black.

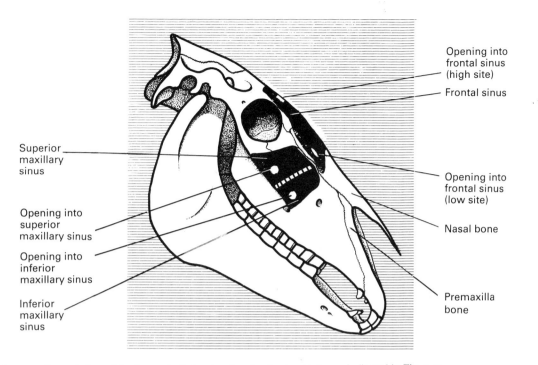

Opening into frontal sinus (high site)

Frontal sinus

Superior maxillary sinus

Opening into frontal sinus (low site)

Nasal bone

Opening into superior maxillary sinus

Opening into inferior maxillary sinus

Inferior maxillary sinus

Premaxilla bone

Fig. 2.21. Lateral view of the horse skull showing the sites for trephining as indicated in Fig. 2.20.

Low site

Take a line joining the inner canthus of the eye and junction of the nasal and premaxilla bones. Trephine 6.5 cm down and 2.5 cm in front of this line. This is the lowest part of the sinus when the head is held vertical.

Superior maxillary sinus

With the head vertical, trephine about 4.0 cm cranially from the distal extremity of the facial crest and about 2.5 cm medially. This position places the lower portion of the trephine hole almost level with the osseous septum separating the superior and inferior maxillary sinuses. This septum provides a natural floor for drainage and prevents the 'pocketing' of purulent material behind the trephine opening.

In young horses it is advisable to select a site 4–5 cm from the facial crest to avoid damaging the alveoli of the molar teeth.

Using these sites there is little chance of injuring the facial vein but the levator labii superioris proprius muscle is exposed and has to be displaced from the site by reflecting it dorsally.

Inferior maxillary sinus

This sinus is opened by trephining about 2.5 cm

medially from the distal extremity of the facial crest.

Following the operation of trephining, the sinuses are irrigated twice daily with normal saline until all infective material has been removed. The trephine opening is kept patent between irrigations with a gauze plug.

Alternative method

An alternative method is to insert a self-retaining catheter for post-operative irrigation (Figs 2.22–

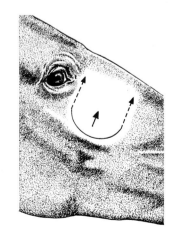

Fig. 2.22. A semicircular flap of skin measuring approximately 4 cm × 4 cm is reflected dorsally.

2.25). When removed, the catheter leaves a fistula between the sinus and the nasal passages providing drainage from the sinus for a further period.

The sinus should be irrigated at least twice daily and the catheter, which can remain in position for up to 3 weeks, should not be removed until nasal swabs are free of bacterial infection.

OPENING THE FACIAL SINUSES — CAT

Chronic rhinitis and sinusitis in the cat are very resistant to medical treatment and radical procedures such as the surgical removal of the turbinate bones have been described. It has been shown that if irrigating fluid is introduced into the frontal sinuses of normal cats it reaches all areas of the turbinate bones and nasal chambers.

The two frontal sinuses are separated by a thin bony septum. In the young cat, under 4 months of age, they are situated on either side of the midline of the skull on a line joining the medial canthus of the eyes. In adult cats, over 1 year old, they are situated more caudally on a line joining the cranial border of the supraorbital processes (Fig. 2.26).

The precise site for trephining will vary with the age of the cat. In cats under 4 months of age, a point is selected slightly to the side of the midline and midway along a line joining the inner canthus of the eye and the supraorbital process. For adult cats over 1 year old, a point is selected slightly to the side of the midline and just above a line joining the cranial borders of the supraorbital processes.

A skin incision about 0.5 cm in length is made to expose the underlying frontal bone which is then penetrated with a bone awl. The sinus and nasal cavity are irrigated with warm normal saline solution, until the fluid flows out free of pus. This is repeated every second day followed by instilling the appropriate antibiotic solution as determined by sensitivity tests.

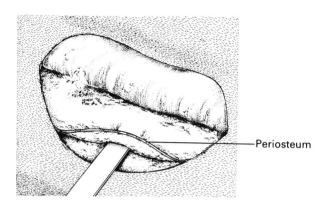

Fig. 2.23. The exposed periosteum is reflected using a periosteal elevator.

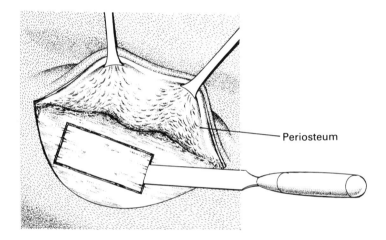

Fig. 2.24. A flap of bone is removed with an osteotome. The sinus is inspected and flushed out with normal saline.

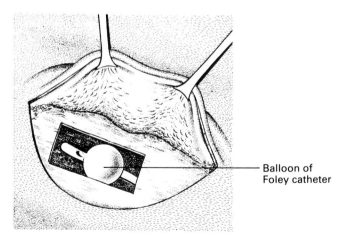

Fig. 2.25. A Foley catheter is inserted via the middle meatus. Injury to the turbinate bones is minimal but may occasion slight haemorrhage. The balloon of the catheter is filled with sterile water to anchor it, and the exposure closed in three layers, the periosteum, fascia and skin. The reflected periosteum should be kept moist to prevent shrinkage which makes suturing difficult.

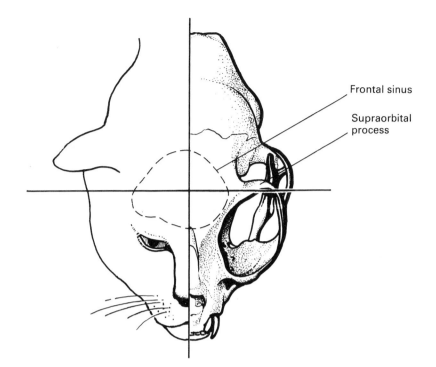

Frontal sinus

Supraorbital process

Fig. 2.26. Dorso-rostral view of the skull of an adult cat showing the site of the frontal sinus.

REPULSION OF TEETH — HORSE

In the horse it is not possible to extract a molar tooth by conventional methods unless it is loose, and so it is necessary to repulse it.

The operation of repulsion comprises removing a disc of bone with a trephine to expose the root of the tooth and then to drive it into the mouth with a punch placed between the two roots of the tooth. It is often necessary when repulsing the molars of the upper jaw, to have to chip away the outer wall of the alveolus, in addition to making a trephine hole, in order to expose the root.

It is essential to trephine exactly over the root of the tooth to be repulsed. To determine accurately this site is not always easy, especially as the natural curvature of the long axis of the teeth varies with age. The site can be located either by taking a radiograph with a hypodermic needle placed in the skin as a marker or by relating the table of the tooth (a) in the upper jaw to the line of the nasolacrimal duct, and (b) in the lower jaw to the ventral edge of the mandible (Tables 2.1–2.2, Fig. 2.27).

The course of the nasolacrimal duct corresponds to a line drawn from the medial canthus of the eye to the angle formed by the nasal and premaxilla

Table 2.1 Sites for trephining to repulse the teeth of the upper jaw.

Tooth	Site	Location of site
Second premolar	Nasal cavity	On a line through centre of tooth
Third premolar	Nasal cavity	
Fourth premolar	Nasal cavity	Along a line from the caudal edge of the crown of the tooth to the line of the nasolacrimal duct
First molar	Inferior maxillary sinus	
Second molar	Superior maxillary sinus	
Third molar	Frontal sinus	On a line joining the medial canthus of the eye and about 4.0 cm from the medial line

Table 2.2 Sites for trephining to repulse the teeth of the lower jaw.

Tooth	Site	Location of site
Second premolar	Ventral border of the mandible	Immediately below table of tooth
Third premolar		Along a line from the caudal edge of the crown of the tooth to the ventral edge of the mandible
Fourth premolar		
First molar	Lateral aspect of the mandible over root of tooth	
Second molar		
Third molar		On a line through centre of tooth to point of greatest curvature of mandible

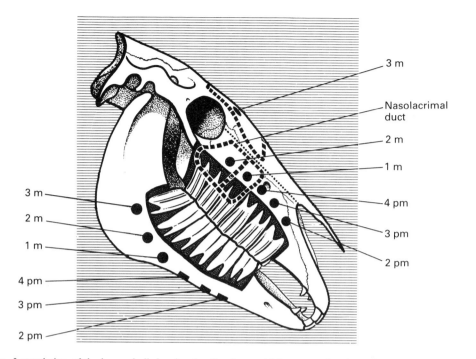

Fig. 2.27. Lateral view of the horse skull showing the sites for trephining to repulse the molar teeth of both the upper and lower jaws. The area of the sinuses are outlined by dashed lines.

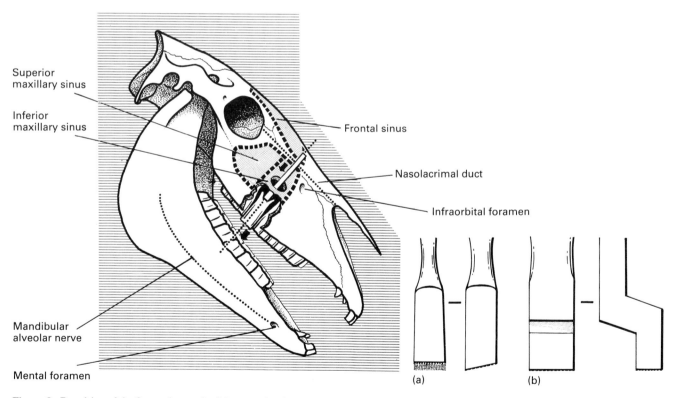

Fig. 2.28. Repulsion of the first molar tooth of the upper jaw by trephining the inferior maxillary sinus and exposing the root. Two types of punch are required for tooth repulsion: (a) standard straight punch, and (b) an off-set punch. This punch is especially useful for inserting through the trephine hole to make contact with the root of the tooth and to commence its repulsion.

bones, and therefore to avoid injuring it the trephine holes must be placed below this line. When trephining to repulse the fourth premolar, care must be taken to avoid the infraorbital nerve and the lateral nasal artery.

The molars of the mandible cannot be repulsed without causing some damage to the mandibular alveolar nerve which fortunately does not appear to have any adverse effects. When exposing the site to repulse the first molar (Fig. 2.28) care must be taken not to injure the facial artery or vein, or the parotid duct, and when exposing the site for either the second or third molar the masseter muscle has to be split and the masseteric artery avoided.

Following repulsion of a tooth the alveolus is searched with a finger and any fragments of bone are removed by curetting. To prevent food from entering the sinuses or alveolus, the alveolus is plugged with gutta-percha. The object is to close the oral entrance to the alveolus without filling the alveolar cavity completely thus allowing healing to take place by granulation. This is accomplished by first softening the gutta-percha in warm water and then, with one finger inserted through the trephine hole to block the depth of the alveolus, the gutta-percha is packed into the alveolus via the mouth and moulded over the gum. In the majority of cases the plug is rejected in 2−3 weeks by which time healing is well established.

EXPOSING THE NASAL CAVITIES − DOG

Exposure of the various compartments of the nasal cavities (Figs 2.29−2.33) is necessary for the removal of foreign bodies, necrotic bone and in the treatment of chronic rhinitis.

Removal of portions of the ethmoid and turbinate bone is always accompanied by severe haemorrhage. Elevation of the head will reduce bleeding. Further control of haemorrhage can be effected by temporary occlusion of the ipsilateral carotid artery. Before suturing the periosteum, haemorrhage is controlled by packing the cavity with tape impregnated with iodoform. The end of the tape is brought out through the nostril and anchored to the edge of the muzzle with a single interrupted suture. The tape pack is carefully removed via the nostril in 5−7 days.

Trephining the frontal sinuses in the dog, followed by placement of irrigation tubes and topical medication with enilconazole (Imaverol) is the most satisfactory treatment of nasal aspergillosis. Trephining is performed at the level of the supraorbital process and the drug is flushed through the nasofrontal ostium into the nasal chambers, twice daily, for 10−14 days.

Rhinotomy may worsen the prognosis for many nasal tumours and, if employed, should be combined with radiation.

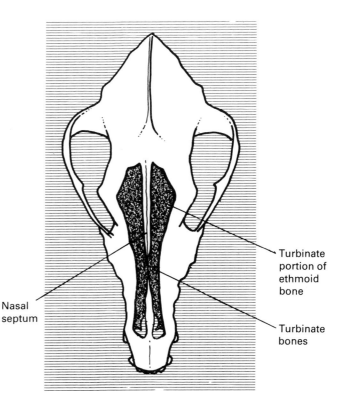

Fig. 2.29. Dorsal view of the dog skull showing the nasal cavity which is divided into left and right compartments by the nasal septum. Each nasal cavity comprises a rostral portion which contains the superior and inferior turbinate bones and a caudal portion which is mainly occupied by the turbinate portion of the ethmoid bone. The shaded area shows the extent to which the nasal bones and portions of the maxillary and frontal bones can be safely removed to expose the nasal cavities.

Nasal septum

Turbinate portion of ethmoid bone

Turbinate bones

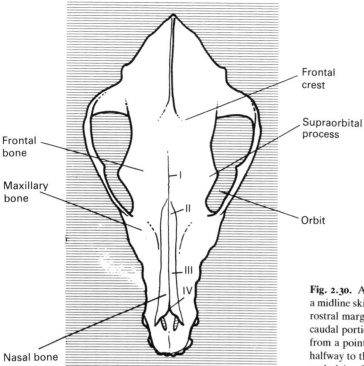

Fig. 2.30. Access to the rostral portion of the nasal cavity is obtained by making a midline skin incision which extends from site II to IV, i.e. from a line joining the rostral margins of the orbit to the caudal edge of the muzzle. Access to the caudal portion is by a midline skin incision which extends from site I to III, i.e. from a point level with the supraorbital processes to a point approximately halfway to the muzzle. The skin is reflected to the appropriate side to expose the underlying frontal and/or nasal bone.

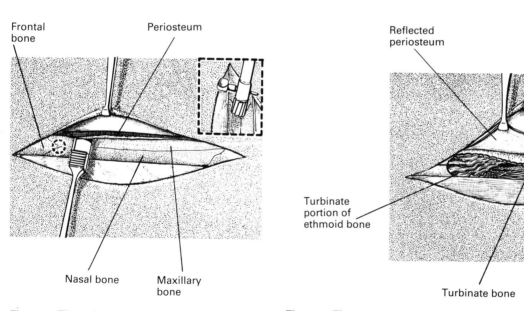

Fig. 2.31. The periosteum is reflected from the nasal and maxillary bones with a periosteal elevator and a hole drilled, using a 0.6-cm trephine, at the junction of the frontal and nasal bone.

Fig. 2.32. The maxillary and nasal bone is removed with Luer bone-nibbling forceps to expose the underlying nasal cavity, the turbinate portion of the ethmoid bone, and the turbinate bones. Alternatively, the bone may be removed with an oscillating saw.

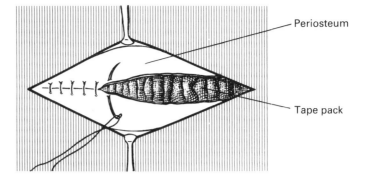

Periosteum

Tape pack

Fig. 2.33. The incision is closed by co-apting the periosteum and subcutaneous tissues with a series of interrupted sutures using a synthetic absorbable material, and closing the skin in the customary manner.

The mouth

TONSILLECTOMY — DOG

The indiscriminate removal of the tonsils is to be deprecated. A persistent cough is sometimes due to a chronic hypertrophic tonsillitis and in these cases tonsillectomy affords relief. Tonsillectomy for carcinoma results in only temporary relief as invariably the neoplasm either recurs locally or metastasizes.

For the operation to be successful all tonsillar tissue must be removed. The very shape of the tonsil, i.e. elongated and fusiform, coupled with the depth of the tonsillar fossa, mitigates against the successful use of the popular 'guillotine' method. To ensure complete removal of the tonsil it must be dissected out (Figs 2.34—2.36).

Haemorrhage, which is always a problem when removing tonsils, is satisfactorily controlled by this method. If diathermy is not available then the vessels must be picked up with artery forceps and tied off using 2 metric synthetic absorbable suture material. Post operation, no special attention is required and complications are rare.

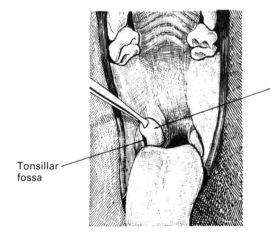

Tonsil

Tonsillar fossa

Fig. 2.34. The tonsil is grasped with Allis forceps and drawn out of its fossa until its pedicle is taut.

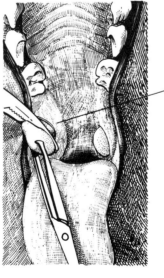

Triangular fold of mucous membrane

Fig. 2.35. The pedicle of the tonsil is clamped with curved Dunhill artery forceps.

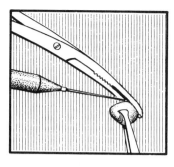

Fig. 2.36. The tonsil is removed by severing it along the blade of the artery forceps with a diathermy needle.

SPLIT PALATE – CAT

A split palate is a common cause of epistaxis in the cat. The injury comprises a central and longitudinal split of the hard palate complicated by a separation of the underlying palatine bones. If this is not immediately suspected by epistaxis it soon becomes evident due to the escape of ingesta from the nostrils.

It is not possible to co-apt satisfactorily the separated palatine bones but the breach can be occluded by co-apting the mucous membrane of the hard palate (Fig. 2.37).

Post operation, no special precautions are necessary except to control infection and to keep the cat on a fluid diet until healing is established.

EXTRACTION OF TEETH – DOG

The extraction of a dog's teeth, with the exception of a canine or carnassial tooth, is accomplished by conventional methods. The basic principles comprise:

Correct adjustment of the forceps

The blades of the forceps must be selected to fit the contour of the tooth (Fig. 2.38).

Rupture of the periodontal membrane

The periodontal membrane binds the root of the tooth to the alveolar wall and in many cases it is necessary to break it down and dilate the socket with a dental elevator before the tooth can be extracted (Fig. 2.39).

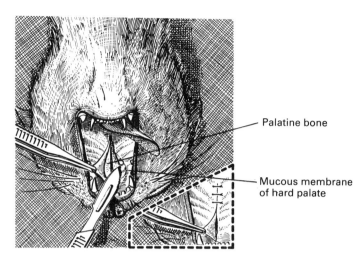

Palatine bone

Mucous membrane of hard palate

Fig. 2.37. By careful dissection the mucous membrane of the hard palate is freed from the underlying palatine bones which permits its edges to be brought together with a series of interrupted sutures using absorbable synthetic suture material.

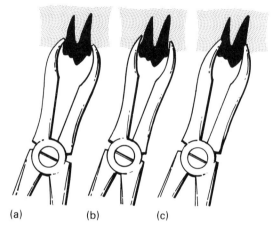

(a)   (b)   (c)

Fig. 2.38. Selection of dental forceps. (a) Forceps with too great a curvature cut the tooth and break off the crown. (b) Forceps with too little curvature crush the crown of the tooth. (c) Correctly shaped forceps accurately grip both the crown and root of the tooth.

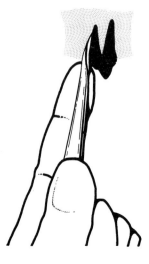

Fig. 2.39. The elevator blade, with the flattened surface towards the tooth, is inserted between the root and the alveolus. The blade is forced as far as necessary into the alveolus. The elevator is then used as a lever which raises the tooth in its socket and displaces it in the required direction. Note the method of holding the elevator and the position of the finger in relation to the top of the elevator blade.

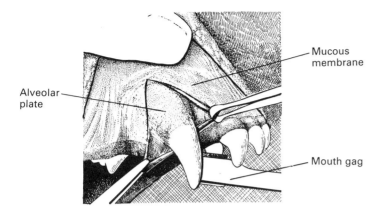

Fig. 2.40. The mucous membrane is incised along the central and lateral axis of the tooth and reflected to expose the underlying alveolar plate.

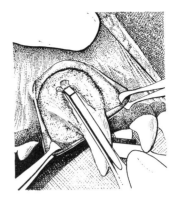

Fig. 2.41. A dental chisel is worked under the lateral alveolar plate which is gradually removed to expose the lateral surface of the tooth.

Removal of the tooth

When using forceps the periodontal membrane is ruptured and the socket dilated by force with either a rotary or lateral movement. Rotary movement is only admissible for those teeth with single conical roots. The blades of the forceps selected are applied parallel to the long axis of the root and pressed under the gum and alveolus, in the direction of the apex of the tooth, until a firm grip of the root is obtained.

The incisors, the first premolar of the upper jaw, the first and second premolars and the third molar of the lower jaw all have single conical roots and therefore are suitable for forceps extraction.

The remaining teeth, with the exception of the fourth upper premolar or carnassial tooth and the canine tooth — which are dealt with as separate problems — have either two or three roots. In consequence these teeth cannot be loosened in their sockets by rotation and the periodontal membrane has to be broken down with a dental elevator before applying forceps.

Sometimes when using forceps the tooth breaks and the roots are left *in situ*. In these cases an attempt should be made to remove them using either a dental elevator or special stump forceps. If they are so firmly embedded that they cannot be extracted without causing local tissue damage it is best to leave them alone for 2 or 3 weeks by which time they will have become loose and can be easily removed.

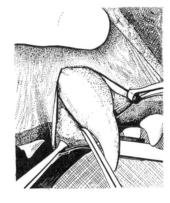

Fig. 2.42. A dental gouge is thrust between the anterior and posterior edges of the tooth and the alveolus to break down the periodontal membrane.

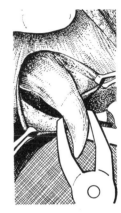

Fig. 2.43. The tooth has been freed and is now easily lifted out of the alveolus with dental forceps.

Excision of a canine tooth

It is extremely difficult to loosen or remove a canine tooth with forceps because it curves caudally, is flattened laterally and its buried central portion is wider than the opening of the alveolus at the jaw margin. For this reason it has to be excised (Figs 2.40–2.43).

Following extraction, the mucous membrane is co-apted with a series of interrupted sutures using 2 metric synthetic absorbable suture material. Haemorrhage is slight and it is seldom necessary to control it by packing the alveolus.

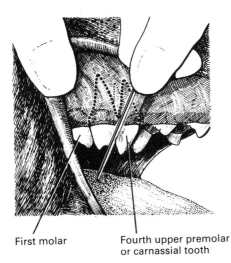

First molar   Fourth upper premolar
                               or carnassial tooth

Fig. 2.44. Using a hack-saw blade the crown is divided by making a cut parallel to the rostral border of the tooth to extend from just behind the main cusp to the space between the rostral and caudal roots.

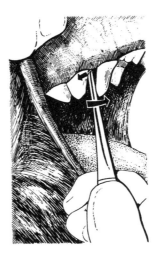

Fig. 2.45. Division of the tooth is completed by thrusting a dental chisel down the saw cut. Next, using the single caudal root as a fulcrum, the double-rooted rostral portion is loosened, elevated and removed with forceps.

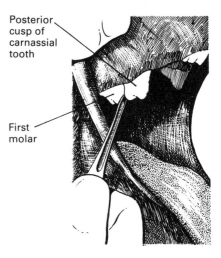

Posterior
cusp of
carnassial
tooth

First
molar

Fig. 2.46. The remaining caudal portion of the carnassial tooth is loosened by thrusting a dental gouge between the caudal edge of the root and the alveolus.

Extraction of an upper carnassial tooth

The extraction of the fourth upper premolar or carnassial tooth presents a difficult problem because of the shape of the tooth and the size and disposition of its three roots, two rostral and one caudal. The most satisfactory method is to divide the tooth between its roots and then to extract each half separately (Figs 2.44–2.47). No special treatment is required following extraction.

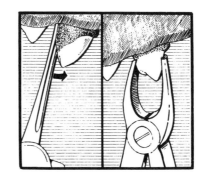

Fig. 2.47. Using the first molar as a fulcrum, the caudal portion which is already loose is elevated with a dental gouge before applying forceps and extracting it.

The poll

DISBUDDING – CALF

Cattle are polled so that they cannot gore one another and are less dangerous to handle. If possible, every effort should be made to disbud calves rather than wait until they are adult and then dehorn them.

Calves should be disbudded when they are between 5 and 10 days old. The application of caustics is an unsatisfactory method and the best method is to remove the horn buds with a disbudding iron under local analgesia (Fig. 2.48).

There are numerous patterns of disbudding irons, but most are heated by calor gas or electricity. The head of the iron is made of copper to retain the heat and its end is hollowed out to form a dome-shaped depression 12 mm in diameter, 8 mm deep and with a rim 3 mm thick.

This method has the advantage that haemorrhage is controlled, no post-operation dressings are required, and healing is complete in 10–14 days leaving little or no scar.

Once calves have begun to grow horns, disbudding is no longer possible, and the rudimentary

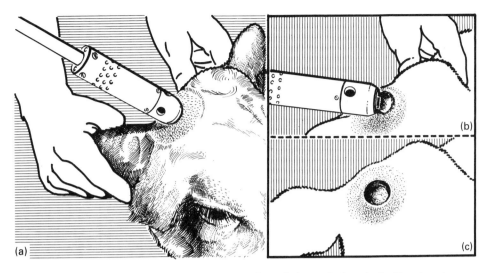

Fig. 2.48. (a) The disbudding iron, heated to a dull red heat, is applied over the horn bud with a stamping movement. Next, with a rotary movement a groove, 3 mm wide, is burnt through the skin at the base of and surrounding the horn bud. (b) The disbudding iron is angled and using the edge of the rim the horn bud is removed by searing it off the underlying frontal bone. (c) Horn bud removed. Note the circle of burnt skin round the base of the horn which has destroyed the corium and prevents any further development of horn.

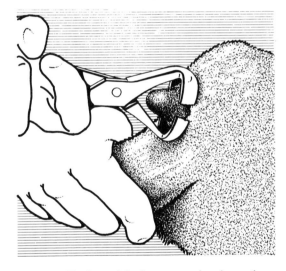

Fig. 2.49. The jaws of the forceps are placed over the horn and pressed well down so as to include the skin around the base. The jaws of the forceps are closed and then with a sharp twist and pull, the horn, including the processus cornus or 'horn core', is neatly separated from the frontal bone, with a fringe of skin attached.

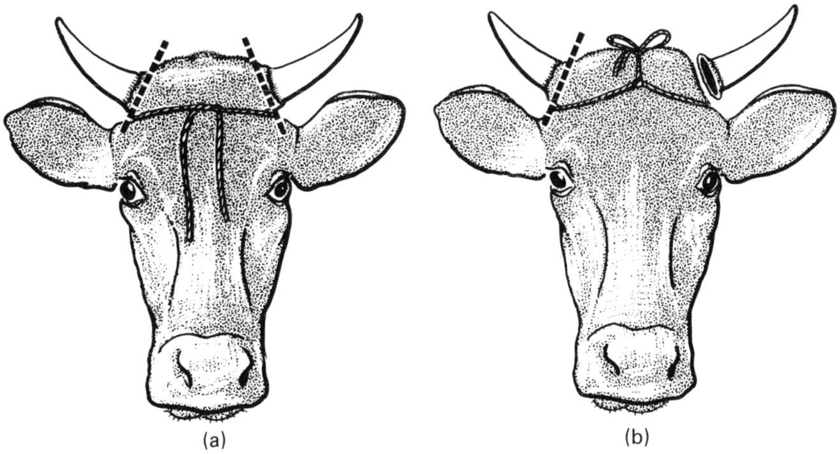

Fig. 2.50. (a) Haemorrhage is controlled by tying a length of string around the base of both horns; in (b) note how the tie is completed to tighten it. The actual method of removing the horn is relatively unimportant provided the corium is removed with the horn. Note the angle of severance which conforms to the contour of the poll and gives the animal the neat appearance of the polled breeds.

horns are removed with special gouge forceps (Fig. 2.49).

In the majority of cases haemorrhage is slight, but if it does not cease within a few minutes the artery should be picked up with forceps and tied off.

DEHORNING — CATTLE

Adult cattle are satisfactorily dehorned standing, under local analgesia and preferably restrained in a crush. The horns can be removed with a hack saw, a dehorning guillotine or embryotomy wire. The method employed is very much a matter of personal preference but whichever method is practised it is essential to remove the horn together with 1.5 cm of the skin around its base (Fig. 2.50). This ensures that the corium is removed and prevents the development of any stumps of distorted horn.

Post-operation complications are rare, the most

troublesome being a purulent sinusitis, due to the inevitable opening of the frontal sinus when the horn is amputated. The condition will frequently clear following irrigation and drainage. This can only be achieved by tilting the head until the accumulated inflammatory exudate drains from the opening at the top of the sinus. Occasionally this opening will heal before the infection is cleared, and this may necessitate draining the pus through a trephine hole placed low in the frontal sinus in order to attain dependent drainage.

The neck

LARYNGEAL VENTRICULECTOMY – HORSE

Paralysis of the left recurrent laryngeal nerve in the horse is followed by paralysis of the intrinsic muscles of the larynx which gives rise to a laryngeal hemiplegia. As a result the affected side of the larynx fails to dilate during inspiration so that the flaccid vocal cord with a relaxed arytenoid cartilage encroaches on the lumen of the larynx. With exercise this obstruction results in the production of a characteristic inspiratory noise which is commonly referred to as 'whistling' or 'roaring'.

Laryngeal hemiplegia may be relieved by performing a laryngeal ventriculectomy, i.e. stripping the mucous membrane of the laryngeal saccule via the lateral ventricle (see Figs 2.51–2.60). Healing is by granulation and cicatrization which anchors the vocal cord and arytenoid cartilage to the thyroid cartilage, thus widening the airways and preventing obstruction on inspiration.

Post operation, the incision is not sutured but left to heal by granulation which is complete in about 3 weeks. The wound is cleansed of all discharges two or three times daily. The only immediate post-operation complication which may develop is a spasm of the larynx and for this contingency an emergency tracheotomy tube (see Fig. 2.72) should be at hand. At a later date a chondroma of either the thyroid or cricoid cartilages may develop if they are injured during the operation.

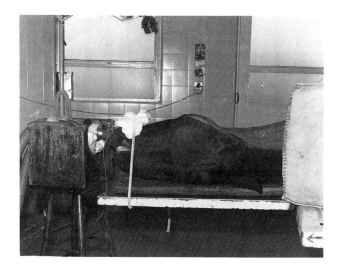

Fig. 2.51. The operation is performed under general anaesthesia with the horse in dorsal recumbency and its head and neck fully extended.

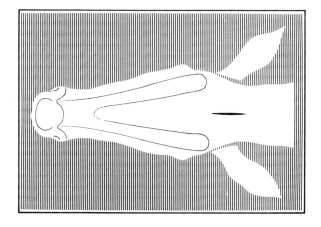

Fig. 2.52. A midline skin incision is made over the larynx from a point just in front of a line joining the angles of the jaws to the level of the first tracheal ring.

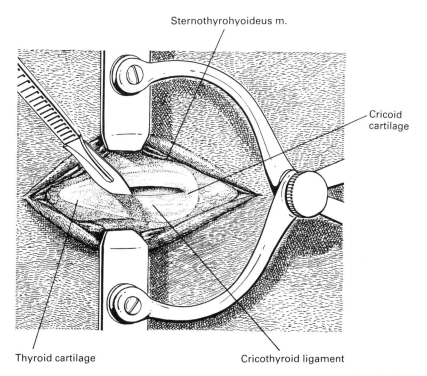

Sternothyrohyoideus m.

Cricoid cartilage

Thyroid cartilage

Cricothyroid ligament

Fig. 2.53. The underlying sternothyrohyoideus muscle is divided and retracted to expose the cricothyroid ligament. This ligament is triangular and its edges are bordered by the wings of the thyroid cartilage which converge to a point cranially. The cricothyroid ligament and underlying mucous membrane are punctured with the point of the scalpel and the incision extended cranially to the body of the thyroid cartilage and caudally to the cricoid cartilage, care being taken not to damage either cartilage.

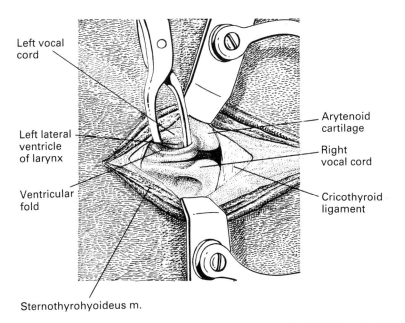

Left vocal cord

Left lateral ventricle of larynx

Ventricular fold

Arytenoid cartilage

Right vocal cord

Cricothyroid ligament

Sternothyrohyoideus m.

Fig. 2.54. The interior of the larynx is inspected and the component structures identified. Note that the lateral ventricle is located under the vocal cord and to obtain a good view of it the vocal cord has to be retracted laterally.

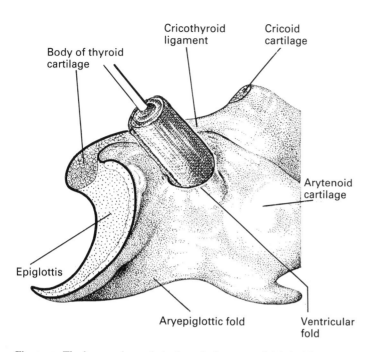

Body of thyroid cartilage
Cricothyroid ligament
Cricoid cartilage
Arytenoid cartilage
Epiglottis
Aryepiglottic fold
Ventricular fold

Fig. 2.55. The laryngeal saccule is cleared of mucus and dried with a gauze swab with the horse in dorsal recumbency. The figure shows the left side of a sagittal section of the larynx.

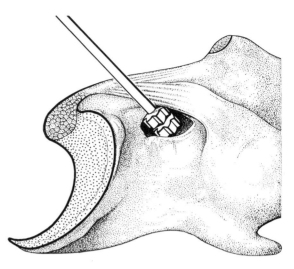

Fig. 2.56. The burr is directed caudo-ventrally into the lateral ventricle making sure that it engages the depth of the laryngeal saccule.

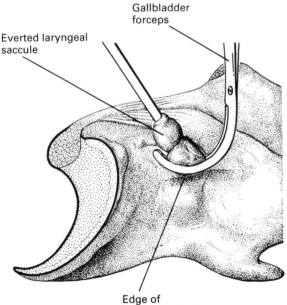

Everted laryngeal saccule
Gallbladder forceps
Edge of ventricular fold

Fig. 2.57. The burr is pushed firmly into the depth of the laryngeal saccule and slowly rotated until it picks up the mucous membrane. Rotation is slowly continued and at the same time the burr is withdrawn from the lateral ventricle, with the mucous membrane attached, thus everting the laryngeal saccule. The base of the saccule is then clamped with gallbladder forceps.

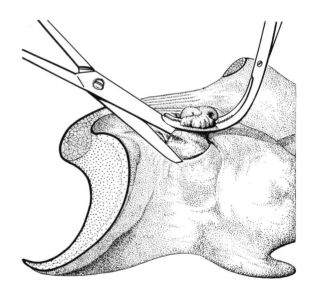

Fig. 2.58. The burr is removed. Traction is applied to the laryngeal saccule to ensure that it is completely everted. It is removed by cutting along its attachment to the edge of the lateral ventricle.

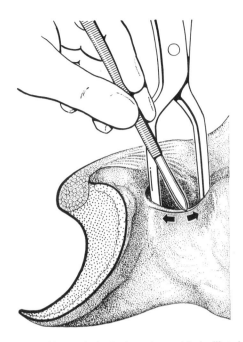

Fig. 2.59. Alternatively the lateral ventricle is dilated with 'glove-stretching' forceps and, using a special scalpel with an edge on each side of its point, an incision is made between the edge of the laryngeal saccule and the length of the ventricular fold. Then, by blunt dissection using a finger, the connective tissue attachments are broken down and the laryngeal saccule everted. It is then grasped with forceps and removed by severing it along the other edge of its attachment to the lateral ventricle.

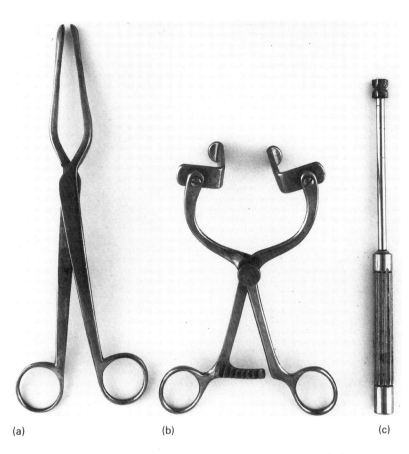

(a)　　　　　　　　　(b)　　　　　　　　　(c)

Fig. 2.60. Special instruments required for performing laryngeal ventriculectomy: (a) 'glove-stretching' forceps, (b) laryngeal retractor, and (c) a burr.

PROSTHETIC LARYNGOPLASTY — HORSE

Laryngoplasty offers the best chance of improving exercise intolerance and reducing the inspiratory noise associated with paralysis of the left recurrent laryngeal nerve. Two sutures placed between the muscular process of the arytenoid cartilage and the caudodorsal aspect of the cricoid cartilage mimic the action of the paralysed cricoarytenoideus muscle and abduct the arytenoid. Although the principle is simple a thorough knowledge of the anatomical landmarks is essential if disappointment is to be avoided.

Laryngoplasty is always augmented by a laryngeal ventriculectomy. If this has been performed previously the ventricle is re-opened to encourage the formation of new adhesions between the repositioned arytenoid cartilage and the thyroid cartilage.

Some horses will cough post-operatively due to the inhalation of food since the lateral fixation of the arytenoid impairs the protective mechanism of the larynx. Coughing has also been associated with faulty placement of the prosthesis; in particular, penetration of the lumen of the larynx has resulted in the formation of granulomas.

The horse is placed in right lateral recumbency with the head and neck extended. A 12-cm incision is made immediately ventral to the linguofacial vein and the underlying omohyoideus muscle is identified (Fig. 2.61).

Blunt dissection is followed by elevation of the fascia from the omohyoideus muscle to expose the lateral aspect of the larynx. The dorsal aspect of the cricoid cartilage is identified and the fascial septum between the thyropharyngeus and cricopharyngeus muscles is divided with scissors to expose the muscular process of the arytenoid cartilage (Fig. 2.62).

A double suture of 7 metric polyester suture (Ethibond) on a half-circle needle is placed through the muscular process. This is made easier if the arytenoid cartilage is grasped with a pair of towel clips to elevate the process (Fig. 2.63).

A tunnel is created with a pair of forceps under

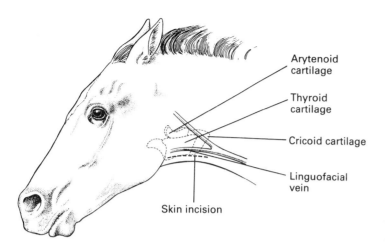

Arytenoid
cartilage

Thyroid
cartilage

Cricoid cartilage

Linguofacial
vein

Skin incision

Fig. 2.61. The horse is placed in right lateral recumbency with the head and neck extended. A 12-cm incision is made immediately ventral to the linguofacial vein and the underlying omohyoideus muscle is identified.

the cricopharyngeus muscle, and fascia is removed from the dorsal caudal portion of the cricoid cartilage to expose its most axial aspect. The double suture is divided so as to produce two separate sutures and one end of each suture is passed under the cricopharyngeus muscle (Fig. 2.64). The notch immediately adjacent to the dorsal midline of the larynx is palpated to indicate the correct placement of the sutures in the cricoid cartilage. The tip of the needle is inserted behind the cricoid in the region of this notch and the needle is carefully advanced submucosally to penetrate the cricoid cartilage 1.5 cm rostral to its caudal border. The second suture is then placed 1 cm lateral to the first and both are tied under moderate tension (Fig. 2.65).

The thyropharyngeus and cricopharyngeus muscles are co-apted with a simple continuous suture of 3 metric synthetic absorbable suture and the fascia and subcutaneous tissues are closed similarly. The skin is closed with interrupted sutures of nylon.

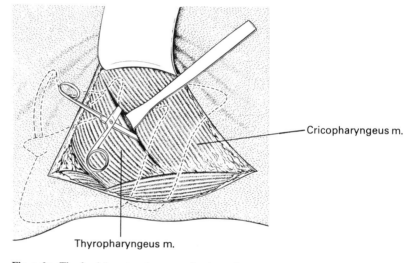

Cricopharyngeus m.

Thyropharyngeus m.

Fig. 2.62. The fascial septum between the thyropharyngeus and cricopharyngeus muscles is divided with scissors to expose the muscular process of the arytenoid cartilage.

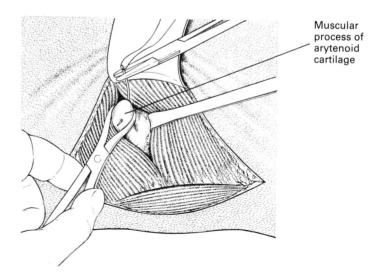

Muscular process of arytenoid cartilage

Fig. 2.63. The arytenoid cartilage is elevated with a pair of towel clips and a double suture of braided polyester is placed through the muscular process.

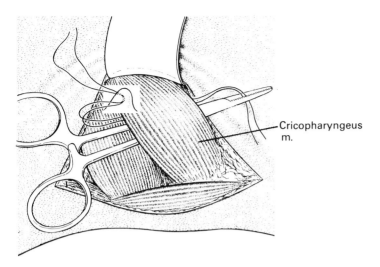

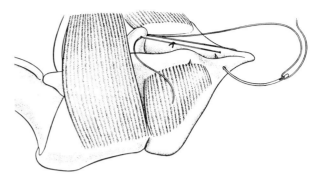

Fig. 2.65. Both sutures are passed through the cricoid cartilage and tied.

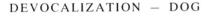
Cricopharyngeus m.

Fig. 2.64. The loop is cut and the needle removed. The double suture is passed under the cricopharyngeus muscle.

DEVOCALIZATION — DOG

Removal of the vocal cords in the dog reduces its bark to a low and husky noise but the vocal cords regenerate very rapidly resulting in a partial recovery within weeks and an almost complete recovery in 6 months. The surgery should only be performed in exceptional circumstances and the reader should be aware of possible ethical implications.

To devocalize a dog it is necessary to remove completely all the vibrating structures within the larynx responsible for voice production. This entails removing the ventricular and vocal folds with parts of the underlying cuneiform and arytenoid cartilages.

An attempt may be made to remove these structures *per os* using a biopsy punch or scissors but the only satisfactory procedure is to perform a laryngotomy and dissect them out (Fig. 2.66).

With the dog in dorsal recumbency a midline skin incision is made extending from the basihyoid bone to the cricoid cartilage. The underlying sternohyoideus muscle is divided and separated to expose the cricothyroid ligament and thyroid cartilage. The cricothyroid ligament is incised throughout its length and the incision continued through the body of the thyroid cartilage. A small self-retaining retractor is inserted which enables the laryngeal cavity to be completely visualized.

Care must be taken to ensure that haemostasis is

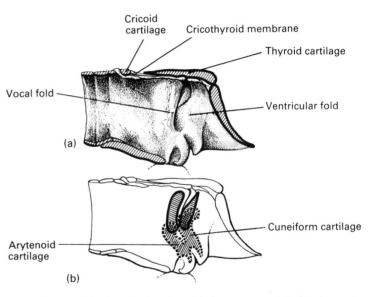

Fig. 2.66. (a) Right side of a sagittal section of the larynx as seen following laryngotomy. Note how the ventricular fold and part of the cuneiform cartilage are situated under the vocal fold. (b) The ventricular fold with part of the cuneiform cartilage and the vocal fold with part of the arytenoid cartilage, as indicated by the dotted lines, are removed by diathermy.

complete before the laryngeal opening is closed using interrupted sutures of synthetic absorbable suture material. The sternohyoideus muscle and skin are co-apted in the customary manner. Although this method does not completely devocalize dogs its results are better than those achieved by removing the vocal cords.

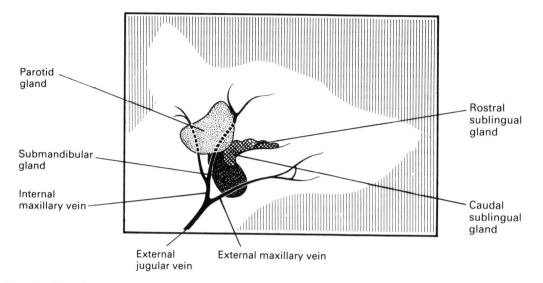

Fig. 2.67. Note the position of the submandibular salivary gland located between the external and internal maxillary veins and its intimate relationship with the caudal sublingual salivary gland.

SALIVARY RETENTION CYSTS – DOG

These cysts develop as painless fluctuating swellings in either the submandibular or cervical region of the neck or sublingually where they are called ranulae. They are generally the result of saliva leaking from a ruptured sublingual gland or duct, or, more rarely, from the submandibular gland. The escaping saliva accumulates under the tongue in the submandibular region or in the dependent part of the neck where it stimulates a local tissue reaction which leads to the development of an organized cyst wall (mucocoele).

The removal of the entire sublingual/mandibular complex is recommended since it is difficult to separate the caudal portion of the sublingual gland from the submandibular gland (Fig. 2.67).

The dog is positioned in lateral recumbency with a sandbag under the neck and the head rotated so that the cyst is uppermost (Figs 2.68–2.71). Following removal of the salivary gland complex the incision is closed by co-apting the parotido-auricularis muscle with interrupted sutures of synthetic absorbable suture material and the skin is repaired in the customary manner. The mucocoele is drained by a stab incision. It is rarely necessary to debride or remove the sac lining.

It is not always obvious on which side of the neck the affected glands are located. If so the gland may be located by opening the cyst and tracing the sinus back to the gland.

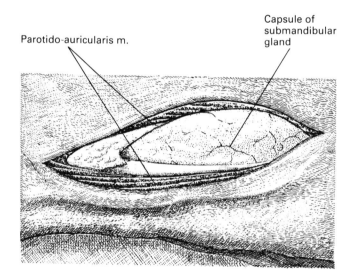

Fig. 2.68. The dog is placed in lateral recumbency with the affected side uppermost and its head and neck extended. A skin incision 7.5–10 cm long is made from the angular process of the mandible to the point of the V formed by the union of the external jugular vein with the internal and external maxillary veins. The underlying parotido-auricularis muscle is incised to expose the capsule of the mandibular gland.

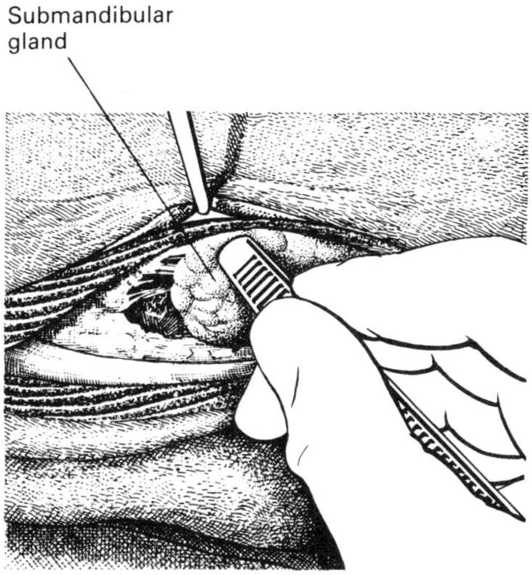

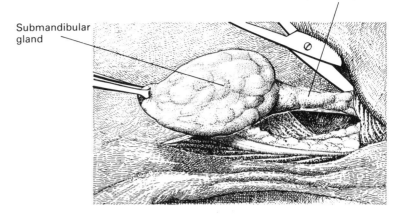

Fig. 2.69. The capsule is incised and the submandibular and caudal portion of the sublingual gland is freed by blunt dissection.

Fig. 2.70. The freed glands are brought out of the incision and the rostral portion of the sublingual gland separated by blunt dissection using scissors.

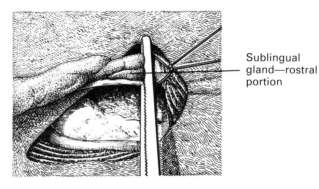

Fig. 2.71. When the rostral portion of the sublingual gland has been entirely freed, its extremity is seized with artery forceps. It is then drawn back to expose the ducts which are tied off and the attachments severed to complete the removal of the glands.

TRACHEOTOMY — HORSE

The operation of tracheotomy is performed to insert either a temporary or permanent tracheotomy tube. Temporary tracheotomy is employed to provide an airway for the relief of an acute high obstruction. The latter is employed when permanent obstructions are present such as ossification of the larynx, neoplasms, a fractured tracheal ring or as a substitute for laryngeal ventriculectomy to relieve the effects of paralysis of the intrinsic muscles of the larynx when a quick result is required.

The operation is satisfactorily performed with the horse standing under sedation and local analgesia (Figs 2.72–2.75). Under sedation the horse lowers its head and it is necessary to have an assistant supporting its jaw to obtain satisfactory exposure of the site.

The tube is composed of four parts, a lower and upper, a central cylindrical portion and a plug, securely held together by small thumbscrews (Fig. 2.76). Each part is introduced separately in its proper order.

For the first few days post operation, there is considerable mucous discharge and the tube has to be removed daily for cleaning. Once the local

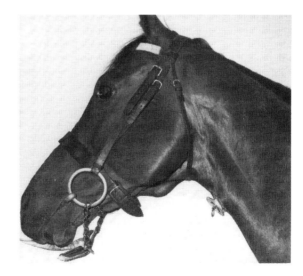

Fig. 2.72. The correct site for inserting a permanent tracheotomy tube is in the midline of the ventral aspect of the neck at the upper and middle thirds. This site is clear of the harness and leaves room for repeating the operation lower down should stenosis of the trachea occur.

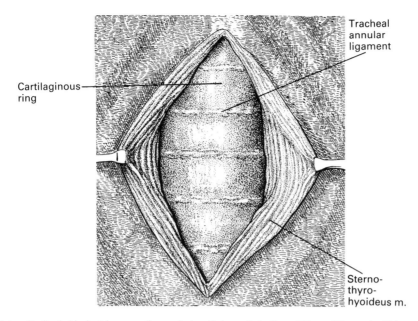

Fig. 2.73. A longitudinal skin incision 5.0–6.5 cm in length is made in the midline of the neck. This exposes the sternothyrohyoideus muscle, which is divided and retracted to expose the trachea.

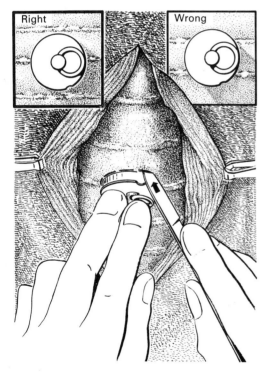

Fig. 2.74. A semi-disc of cartilage is removed from two adjacent tracheal rings. This leaves a strip of each ring intact and prevents the rings from collapsing. The size of the disc to be removed is gauged by using the plug of the tube as a guide. It is important to use a solid scalpel to remove the cartilaginous disc as the tip of a fine detachable blade can easily snap off and disappear down the trachea.

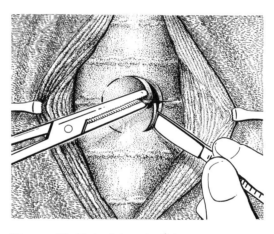

Fig. 2.75. The blade of the scalpel is inserted through the annular ligament and the upper ring partly severed. The disc of cartilage to be removed is then seized securely with Kocher forceps and a circular incision is continued through the cartilage to complete its removal.

inflammation has subsided the tube can be cleaned *in situ* and need only be removed at 10–14 day intervals.

When in the stable the tube is kept closed by its plug to prevent dust, etc. entering the trachea, and care must be taken to ensure there is no place against which it can be rubbed. If the top half of a loose box door is kept open then a grill should be put up to prevent the horse getting his head over the lower half. A horse should never be turned out to grass wearing a tube.

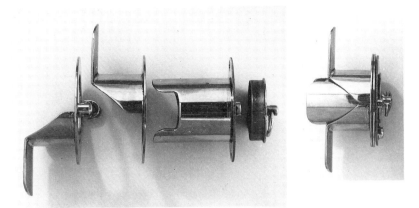

Fig. 2.76. Jones' tracheotomy tube. This is the standard permanent self-retaining tracheotomy tube and is available in the following sizes:

Size	Bore (mm)	Neck (mm)
1	25	25
2	28.5	28.5
3	32	32
4	35	35

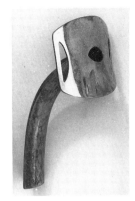

Fig. 2.77. Temporary or emergency tracheotomy tube for a horse. The trachea is exposed in the manner described but instead of removing a disc of cartilage from two adjacent rings an intertracheal annular ligament is divided transversely and the flange of the tube inserted between the two tracheal rings. It is retained in position with tape tied around the neck.

TRACHEOTOMY — DOG

It is sometimes necessary to perform a temporary tracheotomy (Figs 2.78—2.79) in the dog to provide an emergency airway for a high obstruction or in the treatment of intrapulmonary haemorrhage or pulmonary oedema in which the tidal volume has been reduced to that approximating the physiological dead space. It also enables the bronchial tree to be aspirated of mucus and secretions, which is not possible via the larynx.

The tube is retained *in situ* with a tape tied around the neck and has to be cleaned out two or three times daily. When the tube is removed the flap of trachea is repositioned and the overlying muscle and skin closed in the usual manner. The edges of the flap and of the trachea rapidly adhere and prevent stenosis of the lumen.

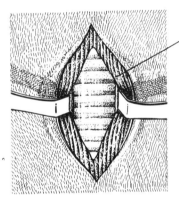

Sterno-hyoideus m.

Fig. 2.78. The dog is restrained in dorsal recumbency with its head and neck fully extended. A longitudinal and midline skin incision 2.5—4.0 cm in length is extended caudally from just below the cricoid cartilage of the larynx. The underlying sternohyoideus muscle is divided and retracted to expose the trachea.

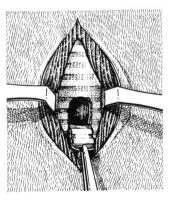

Fig. 2.79. The tracheotomy is performed by severing two or three tracheal rings and reflecting a complete section of the trachea.

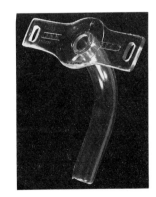

Fig. 2.80. A plastic tracheotomy tube. This type, moulded in transparent non-toxic PVC, is very suitable for dogs and is obtainable in sizes ranging from French Gauge 16 to 42 (9—22 mm external diameter).

OPERATION FOR WINDSUCKING AND CRIB-BITING (FORSELL'S OPERATION) – HORSE

Windsucking and crib-biting can be alleviated and often permanently cured by resecting 15 cm of each pair of the sternohyoideus and omohyoideus, sternothyroideus and sternocephalicus muscles from near their cranial insertions (Fig. 2.81).

The operation is performed with the horse in dorsal recumbency, its neck extended and with its head resting at an angle of 30°. If the head is excessively extended it may stretch the recurrent laryngeal nerve and it also makes dissection more difficult.

A midline longitudinal skin incision is commenced just caudally to the body of the hyoid bone and extended caudally for 25–35 cm to expose the muscles of the neck (Fig. 2.82). First the sternohyoideus and omohyoideus muscles are divided 15 cm caudal to the angle of the jaw, dissected forward and resected near their insertions. This exposes the sternothyroideus, a small flat muscle lying on the trachea, which is divided 15 cm from its insertion, dissected forward off the trachea and resected at its insertion. Next the sternocephalicus is resected as it disappears under the parotid gland and submaxillary vein. This muscle is enclosed in a sheath of fascia which is incised longitudinally from

just behind the point where it passes under the maxillary vein and extended caudally for 15 cm. The muscle is then separated from the fascia by blunt dissection and when it has been completely separated, tension is applied and it is severed about 2.5 cm cranial to the point where it disappears under the maxillary vein. The severed muscle is then reflected about 15 cm and removed together with the fascia, but two points deserve attention: (a) a large artery enters towards the centre of this muscle and requires to be ligated; and (b) a branch from the carotid artery enters the muscle 3.5–5 cm

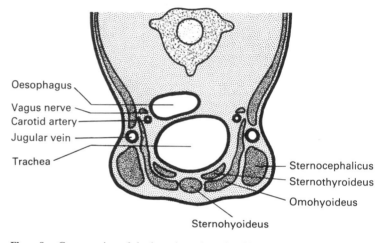

Fig. 2.81. Cross-section of the horse's neck at the third cervical vertebra.

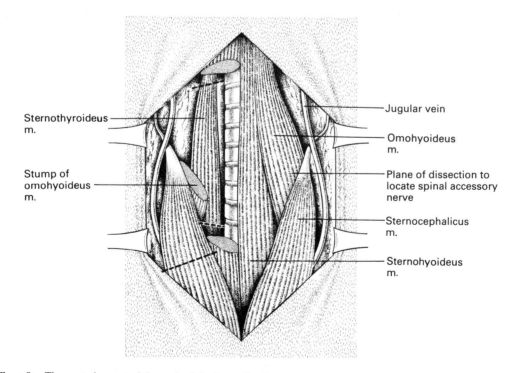

Fig. 2.82. The ventral aspect of the neck of the horse showing the sites of transection of the sternothyroideus and sternocephalicus muscles (dashed lines).

to the point where it disappears under the sub-maxillary vein and so particular care must be taken when it is divided.

Although haemorrhage during the operation is minimal it should be meticulously controlled by forcipressure or diathermy to minimize seroma formation. A 2.5-cm diameter Penrose drain is inserted at both extremities of the wound or, alternatively a continuous suction drain may be employed. Closure of the wound consists of a simple continuous suture in the subcutaneous tissue with synthetic absorbable material and horizontal mattress sutures of nylon in the skin. A stent bandage sutured over the length of the incision helps to eliminate dead space. This is removed 4 days post-operatively and the drainage tubes after 3–7 days.

The not inconsiderable mass of muscle removed, inevitably results in some disfigurement. A modification of the technique in which the sternocephalicus muscle, the largest and most powerful muscle involved in cribbing is denervated rather than resected, improves the cosmetic result without reducing the overall success rate. The sternocephalicus muscle is innervated by the ventral branch of the spinal accessory nerve. Although the neurec-

tomy can be performed after myectomy of the omohyoid and sternothyrohyoideus muscles, the nerve is easier to identify before the surgical field has become obscured by blood. A plane of dissection is established on the medial side of the sternocephalicus muscle about 5 cm caudal to its musculo-tendinous junction. By carefully rotating the muscle laterally, the nerve is identified on its dorsomedial aspect (Fig. 2.82). Gentle pressure on the nerve with forceps evokes sudden contraction of the muscle. Curved haemostats are placed under the nerve which is separated from the underlying muscle using two fingers, allowing at least 12 cm to be removed. The procedure is repeated on the other side.

CANNULATING THE CAROTID ARTERY – DOG

Blood for transfusion is obtained from the jugular vein of the donor unless exsanguination is practised, when the carotid artery is cannulated. The carotid artery has also to be cannulated for cerebral angiography. The procedure is shown in Figs 2.83–2.86.

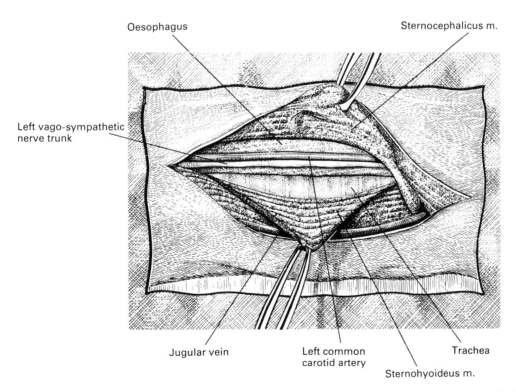

Fig. 2.83. With the dog in right lateral recumbency a longitudinal skin incision is made dorsal to and parallel with the jugular furrow. The line of cleavage between the sternocephalicus and sternohyoideus muscle is located and the muscles separated by blunt dissection to expose the left common carotid artery and left vago-sympathetic nerve trunk lying between the trachea and oesophagus.

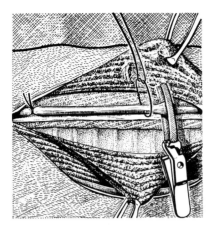

Fig. 2.84. The left common carotid artery is freed by blunt dissection, ligated cranially and clamped caudally with a bulldog clip. A ligature is placed around the artery and left untied.

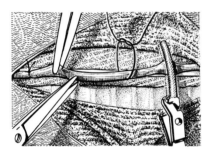

Fig. 2.85. The artery is picked up with dissecting forceps and partially severed with scissors to fashion a V-shaped opening.

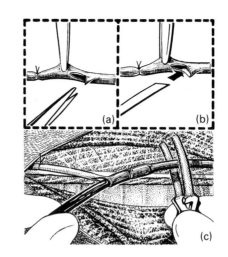

Fig. 2.86. Method of cannulating the artery. (a) V-shaped opening produced by cutting the artery with scissors. (b) The end of the cannula is bevelled. To insert the cannula into the lumen of the vessel the point of the bevelled end is inserted under flap. (c) The cannula is inserted until it encounters the clamp and then retained in position by tying the ligature previously laid. Finally, the clamp is released.

The mandible

FRACTURE OF THE HORIZONTAL RAMUS — DOG

Many methods have been advocated for immobilizing fractures of the horizontal ramus. These include fixation with a bone plate or transfixion by an intramedullary pin but in the majority of cases the easiest and most effective method is to immobilize the fracture with a wire suture supported by interdental wiring (Figs 2.87–2.90). If this method is impractical due to loose, broken or missing teeth then fixation with a bone plate is an alternative method (Fig. 2.91).

A fracture of the ramus is invariably complicated by torn gums and mucous membranes. These are sutured using 2 metric synthetic absorbable suture material. Post operation, particular attention must be paid to mouth hygiene and to the control of infection.

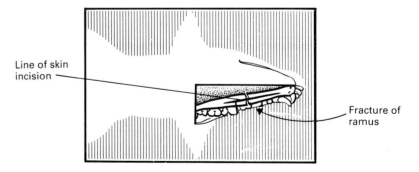

Line of skin incision

Fracture of ramus

Fig. 2.87. The dog is placed in dorsal recumbency with its head and neck fully extended and the skin is incised along the ventral border of the ramus.

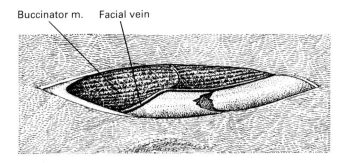

Buccinator m.　　Facial vein

Fig. 2.88. The fracture site is exposed by reflecting the buccinator muscle and facial vein medially.

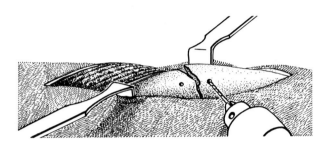

Fig. 2.89. Using a 1.5-mm drill, two holes are drilled through the ramus one on each side of the fracture, making sure they are placed below the alveoli of the adjacent teeth.

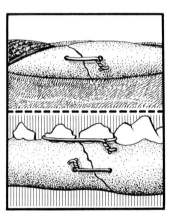

Fig. 2.90. A length of wire is passed through the drill holes, the fracture reduced and then immobilized by twisting tight the ends of the wire. The twisted portion is then cut off short and the end pressed flat against the lateral aspect of the ramus. With the dog turned on its side the immobilized fracture is further supported by wiring together the two teeth adjacent to the fracture.

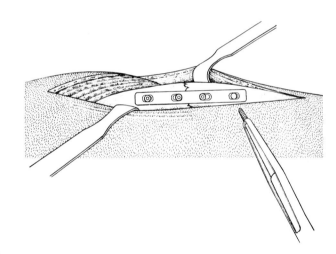

Fig. 2.91. In many cases a bone plate and screws provides more stable immobilization. A 2.7-mm dynamic compression plate is suitable for most sizes of dogs.

An external fixator consisting of multiple percutaneous pins joined by a 'sausage' of methylmethacrylate is a cheap and versatile method of repairing many mandibular fractures (Fig. 2.92). Perfect reduction of all of the fractured fragments is not important provided dental occlusion is achieved.

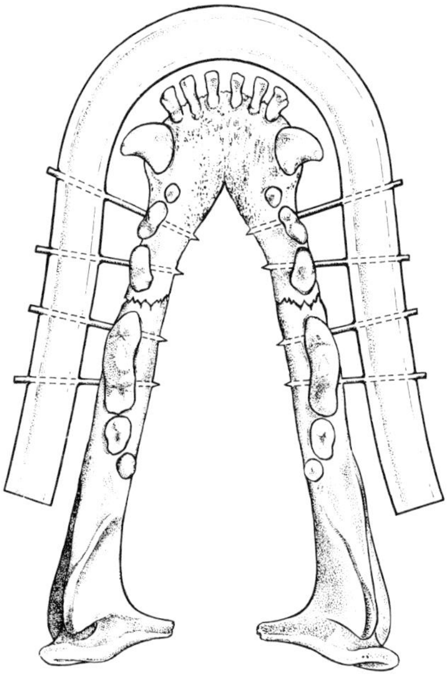

FRACTURE OF THE SYMPHYSIS — CAT

This is a very common fracture in the cat and is best treated by encircling the symphysis with a wire suture (Fig. 2.93).

Healing should be established in about 3 weeks when the wire is removed. A similar fracture in the dog is treated in like manner.

Fig. 2.92. An acrylic external fixator. The jaws are closed and two or more Kirschner wires are inserted percutaneously into each major fracture segment. The ends of the wires are pushed through wide-bore polythene tubing which is then filled with methylmethacrylate. The acrylic is prepared by mixing liquid monomer with a powdered polymer. It sets within a few minutes by an exothermic reaction.

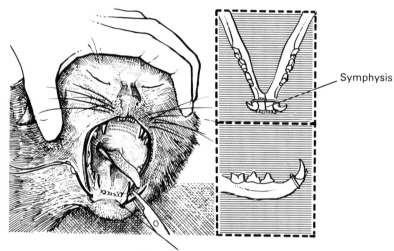

Symphysis

Mucous membrane

Fig. 2.93. Using a full-curved round-bodied needle, a monofilament wire suture is passed beneath the mucous membrane ventral to the incisors, and then around the symphysis behind the incisors, before being twisted tight and cut off.

Section 3
Abdominal Surgery

Laparotomy

In the dog it is normal practice to carry out laparotomy through the linea alba or by variations of this simple approach (Fig. 3.1). This is well tolerated by the patient and gives an excellent surgical exposure to all the abdominal viscera.

During recent years it has become common practice to enter the abdomen of the horse through the linea alba; an incision which allows excellent surgical exposure, reduces post-operative tissue reaction and eliminates the possibility of unsightly scarring of the sublumbar fossa.

In the larger domestic animals, however, incisions near the lower abdomen are subjected to considerable pressure from the weight of the overlying abdominal contents, and wound breakdown is likely to be complicated by a massive prolapse of viscera. For this reason, laparotomy is commonly carried out through a flank incision. As the ox does not tolerate lateral recumbency for any length of time due to ruminal tympany, this, together with the placid temperament of the cow, has led to major abdominal surgery being carried out on the standing animal under regional analgesia. Although there are advantages with this procedure, one must bear in mind that the flank incision considerably reduces the surgical exposure and makes manipulation of the large abdominal viscera very exhausting. Nor is it possible to block all sensory nervous pathways from the abdominal viscera by the commonly used techniques of regional analgesia.

Anatomical considerations

The anatomical distribution of the abdominal muscles follows a common pattern, with only minor species modifications. The external and internal oblique abdominal muscles, and the transverse abdominal muscle all arise as muscle masses each forming a broad fibrous tendon of insertion or aponeurosis. The aponeuroses of the two oblique muscles fuse at the linea alba external to the flat muscle mass of the rectus abdominis muscle, and together form the external sheath of the rectus. The aponeurosis of the transversus muscle forms the internal sheath of the rectus muscle. It fuses at the linea alba deep to the rectus abdominis, together with the peritoneum.

DOG

Linea alba incision

Careful dissection through the fibrous linea alba allows an almost bloodless laparotomy incision. The incision may be closed by a single layer of interrupted sutures. Alternatively, a continuous suture is simple and quick.

To carry out a cranial laparotomy through the linea alba it is necessary to trim the fatty falciform

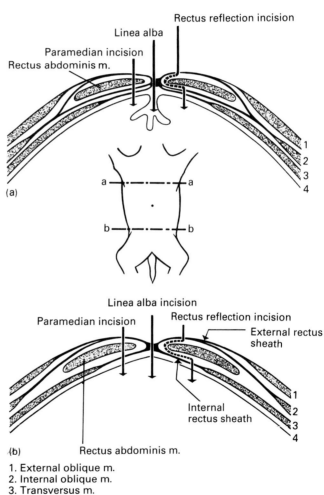

1. External oblique m.
2. Internal oblique m.
3. Transversus m.
4. Peritoneum

Fig. 3.1. The abdominal wall of the dog may be opened surgically from xiphisternum to pubic brim, but this is rarely if ever necessary. Operations on the diaphragm, stomach, spleen and small intestine are normally carried out through an incision anterior to the umbilicus (cranial laparotomy, a), whereas hysterectomy, cystotomy and surgery of the rectum and colon require an incision between the umbilicus and pubic brim (caudal laparotomy, b).

ligament which lies in the midline and extends from the umbilicus forward between the central lobes of the liver.

Rectus-splitting or paramedian incision

This can be conveniently used for both cranial and caudal laparotomies. The incision is made parallel to the linea alba through the external and internal sheaths and the substance of the rectus abdominis muscle. Surgical trauma is not excessive as the fibres of the rectus muscle run in the direction of the incision, but haemorrhage is often considerable and must be carefully controlled. Closure is effected by a continuous suture in the internal rectus sheath and the peritoneum, then by a layer of interrupted sutures in the external rectus sheath.

Rectus reflection

This may again be used for a cranial or caudal laparotomy and if correctly carried out is almost bloodless. The external rectus sheath is incised parallel to and about 1 cm away from the linea alba to expose the rectus muscle. The rectus sheath is blunt-dissected away from the rectus muscle towards the midline until the medial edge of the rectus muscle is exposed along the required length. The edge of the rectus muscle is then lifted away from the internal sheath, which is opened about 5 mm away from and parallel to the linea alba. Closure is effected by a continuous suture in the internal sheath and peritoneum, and interrupted or continuous sutures in the external sheath.

HORSE

Laparotomy is now widely practised in the horse and includes operations to correct disorders of the alimentary tract, surgery of the abdominally placed genital organs and surgery of the urinary bladder. In addition to allowing access to the organ on which surgery is contemplated, the laparotomy incision must fulfil other requirements.

The site of the incision and the materials and methods used to close it, must be able to withstand the great stresses and strains to which it will be subjected, e.g. when the patient regains its feet after surgery. The incision should be simple to perform, produce minimal damage to the abdominal wall and should heal without impairment of function.

A variety of approaches are employed, the most important being: ventral midline, ventral paramedian and flank.

Ventral midline incision

The linea alba approach is the most versatile and is now used almost universally for colic surgery. It is also the approach favoured by most surgeons for Caesarean section and ovariectomy in the mare.

A short exploratory incision in the central midline can be extended in either direction to accommodate any problem encountered. For colic surgery an initial skin incision, 20 cm long, is made commencing at the umbilicus and extending cranially. Separation of the subcutaneous fat and connective tissue for a centimetre or so on either side facilitates closure of the linea alba later.

The incision in the linea alba, which is only a few millimetres wide, is made carefully and precisely commencing at the umbilicus where the exact midline can be identified even when the abdomen is very distended. The underlying retroperitoneal fat, which may be several centimetres thick, is divided exposing the thin peritoneum which is opened along the length of the round ligament of the liver.

Midline incisions heal more slowly than paramedian or flank incisions because of the relative lack of vasculature of the linea alba. Improved anaesthetic and surgical techniques and reliable suture materials allow reconstruction to be accomplished quickly and easily with only minimal risk of herniation and evisceration even in the biggest horses. A wide variety of suture techniques and materials have been used.

The peritoneum is thin and tears easily but providing adequate decompression of bowel has been carried out, it can be sutured using a continuous suture of 3 metric polyglycolic acid or polyglactin 910. Experimental and clinical experience has shown that no detrimental effects result if the peritoneum is left unsutured. The linea alba is closed using a continuous suture of 5 metric coated polyglactin or 5 metric polyglycolic acid doubled (Fig. 3.2a). In extremely large or muscular horses, or when considerable tension is required to approximate the edges of the incision the far and near suture pattern is useful (Fig. 3.2b). Non-absorbable, coated braided polyester suture material may be used.

The subcutaneous tissue is closed with a continuous suture of 3.5 metric polyglactin and the skin with a continuous mattress suture of 8 metric sheathed multifilament polyamide. Although the use of continuous suture patterns and absorbable materials would appear, theoretically at least, to be risky, it has proved a reliable method and has the advantage of significant saving in time (this may be critical in colic cases) and a reduced incidence of sinus formation.

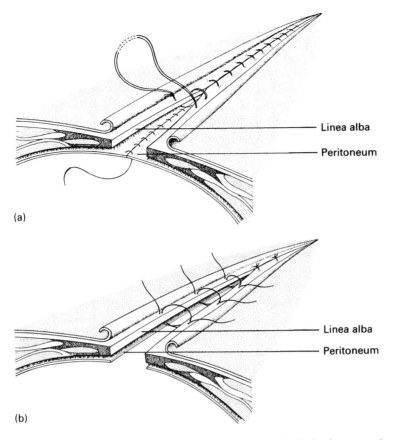

Fig. 3.2. (a) The linea alba is closed using a continuous suture of 5 metric coated polyglactin or 5 metric polyglycolic acid doubled. (b) When considerable tension is required to close the incision the linea may be repaired with a far and near suture pattern.

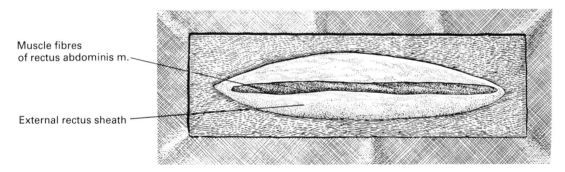

Fig. 3.3. After incision of the skin, the cutaneous trunci muscle and the abdominal tunic, the external sheath of the rectus is incised.

Paramedian incisions

Paramedian incisions (Figs 3.3–3.6) are most useful to gain access to the caudal abdomen in the male horse for cryptorchidectomy, cystotomy and repair of a ruptured bladder.

The skin incision is made along the line of the fibres of the rectus abdominis muscle and is therefore parallel to the midline, if made anywhere from the xiphoid as far back as the entrance to the sheath. Made further caudally, the incision should be angled slightly medially at its caudal end because the fibres are converging on the linea alba.

Closure is effected by a continuous suture in the peritoneum and transversus fascia, which is often difficult if the retroperitoneal fat layer is very thick. The fascia of the external sheath is closed with interrupted sutures.

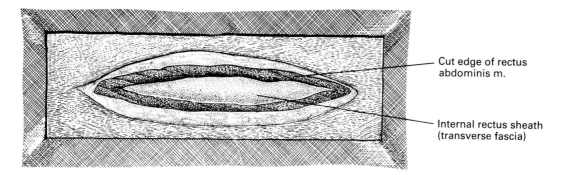

Fig. 3.4. The rectus muscle is gently split longitudinally in the direction of its fibres by blunt dissection to expose the internal rectus sheath. This allows the vessels which traverse the incision to be recognized and ligated before they are cut.

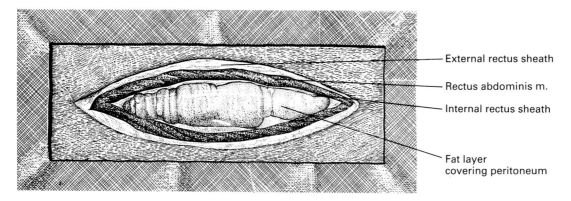

Fig. 3.5. The internal sheath of the rectus is opened to expose the layer of fat which covers the peritoneum.

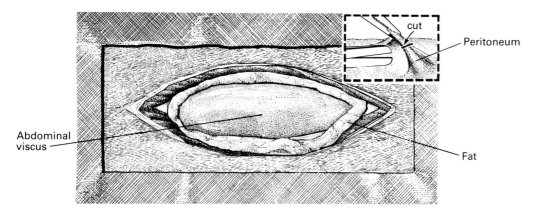

Fig. 3.6. The peritoneum is carefully 'tented' to avoid damage to the underlying viscera, and opened with scissors. Absorbable sutures of polyglycolic acid, polyglactin or polydioxanone are used for all layers other than skin.

Flank incision

The paralumbar fossa in the horse is very small and this site allows only enough room for manual exploration, with little or no visualization of abdominal contents. Therefore, it is more common to make the incision lower in the flank (Figs 3.7–3.10).

This type of muscle-splitting flank incision is sometimes referred to as a 'grid-iron' incision, and has the advantages of causing the minimum of surgical trauma, and once traction is removed from each muscle layer the wound tends to be self closing. It is usual to close the peritoneum and the overlying fat layer with a continuous suture. Interrupted sutures are placed in the internal and exter-

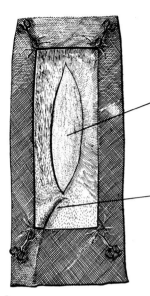

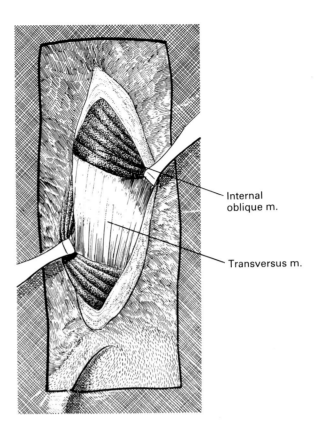

Fig. 3.7. A vertical incision is made through the skin and cutaneous trunci muscle. The incision extends from just cranial to the external angle of the ileum down to the fold of the flank to expose the aponeurosis of the external oblique muscle. This avoids the danger of cutting the lateral border of the rectus abdominis muscle, and its adjacent posterior abdominal artery.

Fig. 3.9. The fibres of the internal oblique are split and retracted to expose the aponeurosis of the transversus muscle whose fibres tend to run in the vertical plane.

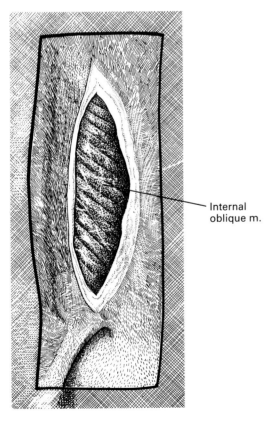

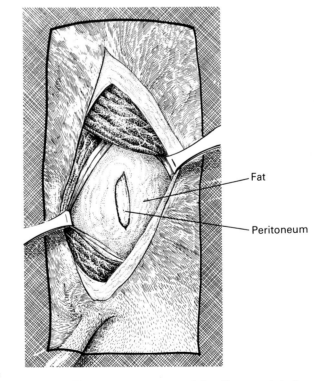

Fig. 3.8. The aponeurosis of the external oblique muscle is opened in the vertical plane to expose the thick origin of the internal oblique muscle, whose fibres are inclined in a cranio-ventral direction.

Fig. 3.10. The transversus aponeurosis is split to reveal the layer of fat covering the peritoneum. This is not usually as thick as in the lower abdomen, but must be 'tented' and opened with care.

nal oblique muscles and the skin is closed separately incorporating the cutaneous trunci muscle.

This approach has been used for cryptorchidectomy and ovariectomy and should be employed in colic cases should a repeat laparotomy be necessary more than 4 days after the initial operation.

Access to a viscus located near the roof of the abdomen sometimes necessitates removal of the 17th and/or 18th rib. Splenectomy, nephrectomy and total resection of the caecum are performed using this approach.

The technique of rib resection is as described for the dog (Section 7).

In some horses with a more caudal attachment of the diaphragm, removal of the 17th rib may result in the thoracic cavity being opened but this presents no problem providing the margin of the diaphragm is included in the sutures used to close the deepest layer of the incision.

CATTLE

The sublumbar fossa of the ox is wider than that of the horse, and flank laparotomy may be carried out either cranially for rumenotomy or caudally either for Caesarean section or to rectify a displaced abomasum. Both of these incisions should be modelled on the 'grid-iron' technique as described for the horse, with the following anatomical variations.

1 The cranial incision will pass through the thick muscular origin of the external oblique, whereas the underlying internal oblique in this region is only an aponeurosis. If the incision is high in the sublumbar fossa it will pass through the muscular origin of the transverse muscle, which lower down blends into an aponeurosis in which may be seen the lumbar segmental nerves.

2 Caudal laparotomy just cranial to the external angle of the ileum is anatomically the same as described for a flank laparotomy in the horse, except that there is no fat layer in the cow between the transversus fascia and the peritoneum.

3 When closing both of these incisions the peritoneum and transversus fascia should be closed together with a continuous suture. The other muscle layers are co-apted by interrupted sutures.

Gastro-intestinal surgery

DOG

The high acid content in the stomach of the dog enables it to digest relatively large pieces of meat which are swallowed after a minimum of chewing and often include large pieces of bone. This predisposes to the ingestion of large and undigestable 'foreign bodies', which will often lie in the stomach for long periods of time without giving rise to symptoms. If they cause gastritis by local irritation, or pass into the pyloric area of the stomach they then stimulate vomiting and other signs suggestive of obstruction. Whilst it is difficult to palpate a foreign body in the stomach, it can usually be demonstrated radiographically.

Gastric dilatation and torsion

This condition is most frequently seen in the larger breeds of dog, and usually follows soon after ingestion of a large meal. The condition is characterized by rapid abdominal distension, accompanied by signs of acute discomfort and frequent attempts at vomiting, which are usually unproductive. Experimental work carried out on cadavers showed that dilatation of the dog's stomach led to a tendency for the stomach to rotate around the fixed point of the cardia, and numerous clinical observers have shown that this rotation is invariably 270° in a clockwise direction, as viewed from the abdominal cavity looking cranially.

Whereas simple dilatation causes extreme discomfort and respiratory embarrassment, torsion of the stomach causes profound cardiovascular changes due to the virtual complete occlusion of the venous return from the gastro-intestinal tract. It is therefore vitally important to differentiate dilatation from torsion.

The immediate action of the clinician must be to pass a stomach tube. If this enters the stomach through the cardia it not only relieves the dilatation but also shows that no torsion is present. In cases of simple dilatation it is important to drain the stomach of its contents, if necessary rotating the dog in its long axis several times in order to release all the possible residual pockets of gas and ingesta. This drainage procedure should be repeated frequently during the first 24 hours to guard against the recurrence of the dilatation.

If it proves impossible to insinuate the stomach

tube through the cardia, then the distension must be relieved as a matter of urgency. In cases of extreme distress, where respiratory and circulatory collapse are imminent, the distension can be relieved by trocharization of the stomach through the abdominal wall just caudal to the costal arch in the lower right flank. The trochar will enter the dilated fundus of the stomach, which following a clockwise torsion will be lying in the right epigastrium. Emptying the stomach by paracentesis, followed by warm saline lavage, sometimes leads to spontaneous resolution of the torsion and is confirmed by the ability to pass the stomach tube through the cardia.

An alternative method of decompression is temporary gastrostomy performed under local analgesia. This is a more time-consuming technique but has the advantage over trocharization that there is less likelihood of peritonitis developing. A 5-cm grid incision is made through the previously desensitized abdominal wall 2 cm behind and parallel to the right costal arch. The distended stomach wall is picked up and anchored by two temporary stay sutures before stitching it to the edge of the skin wound with a continuous suture of a synthetic absorbable suture. The stomach wall is incised within the sutured area and its edges oversewn to control bleeding. The stomach can now be emptied and lavaged with warm saline with little risk of contaminating the abdominal cavity. After 24 hours of drainage a laparotomy is performed to excise the gastrostomy and repair the stomach wall.

If decompression fails to relieve the torsion it is necessary to reposition the stomach surgically. In the past this has been done via a laparotomy as an emergency procedure. However, such surgery was invariably carried out on a severely shocked patient and, in spite of vigorous transfusion, the mortality rate was unacceptedly high. It is wiser to defer surgery until the animal is fit for general anaesthesia. This generally means maintaining decompression for 24 hours while cardiovascular and respiratory function improve.

Tube gastrostomy and gastropexy is the surgical procedure of choice to reposition the rotated stomach. This technique can also be used to prevent recurrence of the torsion at a later date. The dog is placed in dorsal recumbency and a midline laparotomy performed. Roberts' forceps are pushed through the parietal peritoneum and musculature of the abdominal wall of the right paracostal region near the tip of the 13th rib. The points of the forceps are directed dorsally so as to emerge half-way between the vertebral column

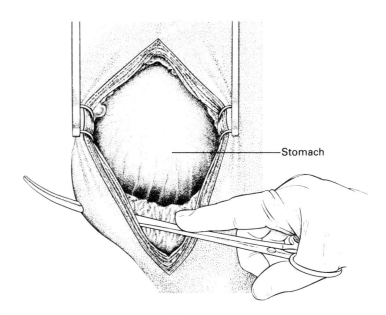

Fig. 3.11. Roberts' forceps are pushed through the abdominal wall ventral to the tip of the 13th rib. The exit hole in the skin is situated dorsally and is of a smaller diameter than the catheter which is to be used.

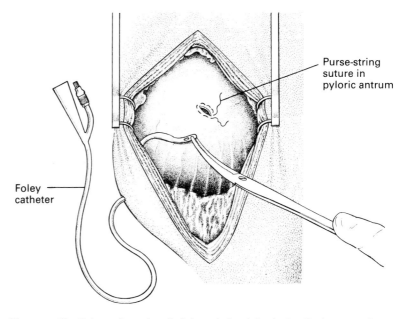

Fig. 3.12. The Foley catheter is pulled through the abdominal wall. A purse-string suture of non-absorbable material is placed in the pyloric antrum and a small incision made within it.

and the linea alba. A small incision is made in the skin to permit the points of the forceps to exit (Fig. 3.11). The end of a 26 French gauge Foley catheter is grasped by the forceps and pulled into the abdomen. The catheter is passed through the greater omentum of the stomach and through an incision in a previously placed purse-string suture in the pyloric antrum. This suture is placed two-thirds of the way from the fundus to the pylorus and should be of non-absorbable material such as polypropylene (Fig. 3.12).

The balloon of the Foley catheter is inflated with saline and the purse-string suture tightened around its body. The inflated catheter is pulled up so that the stomach lies against the abdominal wall and the two are sutured together with interrupted non-absorbable sutures. A purse-string suture is placed in the skin around the Foley catheter (Fig. 3.13) and the laparotomy incision closed in the usual way.

The abdomen is bandaged to prevent the dog from interfering with the catheter. This must be left *in situ* for at least 5 days to minimize the development of peritonitis. Before withdrawing the catheter the balloon is deflated and the purse-string skin suture is removed. The gastrostomy heals by granulation within a few days, during which time the area is kept clean and bandaged.

The significance of delayed gastric emptying in the aetiology of the gastric dilatation/torsion complex is unclear but it is recommended that pyloric myotomy (see Fig. 3.17) is performed as a prophylactic measure. In contrast, there is no indication for splenectomy unless the organ is infarcted.

Gastrotomy

The stomach is approached through a caudal laparotomy incision to the left of the linea alba. The foreign body is readily palpable through the intact stomach wall and can be manipulated into the fundus of the stomach which is then drawn up to the incision by gentle traction. The portion of stomach containing the foreign body is isolated by means of a bowel clamp (Figs 3.14–3.16).

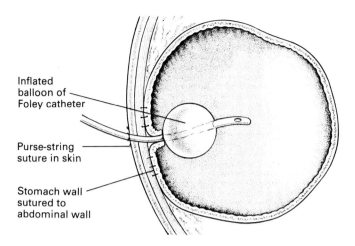

Inflated balloon of Foley catheter

Purse-string suture in skin

Stomach wall sutured to abdominal wall

Fig. 3.13. The Foley catheter is introduced into the stomach and its balloon inflated with saline. Traction is applied to the inflated catheter to appose the stomach and adjacent body wall. A series of gastropexy sutures of silk or polypropylene are placed to anchor the gastric wall to the peritoneum, taking care not to put the needle through the inflated balloon. A purse-string suture is placed in the skin around the Foley catheter.

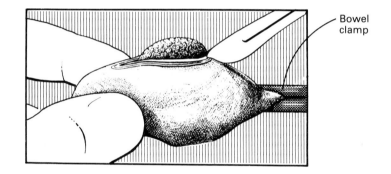

Bowel clamp

Fig. 3.14. The exposed portion of stomach is carefully packed off with moist and warm isolation towels to avoid peritoneal contamination. The stomach wall is opened by cutting down onto the foreign body which is immobilized by gripping it through the stomach wall. It will be noted that the mucous membrane of the stomach is extremely vascular and is freely movable owing to the very loose texture of the submucous connective tissue. After removing the foreign body the stomach wall is closed in two layers.

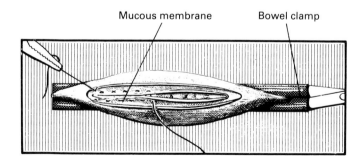

Mucous membrane   Bowel clamp

Fig. 3.15. The mucous membrane is closed by a continuous mattress suture of 2 metric synthetic absorbable material which not only co-apts the edge of the incision but also has a haemostatic effect. If haemorrhage from the mucous membrane is not controlled a large submucous haematoma may form which can lead to complete disruption of the gastrotomy incision.

Interrupted Lembert inversion sutures

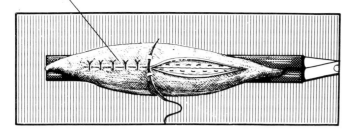

Fig. 3.16. The muscle layer is closed by interrupted sutures which invert the wound edges and bring the peritoneal surfaces into apposition, thus ensuring rapid adhesion of the superficial muscle layer.

Pyloric stenosis

This condition is either congenital or acquired. It may be caused either by spasm of the sphincter or hypertrophy of the pyloric musculature both of which interfere with the passage of food from the stomach into the duodenum. This leads to retention of food in the stomach giving rise to gastric dilatation which is accompanied by vomiting. This is often very forceful in nature and is referred to as 'projectile vomiting'.

Acquired hypertrophic pyloric stenosis appears to be most frequent in young Boxer dogs. Both the congenital and acquired conditions are benign in nature and respond to surgical correction.

The operation of choice is pyloric myotomy using the Fredet–Ramstedt technique which aims to divide the encircling pyloric musculature and thus to relieve the obstruction to the pyloric canal (Fig. 3.17). The area is exposed through a cranial laparotomy to the right of the midline. The thickened pylorus is readily palpable but is relatively immobile, being fixed by the hepatoduodenal ligament, and care must be taken when applying traction to avoid damage to the common bile duct.

An alternative technique is to insert the forefinger into the pyloric canal through a small gastrotomy incision. Once the pyloric sphincter is completely divided the lack of resistance is appreciated by the examining finger.

Gastro-jejunostomy

Some cases of pyloric obstruction are neoplastic and will not therefore be relieved by simple myotomy. In cases where the lesion involves the

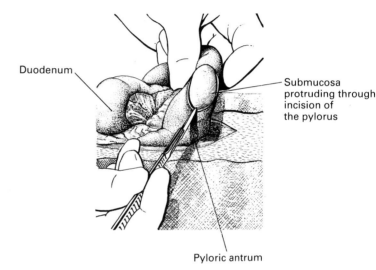

Duodenum

Submucosa protruding through incision of the pylorus

Pyloric antrum

Fig. 3.17. Once the pylorus is adequately exposed an incision is made transversely across the complete depth of the pyloric sphincter, extending 1–2 cm in either direction, to expose the submucous layer which should not be cut. If the technique is carried out correctly the submucosa will protrude through the incision, which is left unsutured, thus relieving the obstruction to the pyloric canal. Should the submucous layer be inadvertently opened, it must be accurately sutured to avoid leakage of ingesta into the abdominal cavity.

pylorus and pyloric antrum the most satisfactory treatment is by gastro-jejunostomy (partial gastrectomy) (Fig. 3.18). Whilst this re-routing of ingesta from the stomach direct into the jejunum does have its disadvantages, it is generally a more satisfactory technique than a direct gastroduodenostomy following resection of the pylorus.

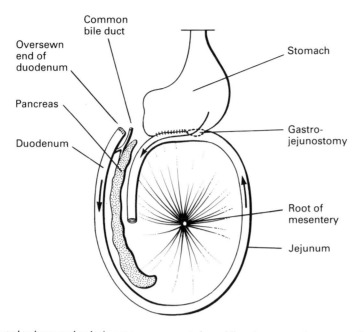

Fig. 3.18. The affected pylorus and pyloric antrum are resected, avoiding damage to the common bile duct. The proximal end of the duodenum is oversewn, and starting at the lesser curvature, the defect in the fundus of the stomach is closed, until a stoma is left on the greater curvature which approximates in size to the lumen of the jejunum. This stoma is then anastomosed to the conveniently adjacent jejunum by an end-to-side anastomosis, so that food leaving the stomach passes into the jejunum direct, and receives bile and pancreatic secretions from the duodenum. The arrows indicate the direction of peristalsis.

Intestinal obstruction

Enterotomy

Foreign bodies which pass through the pylorus into the duodenum often become held up in their passage through the small intestine and cause intestinal obstruction. This is an extremely serious condition and unless it can be quickly relieved death is the inevitable end result. It must be remembered that during normal digestion the fluid and electrolytes which are secreted into the intestine from the duodenum and pancreas are mostly reabsorbed in the lower small intestine, so that the loss of these constituents in the faeces is minimal. In the average animal this turnover of fluid represents about 2.5 times the plasma volume in 24 hours, and thus any interference with the normal cycle as occurs in intestinal obstruction will rapidly lead to extreme dehydration. An obstruction that occurs high in the small intestine completely prevents this cycle of reabsorption and therefore produces a far more rapid and dangerous syndrome than an obstruction which occurs low in the terminal ileum, but both will end fatally if they are not relieved. In addition, the loss of electrolyte occasioned by vomiting further aggravates the dehydration and also gives rise to a metabolic acidosis. It is not difficult to

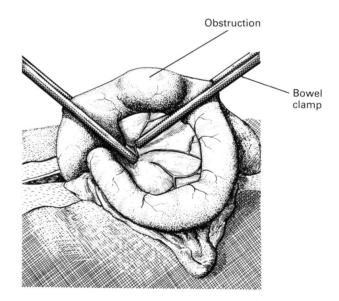

Fig. 3.19. Locate the obstruction, milk the ingesta away from the foreign body and apply bowel clamps to the intestine just above and below the site of obstruction in order to avoid spillage of intestinal contents when the bowel wall is opened. The intestine proximal to the obstruction is invariably distended with fluid which continues to be secreted into the bowel lumen after the obstruction has occurred. Ideally the foreign body should be manipulated distally into a piece of undevitalized bowel before the incision is made, but this is not always possible.

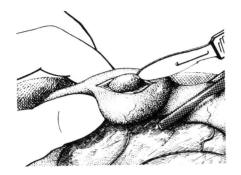

Fig. 3.20. Cut through the wall of the intestine onto the foreign body and remove it.

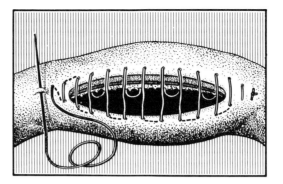

Fig. 3.21. Aspirate any intestinal contents and close the incision with an inversion suture which penetrates the full thickness of the intestinal wall, using an atraumatic needle with 2 metric synthetic absorbable suture material.

appreciate that any case of intestinal obstruction requires a careful pre-operative assessment and that surgery should never be undertaken until replacement has been made of the lost fluid and electrolyte, and the pH has been restored to normal. In the majority of cases the condition can be cured by enterotomy, in which the bowel wall is opened and the foreign body removed (Figs 3.19–3.21), but this should only be attempted after adequate preparation of the patient.

Enterectomy

In cases where intestinal obstruction has occurred and there has been delay in seeking treatment, the bowel wall adjacent to the foreign body undergoes ischaemic necrosis and may actually perforate. In these circumstances it becomes necessary to excise the segment of necrotic intestine and to anastomose the free ends (Figs 3.22–3.29). In the majority of cases the necessity for enterectomy will be obvious due to the devitalized nature of the obstructed bowel wall, but it must be remembered that the intestinal wall has remarkable powers of recovery, and enterectomy is never undertaken without due consideration. In cases in which the intestinal wall will not support sutures without tearing, it is almost certain that the tissue is too devitalized to undergo repair, and therefore enterectomy rather than enterotomy must be performed.

Intussusception is also a frequent indication for enterectomy. The intussuscepted bowel can usually be reduced until the last 2–3 cm when it invariably tears. The technique of making a longitudinal incision through the muscle coat to relieve pressure and overcome tearing during the final stage of reduction has not proved successful in the authors' hands.

The amount of bowel removed is dependent partly on the macroscopic damage and partly on

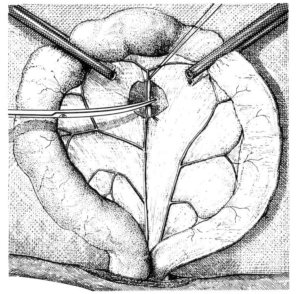

Fig. 3.22. The site of resection is isolated by bowel clamps and the mesenteric blood supply to the devitalized area is isolated and ligated.

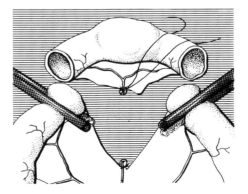

Fig. 3.23. The damaged section of bowel is removed together with the immediately adjacent mesentery.

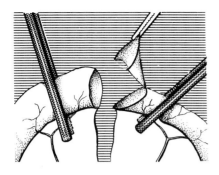

Fig. 3.24. After resection there is often a marked difference in the lumen of the two ends of the bowel and the smaller piece must be trimmed off at an angle to reduce the disparity.

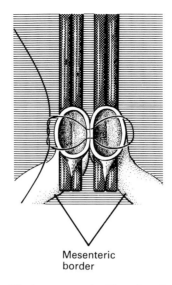

Mesenteric border

Fig. 3.25. The two open ends of bowel are held side by side by bowel clamps and are sutured together by a single mattress-type stitch, which is tied so that the knot lies within the lumen of the intestine, leaving at least 15 cm of synthetic absorbable suture material free on the end which is not attached to the atraumatic needle.

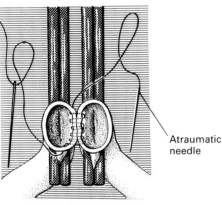

Atraumatic needle

Fig. 3.26. The suture material not attached to the atraumatic needle must now be threaded onto a needle and drawn through the intestinal wall so that it lies outside the bowel lumen. Closure is carried out using the atraumatic needle and a through-and-through stitch until it is no longer possible to continue stitching with the intestinal ends held side by side.

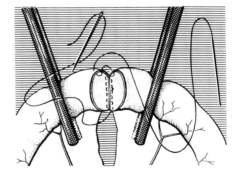

Fig. 3.27. The bowel ends are now rotated until they lie in continuity and the suturing is continued making certain that the needle penetrates the whole thickness of the bowel wall with each stitch.

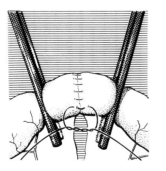

Fig. 3.28. Once the anastomosis is completed the two ends of suture material are tied. The bowel clamps are removed and ingesta is squeezed from proximal to distal bowel across the anastomosis to test both its patency and integrity. Alternatively, simple interrupted appositional sutures allow for easier tissue approximation and less constriction at the anastomosis site.

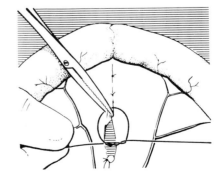

Fig. 3.29. The tear in the mesentery is carefully closed with 2 metric synthetic absorbable suture material.

the distribution of the mesenteric blood supply. It is essential to make the resection at a point where a major mesenteric vessel lies adjacent to the intestinal wall.

An alternative approach to intestinal anastomosis is to employ a simple approximating type of suture pattern such as the simple interrupted appositional suture. This suture is passed through all the layers of the bowel and tied without crushing them. It requires accurate and a traumatic placement of the sutures so that the two ends of the bowel are closely apposed without being under tension, but permits more rapid mucosal healing.

Whichever technique is employed, the anastomosis site should be wrapped with omentum to encourage healing.

HORSE

Side-to-side anastomosis is necessary in horses with chronic, slowly occlusive lesions of the small intestine which result in a great disparity between the diameters of the intestine proximal and distal to the lesion. Some surgeons prefer to use side-to-side routinely for all small intestinal anastomoses.

After closure of the two ends of the intestine by a double inverting suture, the two ends are laid alongside one another so that they overlap by 10 cm. They are united near their mesenteric border with a continuous over-and-over suture of 3 metric polyglycolic acid (Fig. 3.30a).

The lumen of each segment is opened by a longitudinal incision 8 cm long extending as close to the blind ends as possible (Fig. 3.30a).

The lumena of the bowel are united using a Connell suture of 3 metric polyglycolic acid (Fig. 3.30b–d).

Finally the closure is completed by continuing the over-and-over serosal suture to its origin where it is tied. The overlapped mesentery is sutured with a row of interrupted sutures along each free edge (Fig. 3.30e).

Ileocaecal and jejunocaecal anastomosis

The ileum is frequently the site of small intestinal obstruction in the horse. The terminal portion of the ileum is inaccessible via a ventral midline incision making resection and end-to-end anastomosis at that level technically very difficult if not impossible.

To overcome this problem and the limited blood supply at the ileum, side-to-side jejunocaecal anastomosis is now used routinely (Fig. 3.31).

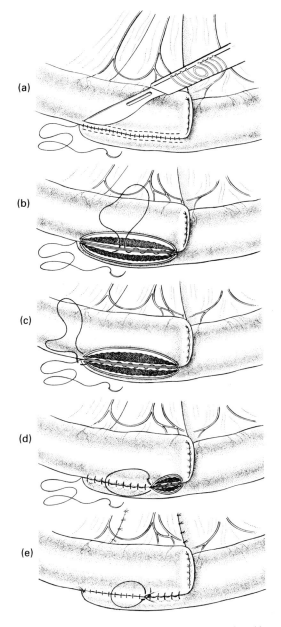

Fig. 3.30. (a) The two ends of the intestine are closed by a double inverting suture and overlapped. They are joined by a continuous over-and-over suture and their lumena opened. The two incisions should extend as close to the blind ends of the segments as possible. (b–d) The lumena of the bowel are united using a Connell suture of 3 metric polyglycolic acid. (e) The closure is completed by continuing the first over-and-over continuous suture back to its origin where it is tied.

The necrotic intestine is resected and the end is closed with an inversion suture. The jejunum is now placed between the dorsal and medial bands of the caecum with its closed end pointing towards the base of the caecum. The anastomosis is carried

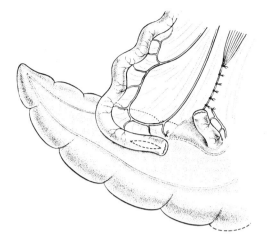

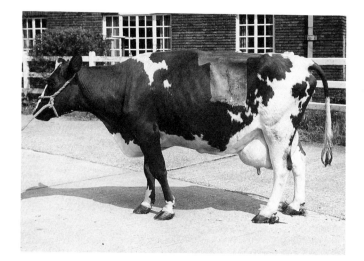

Fig. 3.31. To overcome the problem of poor access to the terminal ileum, a side-to-side jejunocaecal anastomosis is performed. The ileum is incised and its ends closed with an inverting suture. A side-to-side jejunocaecal anastomosis is then performed, as in Fig. 3.30. The blind end of the jejunum must point to the base of the caecum. The defect in the mesentery is closed to prevent other portions of bowel becoming trapped.

Fig. 3.33. Site of left cranial flank incision for rumentomy.

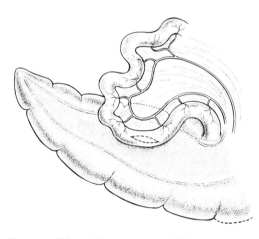

Fig. 3.32. Side-to-side anastomosis of the jejunum to the caecum bypassing the terminal ileum. The anastomosis is performed as in Fig. 3.30.

CATTLE

Rumenotomy

Rumenotomy is indicated either for the relief of rumenal impaction, or as an approach to the examination of the reticulum and its contents. The left dorsal sac of the rumen lies conveniently adjacent to the left sublumbar fossa and can be easily exposed through a cranial flank incision (Fig. 3.33). This approach is well tolerated in the standing animal using paravertebral analgesia or the less specific techniques of local analgesia of the sublumbar fossa. To avoid the danger of peritoneal contamination from spilled ingesta once the rumenal wall is opened, at one time it was common practice to suture the rumenal wall to the edge of the incised peritoneum before it was opened, or as an alternative the rumenal wall was 'tented' through the abdominal incision by means of stay sutures and held by two or more assistants. Both of these techniques had their disadvantages, but have largely been overcome by a set of instruments designed by McLintock, which consist of a rubber covered hook, a reinforced rubber sleeve, and a large adjustable clamp (Figs 3.34–3.36).

out as previously described for side-to-side anastomosis.

The mesenteric defect is closed by suturing the cut edge of the jejunal mesentery to that of the ileum and to the ileocaecal fold.

A modification of this technique, in which the ileum is anastomosed side-to-side to the caecum, without resection, can be used to bypass non-strangulating obstructions of the terminal ileum caused by hypertrophy or ileal–ileal intussus-ceptions (Fig. 3.32).

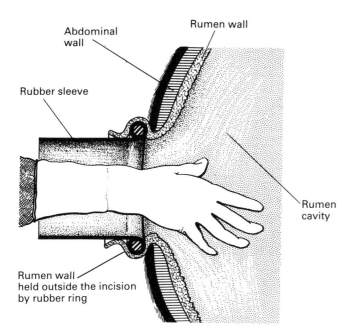

Fig. 3.34. Once the abdominal wall is opened, the rumenal wall is grasped and an incision approximately 12 cm long is made in the left dorsal sac. The rubber-covered hook is inserted into the upper commissure of the incision to hold it until the sleeve is inserted. This rubber sleeve is reinforced at one end by a flexible but firm rubber ring, which enables the sleeve to be compressed, but which immediately springs open when the compression is removed. This ring is compressed and inserted into the rumenal incision, and once released it expands to firmly grip the walls of the incision. The sleeve and adjacent rumen are then manipulated through the abdominal incision, so that the ring holds a portion of rumen firmly against the body wall, and prevents peritoneal soilage. The rumen and reticulum may then be explored by inserting the hand and arm through the cuff.

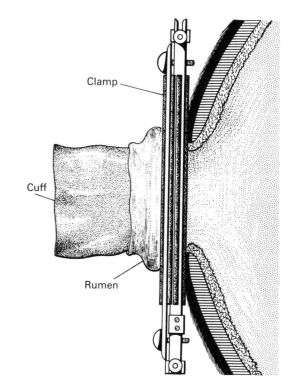

Fig. 3.35. Following the necessary exploratory procedures, the cuff must be removed before the rumenal incision can be sutured. The clamp that is used to hold the rumen during closure consists of a hinged metal frame which incorporates two soft rubber rollers along each arm. The jaws of the clamp are opened and insinuated between the ring of the rubber cuff and the abdominal wall. Once the clamp is in position the rubber cuff can be removed, and the clamp then seals the rumen against spillage of its contents, and at the same time holds the rumen in a convenient position for suturing, free of tension.

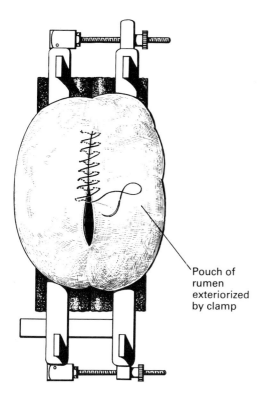

Fig. 3.36. The rumen is closed by a continuous inversion suture of 4 metric synthetic absorbable suture material and this layer is reinforced by a layer of interrupted inversion sutures. The clamp is then removed and the abdominal wall closed.

Left displacement of the abomasum

The abomasum normally lies on the abdominal floor slightly to the right of the midline. Its greater curvature gives attachment to the superficial part of the greater omentum which arises from the left longitudinal groove of the rumen. In left-sided abomasal displacement (LDA) the abomasum becomes trapped between the left side of the rumen and the left abdominal wall, and this in turn leads to a change in position of the omasum and a downward displacement of the duodenum mediated through the omental attachment between the lesser curvature of the abomasum and the duodenum.

The prime objectives of any surgical methods of correction of LDA should be to restore it to its normal position, after reducing its size if necessary, and to stabilize it in this position to prevent recurrence. A variety of techniques carried out in the standing or recumbent animal is commonly used. There is little significant difference between the success rates reported for the different techniques, consequently the method employed will largely depend on the surgeon's experience and preference, and on the facilities and assistance available at the time. It is beyond the scope of this book to give a detailed description of all these techniques.

Standing techniques

These may be carried out via left or right, or both left and right, flank incisions.

Bilateral flank approach. This has the disadvantage of requiring two operators working through incisions in the right and left flanks respectively (Figs 3.37–3.39), but it has several advantages, particularly for those who have little or no experience of the surgical correction of LDA. Identification of the abomasum is made easy for the operator on the right side; decompression of the abomasum by pressure or tapping with a needle can be safely accomplished and any adhesion between the abomasum and left abdominal wall may be assessed and a decision made whether or not to break them down.

Right flank approach. Once the operator is familiar with the bilateral technique, he or she can change to a right paralumbar technique thereby dispensing with the need for a second surgeon (Fig. 3.40). When this single flank approach is adopted, replacement of the abomasum is facilitated by evacuating the gas using a 16-gauge needle

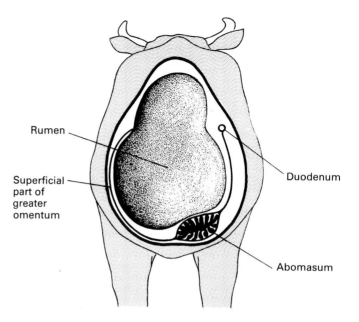

Fig. 3.37. The normal relationship of the rumen and abomasum. The rumen occupies the majority of the left side of the abdominal cavity, but its ventral sac extends to the right of the midline. The superficial part of the greater omentum extends from the left groove of the rumen ventrally around the ventral sac and inserts partly onto the greater curvature of the abomasum, and partly along the second or horizontal portion of the duodenum.

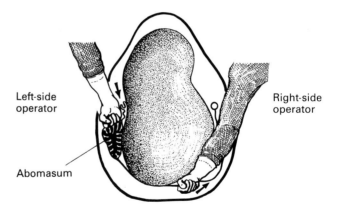

Fig. 3.38. The abomasum is reduced by the left-side operator exerting downward pressure on the abomasum by means of the hand and forearm in order to avoid penetrating the wall, remembering that the abomasum must pass beneath the ventral sac of the rumen. Difficulty may be experienced by the right-side operator in identifying the abomasum. He must largely rely on being 'handed' a piece of abomasum underneath the rumen by his colleague on the left side.

The final reduction from the left to right usually occurs quite suddenly, and this can be judged as complete when the great omentum, between the left rumenal groove and the greater curvature of the abomasum, can be seen lying closely applied to the ventral rumenal sac.

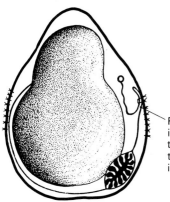

Fold of omentum incorporated in the closure of the right flank incision

Fig. 3.39. The abomasum is anchored by incorporating a fold of greater omentum, 3 cm from the pylorus, in the continuous suture used to close the transversalis muscle and peritoneum. Chromic catgut is preferred for this suture because it is less likely than polyglycolic acid to cut through the omentum and also creates a greater degree of reaction thereby enhancing the adhesion between the omentum and the parietal peritoneum.

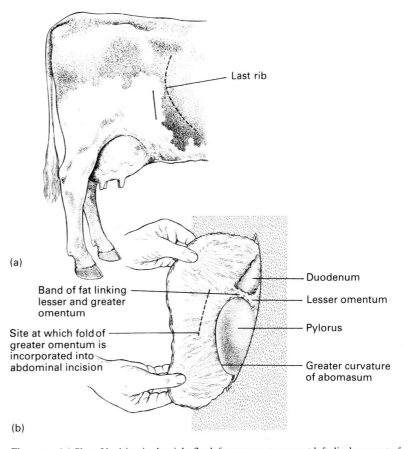

Last rib

(a)

Band of fat linking lesser and greater omentum

Site at which fold of greater omentum is incorporated into abdominal incision

Duodenum

Lesser omentum

Pylorus

Greater curvature of abomasum

(b)

Fig. 3.40. (a) Site of incision in the right flank for surgery to correct left displacement of the abomasum. Although the pylorus can be identified by palpation due to its indurated nature, a simpler method is to grasp the relatively thin caudal part of the greater omentum just cranial to the abdominal incision and gently withdraw it, hand-over-hand, until the pylorus appears at the incision. The omentum will be seen to contain progressively more fat as its attachment to the abomasum is approached. (b) The pylorus can be identified as an apparently blind pouch separated from the thinner-walled duodenum by a narrow band of fat which covers its lateral surface.

on a long length of sterile tubing. This is taken around the caudal aspect of the rumen and inserted through the greater curvature of the abomasum. Once the abomasum is significantly reduced in size, the needle is withdrawn and replacement and fixation are carried out as previously described.

Recumbent technique

A right paramedian approach is performed with the cow cast and restrained in dorsal recumbency. The use of xylazine sedation and local infiltration has now largely superseded general anaesthesia for this operation. The abdomen is entered via a 15-cm incision running parallel to, and 10 cm from, the midline starting just behind the xiphisternum (Fig. 3.41).

Right dilatation and torsion of the abomasum

Torsion of the abomasum, an abdominal catastrophe, is preceded by a period of milder illness corresponding to the progressive dilatation of the organ. The mechanical movements involved are not fully understood. Clockwise and anticlockwise rotation viewed from the right have been described, while in other cases the initial movement is a 180° anticlockwise rotation viewed from behind which is followed by a similar rotation viewed from the right (Fig. 3.42).

Surgery to correct the torsion is carried out in the standing animal via a right flank paracostal incision starting 15 cm below the lumbar transverse processes. Care should be taken to avoid accidental perforation of the grossly distended abomasum which lies in close contact with the peritoneum. Evacuation of gas from the dorsal part of the abomasum by needle suction produces sufficient relaxation to enable it to be grasped and brought to the incision. After insertion of a purse-string suture, a 2-cm diameter tube is introduced to allow partial evacuation of the abomasum of several litres of foul-smelling fluid contents (Fig. 3.43). After removal of the drainage tube the suture is tied and oversewn.

If the direction of the torsion can be determined, it is corrected by counter-rotation using the palm of the hand and the forearm. In cases where the

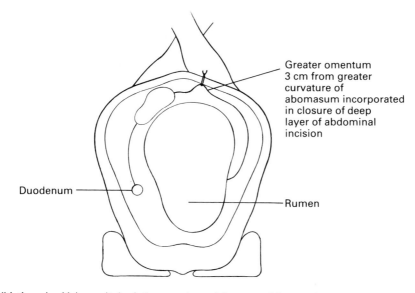

Fig. 3.41. With the animal lying on its back the ventral sac of the rumen falls away from the abdominal floor and thus it does not impede manipulation and drainage of the displaced abomasum. The abomasum is anchored in its correct position by incorporating greater omentum 3 cm from the greater curvature in the abdominal incision as the peritoneum and sheath of the rectus are sutured. Six metric chromic catgut is used for this purpose, while the remainder of the closure is carried out using 5 metric polyglycolic acid.

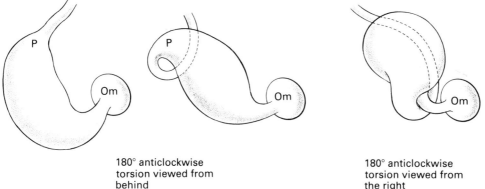

Fig. 3.42. Torsion of the abomasum. Om, omentum; P, pylorus.

nature of the torsion is not immediately apparent, correction is achieved by trial and error and is often signalled by the sound of fluid passing into the duodenum which now appears at the abdominal incision as a distended tube running dorsally and cranially. Further confirmation that the abomasum is in its correct position can be obtained by checking its relationship to the omasum and by identifying the pylorus in its normal position.

In order to reduce the risk of recurrence of the torsion, the greater omentum adjacent to the pylorus is anchored to the abdominal wall.

Supportive therapy in the form of intravenous 0.9 per cent saline (10−30 litres) is necessary to correct the severe hypochloraemia, hypokalaemia and alkalosis resulting from the massive seques-tration of fluid in the abomasum.

The prognosis is favourable if the abomasum is seen to contract vigorously after it is decompressed. However, if it remains flaccid, impaction frequently develops within a few days because of irreversible damage to the ventral vagus nerve supply at the site of the torsion. In the authors' opinion per-forming a pyloromyotomy at the time of the initial surgery does not prevent the impaction from developing.

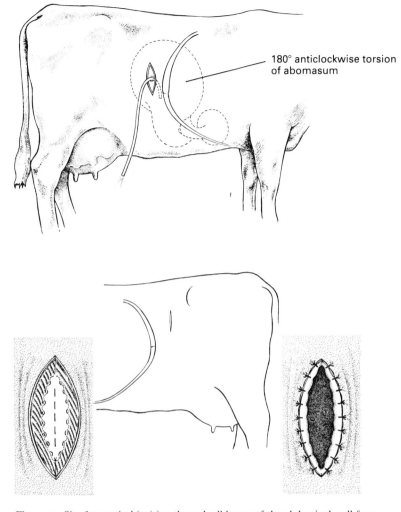

180° anticlockwise torsion of abomasum

Fig. 3.43. Partial evacuation of the abomasum by release of the gas from its dorsal part provides sufficient relaxation to enable it to be grasped and brought to the surface.

Semipermanent rumenal fistula

A semipermanent fistula provides a simple but effective means of treating calves with chronic recurrent ruminal tympany. It is also of value in cattle with tetanus where it provides a means of administering food and water as well as allowing gas to escape.

The site for the operation is the left sublumbar fossa at the point of maximum distension. A vertical incision 10 cm long is made through all the layers of the abdominal wall to expose the rumen which is sutured to the peritoneum and aponeurosis of the transversalis muscle in an oval fashion using a continuous suture (Fig. 3.44). A vertical incision is made into the lumen of the rumen within this area and the margin folded back and sutured to the skin.

Alternatively, the abdominal incision can be made in grid-iron fashion, splitting each layer along the direction of its fibres. A pouch of rumen is brought through the incision, sutured to the skin alone using a number of mattress sutures and opened by removing a portion of its wall (Fig. 3.45). The natural tendency for the incisions in the various layers to close when there is no tension on the abdominal wall acts as a valve reducing leakage of rumen contents but allowing any gas which builds up to escape.

Fig. 3.44. Site for vertical incision through all layers of the abdominal wall for a semipermanent rumenal fistula. The rumen is first sutured to the peritoneum and aponeurosis of the transversalis muscle in an oval fashion, before it is incised vertically. The cut edges are then sutured to the skin.

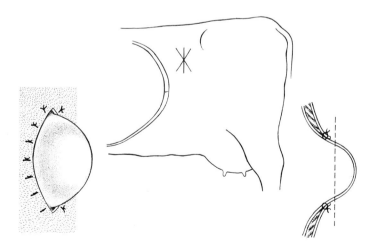

Fig. 3.45. Site for grid-iron incision for a semipermanent rumenal fistula. A pouch of rumen is brought through the incision and sutured to the skin with a number of mattress sutures. The fistula is created by removing a portion of the rumenal wall.

SPLENECTOMY – DOG

The spleen lies parallel to the greater curvature of the stomach in the left hyogastric region, and is supported by the gastrosplenic omentum which runs from the greater curvature of the stomach to invest the spleen. It is a mobile structure and can readily be exteriorized through a left cranial laparotomy incision (Fig. 3.46). The major blood supply is from the splenic artery which is a branch of the coeliac artery. The splenic vein drains into the gastrosplenic vein. The splenic artery runs in the fatty gastrosplenic omentum and then divides into numerous splenic branches which enter the substance of the spleen along the longitudinal hilus.

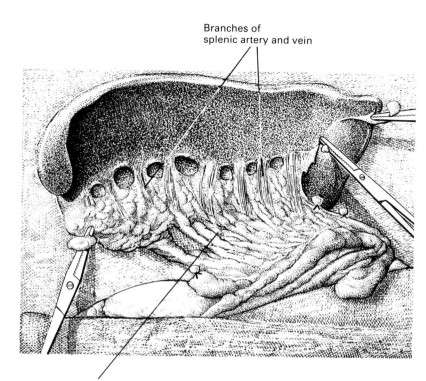

Branches of
splenic artery and vein

Gastrosplenic omentum

Fig. 3.46. Splenectomy is not a difficult operation, but requires patience and careful haemostasis. The rather complex vascular structure necessitates the identification and separate ligation of the numerous splenic branches before they can be divided.

Section 4
Surgery of the Genito-urinary System

Castration

During embryonic development, the testicle arises retroperitoneally from the gonadal ridge, and receives its excretory duct system (epididymis and vas deferens) from the remnants of the mesonephric (Wolffian) duct. It migrates from the dorsal aspect of the abdominal cavity into the scrotum due to the pull of the inguinal ligament of the mesonephros (gubernaculum) which is attached to the tail of the epididymis. The scrotum is lined by the tunica vaginalis, a direct outpouching of the peritoneum through the inguinal canal, and so for the testicle to descend retroperitoneally into the scrotum it is necessary for it to push a double fold of the tunica vaginalis into the lumen of the scrotal sac. The testicle thus lies within the lumen of the tunica vaginalis enclosed in the tunica vaginalis reflexa, and these two serous layers (often referred to as 'the coverings') are joined at the tail of the epididymis by the remains of the gubernaculum, the so-called 'attached portion'. This structure is of significance when considering the techniques of castration.

Haemostasis is an important aspect of castration, and may be considered under three headings.

1 *Haemostasis by traction*. This relies upon rapid blood clotting due to the elastic recoil of the artery wall, which is exacerbated when the artery is torn rather than cut. This is an effective method, but should be limited to very young animals.

2 *By ligature*. This is the most effective method but in the field it raises problems of asepsis and is usually confined to castration carried out under hospital conditions.

3 *By emasculator*. In this method the cord is severed by an instrument which at the same time crushes the cord tissue proximal to the cut end, and thus encourages natural clotting, similar to the effects of traction. A good emasculator is very efficient and easy to use, but is not so reliable as a ligature.

Open technique

In this method all the tissues of the scrotum and tunica vaginalis are incised and the testicle and spermatic cord are removed without their coverings. This method is easily carried out under field conditions, and may be used in the standing colt or bull, under local analgesia. The main disadvantage is that it opens the tunica vaginalis and thus makes a potential connection between the peritoneal cavity and the outside. This means that if an undetected weakness exists in the form of an incipient hernia

there is a danger of intestine escaping through the inguinal canal resulting in an intestinal prolapse.

Closed technique

This technique involves cutting through the scrotal skin and exposing the testicle, complete in the unopened tunica vaginalis. The neck of the tunica vaginalis is then either ligated and severed, or removed by means of an emasculator (Fig. 4.1). This technique involves blunt dissection and, under

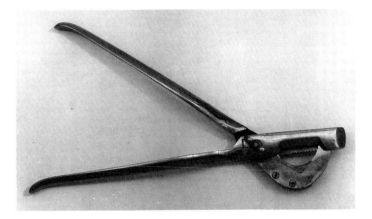

Fig. 4.1. The emasculator.

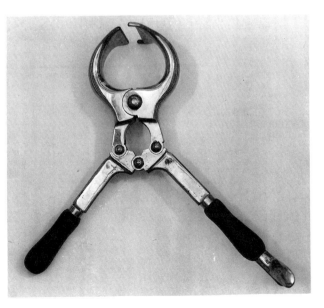

Fig. 4.2. The Burdizzo. Note that one jaw of the Burdizzo is extended laterally so that it overlaps at each end (the cord stop). This is to prevent the spermatic cord slipping from between the jaws when they are closed.

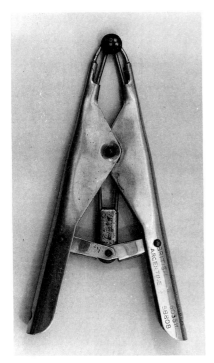

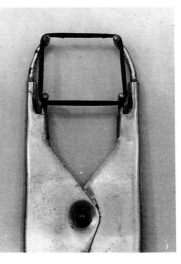

(b)

(a)

Fig. 4.3. The Elastrator: (a) closed, and (b) open.

field conditions, potential contamination of the scrotal area. It does not involve opening the tunica vaginalis and thus avoids the very real danger of intestinal prolapse. It is the method that is used to castrate any animal with an actual or suspected scrotal hernia (see Section 6).

'Bloodless' castration

This method is suitable for use in cattle and sheep, both of which have pendulous scrotums. It involves the use of an instrument which will crush the spermatic cord without opening the scrotum, and this eliminates, to a very great extent, the dangers of post-operative sepsis. In cattle and sheep, the Burdizzo bloodless castrator is used (Fig. 4.2), whereas in young lambs, it is popular to apply a tight elastic band around the neck of the scrotum, using an Elastrator (Fig. 4.3). The pressure of the elastic band causes as ischaemic necrosis of the neck of the scrotum and its contents, all of which separate and drop off after 10–14 days.

HORSE

Open technique

See Figs 4.4–4.8.

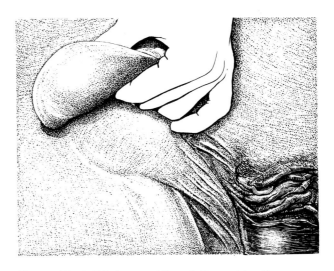

Fig. 4.4. The testicle is grasped through the scrotal wall, so that it is firmly immobilized and the scrotal skin is tightly stretched. The scrotum is opened by a single, firm incision which penetrates the skin, the tunica vaginalis and the testicle.

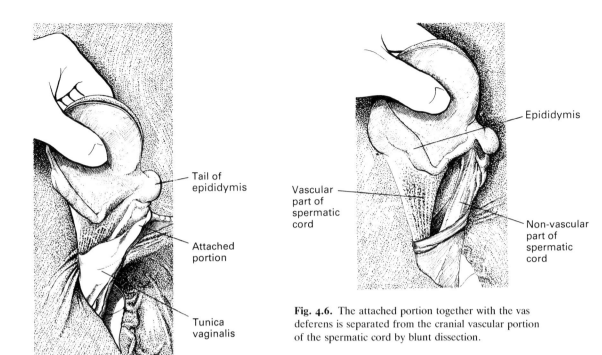

Tail of epididymis

Attached portion

Tunica vaginalis

Epididymis

Vascular part of spermatic cord

Non-vascular part of spermatic cord

Fig. 4.6. The attached portion together with the vas deferens is separated from the cranial vascular portion of the spermatic cord by blunt dissection.

Fig. 4.5. The opened tunica vaginalis retracts to expose the testicle, except for the single area of attachment which unites the tail of the epididymis to the tunica vaginalis by means of the vestigial gubernaculum.

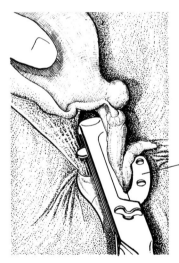

Emasculator severing the non-vascular portion

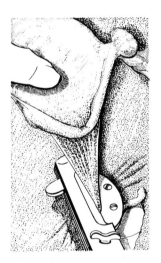

Fig. 4.8. The vascular portion of the spermatic cord is also severed with an emasculator, which should be held tightly clamped to the severed vascular portion for at least 30 seconds in order to ensure adequate haemostasis. It should then be opened sharply, to avoid interference with the crushed vascular tissue.

Fig. 4.7. The attached portion is severed with an emasculator. This reduces post-operative haemorrhage from small blood vessels in the vas deferens.

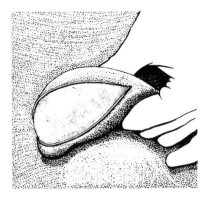

Fig. 4.9. The skin of the scrotum is opened without incising the tunica vaginalis.

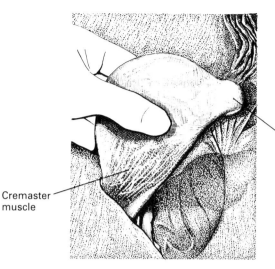

Fig. 4.10. The testicle within the unopened tunica vaginalis is separated from the scrotal sac by blunt dissection. The insertion of the cremaster muscle into the tunica vaginalis is seen on its caudo-lateral surface.

Tail of epididymis

Cremaster muscle

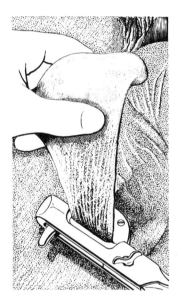

Fig. 4.11. The spermatic cord, together with the tunica vaginalis and cremaster muscle, is severed by using an emasculator as close to the inguinal canal as possible.

DOG

Open technique using a ligature

See Figs 4.12–4.15. Complications of prescrotal castration include haemorrhage from scrotal tissue and bruising of the scrotum. These may be reduced or eliminated by ablation of the scrotum at the time of castration.

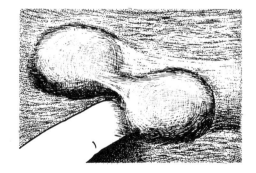

Fig. 4.12. The testicle is pushed forwards so that it can be exposed by a midline skin incision cranial to the scrotum. This allows both testicles to be removed through the same incision and lessens the possibility of post-operative interference by the dog.

Closed technique

See Figs 4.9–4.11.

It is customary to leave the scrotal incisions unsutured to allow drainage, following both the open or closed techniques, but this is a matter of personal preference. In cases of actual, or suspected scrotal hernia, it is normal practice first to obliterate the neck of the cord with 4 metric synthetic absorbable suture material before severing the cord with an emasculator. See Section 6 which deals with the treatment of scrotal hernia.

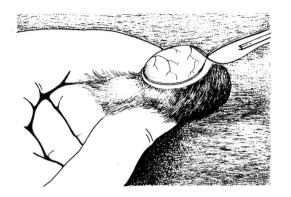

Fig. 4.13. The skin and tunica vaginalis are opened by a single incision.

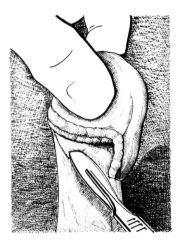

Fig. 4.14. The 'attached portion' of the tunica vaginalis is severed.

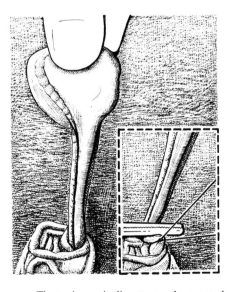

Fig. 4.15. The tunica vaginalis retracts, the exposed spermatic cord is clamped and ligated, and severed above the ligature. The pre-scrotal incision is closed with interrupted sutures.

CALF

Castration by Burdizzo

The calf is restrained against a wall with its tail held vertically. The spermatic cord is palpated, and the scrotal neck is held between the finger and thumb so that the cord is firmly anchored in a fold of scrotal skin. The Burdizzo is applied to the fold of the scrotal skin and the underlying spermatic cord, and the jaws of the instrument are closed (Figs 4.16–4.17).

This is repeated on the same side below the original crushed area. It is important to ensure that the minimum amount of scrotal skin is included in the crush and great care must be taken to ensure that the cord is included in the crushed tissues, otherwise the operation will be a failure, and this may not be noticed until several weeks have elapsed.

Care must also be taken to avoid the crush marks in the scrotal neck coalescing in the midline, otherwise there is the danger that the scrotum will slough.

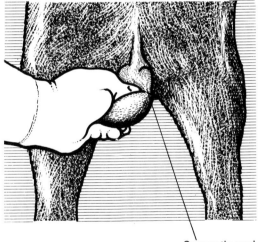

Spermatic cord anchored in a fold of the scrotal neck

Fig. 4.16. The spermatic cord is palpated, and the scrotal neck is held between finger and thumb so that the cord is firmly anchored in a fold of scrotal skin.

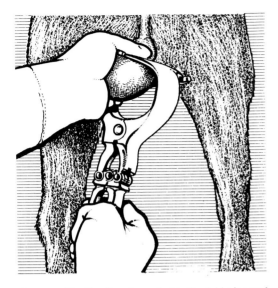

Fig. 4.17. The Burdizzo is applied to the fold of scrotal skin and the underlying spermatic cord, and the jaws of the instrument are closed.

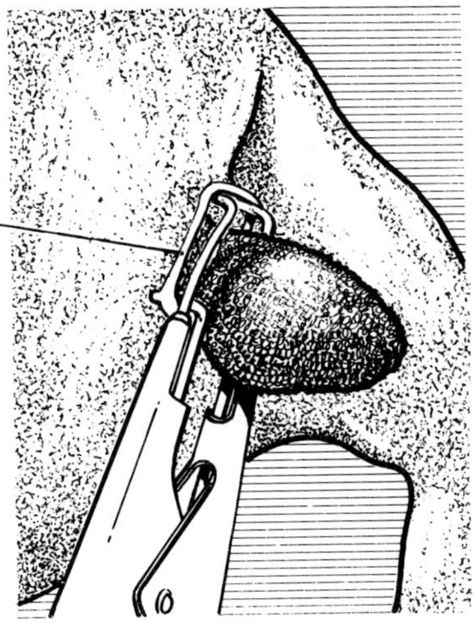

Fig. 4.18. Traction is gently applied to the scrotum after making certain that both testicles are within the scrotal sac. The Elastrator jaws are opened by closing the handles and the stretched rubber ring is manipulated onto the neck of the scrotum.

LAMB

Castration by Elastrator

When using the Burdizzo and Elastrator (Figs 4.18–4.19), great care must be taken to avoid damage to the sigmoid flexure of the penis. Should this happen, the urethra may be irreparably damaged, leading to death from urethral obstruction or necessitating an ischial urethrostomy or amputation of the penis to enable the damaged area to be by-passed (see Figs 4.75–4.76).

RIG CASTRATION (CRYPTORCHIDECTOMY)

Partial or complete retention of the testicle within either the abdominal cavity or the inguinal canal is encountered in all animals, but its incidence is highest in the horse. This is predisposed by the remarkable growth of the equine fetal gonad between 4 and 9 months of gestation, which in the case of the male fetus, makes the gonad too large to negotiate the inguinal canal until shrinkage occurs late in gestation. If the reduction in size of the gonad does not coincide with the period of resorption and shortening of the gubernaculum, then some degree of retention occurs. Although the undescended gonad is incapable of spermatogenesis, it still elaborates male sex hormone, and so the rig or cryptorchid horse develops male behavioural characteristics which makes it unsuitable

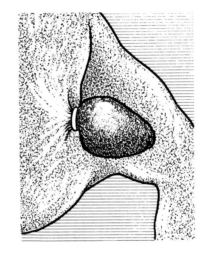

Fig. 4.19. The Elastrator is released and removed, so that the rubber ring tightly encircles the scrotal neck.

for handling and normal work. The type of retention falls into three categories:

1 *Abdominal*, in which the testicle and its complete duct system are retained in the abdominal cavity.

2 *Partial abdominal*, in which the tail of the epididymis is drawn into the inguinal canal by the pull of the gubernaculum, but the testicle remains within the abdominal cavity adjacent to the internal inguinal ring.

3 *Inguinal*, in which the testicle is located within the inguinal canal or just inside the external inguinal ring but has not descended completely into the scrotum.

This pattern of retention dictates a standard

procedure which should be adopted in all cases in which a retained testicle is suspected.

The horse is restrained on its back under general anaesthesia. The scrotal skin is tented by tissue forceps and incised with scissors. In this way it is possible to avoid injury to the large veins which run in the subcuticular tissues. The subscrotal connective tissue is broken down by blunt dissection, and the inguinal canal is located cranio-lateral to the scrotum. It is easily recognized as it offers no resistance to blunt dissection and the fingers readily enter the external ring. If the testicle is in the inguinal canal it is either visible or palpable, and should be grasped by tissue forceps and drawn out of the canal, when it can be removed by an emasculator or any method of choice. Not every horse that is suspected of being a cryptorchid has a retained testis. The owner of a horse bought as a gelding may suspect that the animal is a cryptorchid if it has an intractable disposition, or shows interest in a mare which is in oestrus. In the past if the surgical history of the horse was unknown, it was necessary to explore the inguinal canals in order to eliminate the possibility of a retained testicle. If the horse had already been satisfactorily castrated, the remains of the spermatic cord would be found either adherent to the scrotal skin or to the side of the external inguinal ring. It can be readily recognized by the presence of the cremaster muscle emerging from the inguinal canal and blending with the cord tissue.

The need for such surgery has been eliminated by the introduction of a diagnostic laboratory test for cryptorchidism. Measurement of testosterone levels in blood just prior to, and from 40 minutes to 2 hours of administering 6000 i.u. of human chorionic gonadotrophin (HCG) intravenously, or alternatively, measurement of oestrone sulphate in a single sample (provided the animal is over 3 years of age and is not a donkey) will allow the animal which has not had both testes removed to be identified.

If the testicle cannot be readily palpated within the inguinal canal then it is necessary to carefully explore the depths of the canal. In partial abdominal rigs the tail of the epididymis, enclosed in a small vaginal sac, is palpable and should be grasped with forceps so that gentle traction can be applied. On incising the vaginal sac it will be seen to contain only the tail and body of the epididymis together with the vas deferens (Fig. 4.20). These structures must not be mistaken for a small testis. Further traction on the epididymis will usually draw the testis into the canal but in some cases it is too large to pass through the internal inguinal ring. In these

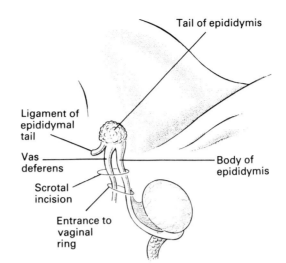

Fig. 4.20. Partial abdominal retention.

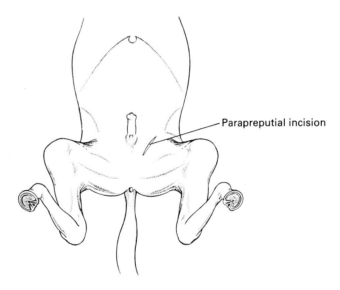

Fig. 4.21. Parapreputial incision.

cases and those with complete abdominal retention in which careful exploration of the inguinal canal fails to locate anything, this approach is abandoned and preparation made to open the abdominal cavity through a parapreputial (paramedian) incision (Fig. 4.21).

Once the abdomen is opened the testis which is usually small and flabby, is often found adjacent to the caudal canthus of the internal inguinal ring. If it cannot be palpated, then search should commence systematically by locating the vas deferens as it enters the prostatic urethra at the neck of the bladder, and then tracing this forwards until the tail of the epididymis and testis are located. One of the most important factors in accurate localization

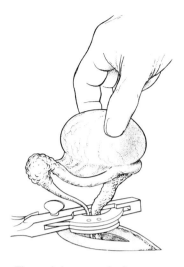

Fig. 4.22. The testis is removed using an emasculator.

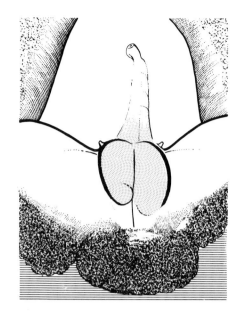

Fig. 4.23. The ram is positioned on its back, and the hair clipped from the abdominal wall. Local or general anaesthesia may be used.

of the testis is recognition of the flabby nature of the majority of the abdominal testes. Once grasped, the testis is brought out through the incision and removed using an emasculator (Fig. 4.22). It is not always possible to exteriorize completely the epididymis through the laparotomy incision and in these cases the emasculator should merely be applied as high up as possible. In cases of bilateral abdominal retention both testes can be found and removed through a single abdominal incision.

Rarely, the abdominally retained testis may be abnormally large because it is teratomatous. In its cystic form the testis can be reduced in size quickly and simply by aspiration of its fluid contents. This is not possible in the case of firm teratomas which require a larger than normal incision for their removal.

VASECTOMY — RAM

The presence of a ram is known to stimulate the onset of oestrus in a flock of ewes during the early stages of the breeding season. Modern methods of sheep husbandry, particularly those related to the artificial control of oestrus by the use of progestagens, aim at the synchronization of oestrus in a flock in order to obtain a compact lambing period in the spring. Vasectomized rams are commonly used to detect early oestrus in ewes, which are then synchronized and served by fertile rams.

Vasectomy renders the ram infertile by obliterating a portion of the vas deferens, but does not make it impotent (Figs 4.23–4.25).

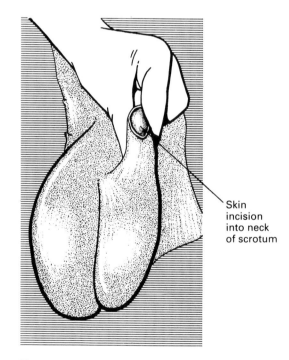

Skin incision into neck of scrotum

Fig. 4.24. The spermatic cord is located above the testicle, and an incision made through the skin to expose the glistening tunica vaginalis.

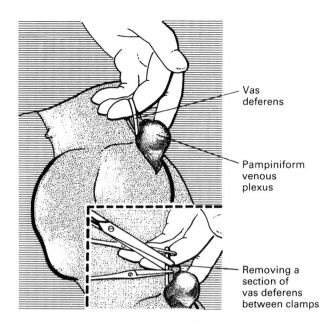

Vas
deferens

Pampiniform
venous
plexus

Removing a
section of
vas deferens
between clamps

Fig. 4.25. The tunic is opened, taking great care to avoid damage to the large venous pampiniform plexus. The vas deferens is recognized as a hard, non-pulsating white tube. It is easily separated from the other tissues of the cord, after which it is double clamped, and a segment at least 2.5 cm long removed from between the clamps. It is not essential to close the tunica vaginalis, and the incision is adequately closed by a series of interrupted sutures in the skin.

OVARIECTOMY — MARE

The indications for ovariectomy in the mare are limited. Unilateral ovariectomy is indicated for the removal of an ovarian tumour. Bilateral ovariectomy is sometimes carried out in an attempt to improve the temperament of a vicious mare, but the results are by no means encouraging and various reports indicate that improvement is only likely to occur in mares that become vicious when in oestrus or in animals which recently have acquired nymphomaniacal symptoms.

Ovariectomy may be carried out through a flank or a midline incision (Section 3, p. 64). The flank approach makes removal of a lower ovary extremely difficult, due to the short length of the mesovarium, and the authors favour a midline approach for either unilateral or bilateral ovariectomy. In addition to the ease of approach to both ovaries through a midline incision, the mare is not left with an unsightly scar in the flank.

The mare is fully starved for 24 hours to reduce the bowel contents. With the mare placed in dorsal recumbency a midline incision is made extending from the mammary gland caudally, to as far forward as is necessary.

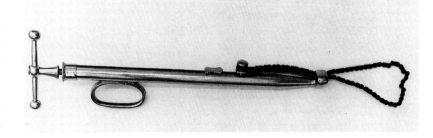

Fig. 4.26. The ecraseur.

The ovary is located and brought to the incision. Normal-sized or small ovaries can be removed solely using an ecraseur (Fig. 4.26). It is important that the ecraseur is tightened slowly by an assistant while the surgeon ensures that bowel or omentum does not become trapped between the chain and the ovarian pedicle. The pedicle should not be stretched while the ecraseur is tightened or haemostasis may be inadequate.

In the case of large granulosa cell tumours of the ovary, it is helpful to reduce the size of the pedicle by ligating the blood vessels nearest the uterine horn, reserving the ecraseur for the major vessels.

OVARIOHYSTERECTOMY — BITCH

Ovariectomy on its own is an uncommon operation in the bitch, and it is invariably combined with removal of the uterus, i.e. ovariohysterectomy. The operation is performed either to neuter the animal in order to avoid the twice yearly oestrus cycle, or for the removal of a diseased uterus affected with cystic hyperplastic endometritis or pyometritis.

The neutering operation, which is normally performed on a young animal, should carry a negligible risk. Technical difficulties arise from an almost universal tendency to attempt the operation through too small an incision, and the use of various forms of non-absorbable ligature material within the abdominal cavity which give rise to chronic fistulae discharging in the flank from a site below the external angle of the ilium.

The operation for pyometritis, on the other hand, often requires extensive treatment for fluid imbalance before surgery may be safely undertaken, but the technique for either operation is basically the same, and will be considered under a common pattern (Figs 4.27–4.32).

A caudal laparotomy incision is made, extending from the pelvic brim to a point just cranial to the umbilicus. The ovarian blood supply in the bitch is homologous to the testicular blood supply in the male, and each ovary receives its arterial supply direct from the aorta. The uterus is supplied by the uterine artery, which is a branch of the internal iliac artery. The uterine artery runs close to the lateral vaginal wall and at the level of the cervix it enters the broad ligament, through which it runs almost parallel to the uterine horn until it reaches the ovarian extremity, where it anastomoses with the ovarian artery. Ovariohysterectomy therefore entails the control of haemorrhage from both the ovarian and the uterine arteries before excision of the ovary and the uterine horns.

The right uterine horn and ovary are exposed by elevating the duodenum towards the midline, thereby using the mesoduodenum as a retractor. The left uterine horn and ovary are similarly exposed by retracting the descending colon.

The right ovary is exposed by gentle traction on its suspensory ligament. The ovarian artery and the tortuous ovarian vein are identified as they run through the cranial border of the broad ligament, and a small hole is made in the broad ligament behind the ovarian vessels, to make an ovarian pedicle.

Ligation of the ovarian blood vessels is always difficult, as the ovaries cannot be easily exposed,

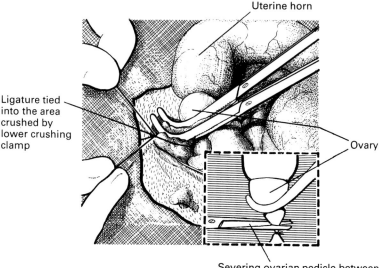

Fig. 4.27. The pedicle containing the ovarian vessels is double clamped and a synthetic absorbable ligature threaded below the lower clamp, which is removed as the ligature is tightened so that the suture material ties into the crushed tissue. The pedicle is severed between the ligature and the ovary. The second clamp is left attached to the ovarian pedicle to prevent 'back-bleeding' from the anastomosis to the uterine artery.

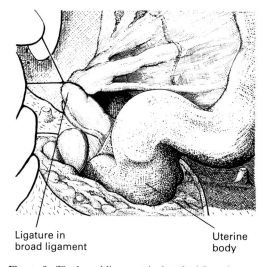

Fig. 4.28. The broad ligament is detached from its connection to the cervix, taking care to avoid tearing the uterine artery and vein. A synthetic absorbable ligature is tied across the base of the broad ligament.

even with maximum abdominal relaxation. The procedure is greatly simplified by the use of the curved gallbladder forceps as illustrated (Geary Grant cholecystectomy forceps).

This procedure is then repeated on the left ovary and broad ligament, so that both ovaries and uterine horns are free, but still attached to the cervix and vagina.

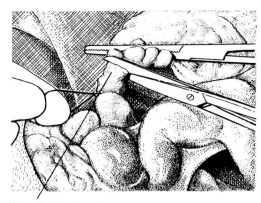

Severing the broad ligament
between ligature and clamp

Fig. 4.29. The broad ligament is clamped on the uterine side, and divided between the clamp and the ligature.

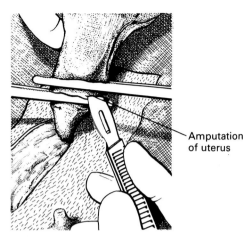

Amputation
of uterus

Fig. 4.31. The cranial vagina is double clamped above the ligatures, and transected as close as possible to the lower clamp.

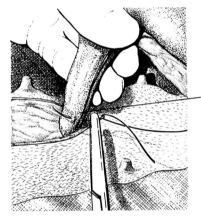

Ligature
encircling
uterine artery
and vein on
one side

Fig. 4.30. The cervix and vagina are exposed by reflecting the uterine horns caudally. A synthetic absorbable ligature is applied to the uterine artery and vein on either side, below the level of the cervix.

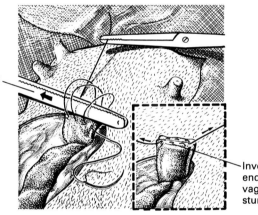

Oversewing
the vaginal
stump

Inverted
end of
vaginal
stump

Fig. 4.32. The clamp may be oversewn using the Parker–Kerr technique. A continuous synthetic absorbable suture is inserted across the crushed end of the stump by picking up a small piece of tissue below the clamp on one side, and then alternating progressively so that the loop of suture material between each stitch loops over the jaws of the clamp. The clamp is then slightly opened to release the crushed tissue, and as it is withdrawn, each end of the suture material is gently pulled. This has the effect of inverting the crushed tissue and sealing the stump. On a small stump, the ends of the inversion suture are tied together, but in a large stump it is advisable to stitch back across the inverted stump so that the suture ends are adjacent before tying them.

OVARIOHYSTERECTOMY — CAT

This operation (Figs 4.33–4.35) is usually carried out through a small incision in the left sublumbar fossa. The cat is restrained on its right side, under general anaesthesia, and fully extended by tapes placed on its front and hind legs. The urinary bladder should be emptied by manual pressure, and it is not facetious to suggest that a check should be made to ascertain that the cat is female.

The site of the incision is mid-flank, below and slightly cranial to the external angle of the ilium. It is important to check this landmark, which can be confused with the great trochanter of the femur.

The uterine horn is sometimes seen lying adjacent to the incision, but in most cases it must be found. This is easily accomplished by identifying the sublumbar fat, and then gently drawing it out of the incision and at the same time displacing it upward when the uterine horn will be drawn into the incision. The sublumbar fat is solid and dark in colour, whereas the omental fat is thin, lace-like in consistency and highly vascular.

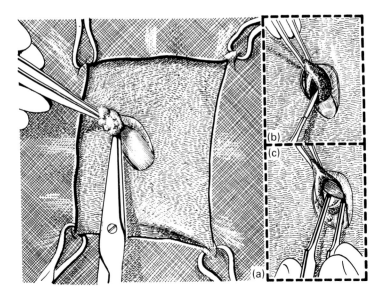

Fig. 4.33. (a) The skin below the external angle of the ilium is incised and a portion of subcutaneous fat removed. (b) The thin aponeurosis of the external oblique is split, and the thick internal oblique is nicked with a scalpel. (c) The nick is enlarged with forceps making certain that the thin peritoneum is also included. This produces a small, almost self-closing, grid-iron incision.

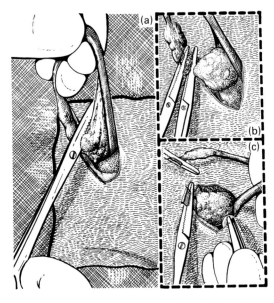

Fig. 4.34. (a) The uterine horn is drawn through the incision and the thin broad ligament is broken down. Further traction will expose the ovary. (b) The ovarian pedicle is double clamped. In a young cat the pedicle is broken by traction. In a mature cat, or one that is near the beginning or end of oestrus, it is safer to ligate the pedicle as described in the bitch. (c) The lower uterine horn is picked up at its junction with the uterine body by traction on the detached horn. The ovary is drawn into the incision, but this is slightly more difficult and requires greater traction than was necessary for the upper ovary.

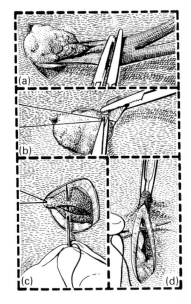

Fig. 4.35. (a–b) The operation is completed by double clamping the cranial vagina, and ligating into the crush of the lower clamp. Clamping the cranial vagina in the mature cat may result in complete amputation, as the tissue tends to be rather friable. In these circumstances the cranial vagina should be transfixed and ligated, without prior crushing. (c) Closure is made with simple interrupted sutures in the internal oblique muscle, and occasionally two to three sutures in the aponeurosis of the external oblique. (d) The skin is closed with interrupted nylon sutures.

Caesarean section

BITCH

The delivery of a litter of puppies by Caesarean section is extremely well tolerated in the bitch (Figs 4.36–4.40), and carries less hazard to both bitch and puppies than does a prolonged vaginal delivery using forceps. Subsequent fertility is unimpaired, and therefore the operation should be considered during the early stage of dystocia, and not put off as a last desperate measure when all else has failed. It is normal to open the abdomen through a linea alba incision in order to avoid damage to the active and highly vascular mammary tissue.

The procedure of removing puppy fetal membranes is continued until all have been delivered. It is important to check that no fetus has been overlooked, especially in the larger breeds which often have numerous puppies in a litter.

Once the uterus is empty, an ecbolic such as ergometrine is injected into the bitch, preferably by the intravenous route, in order to stimulate rapid and effective uterine involution. The uterine incision is closed with a continuous synthetic absorbable inversion suture.

Fetal resuscitation

Normal birth is a traumatic episode in the life of the fetus, whereas delivery by Caesarean section is relatively atraumatic. In cases of prolonged labour necessitating Caesarean section, however, the fetus is frequently hypoxic and may show respiratory depression due to the effect of the anaesthetic drugs that were necessary for the Caesarean operation. All these factors may add up to the need for fetal resuscitation after surgical delivery. This falls into three distinct categories.

1 Ensure an open airway. Always hold the newborn puppy in a head-down position to promote drainage. If necessary, apply suction to the nasopharynx by means of a fine catheter attached to a sucker.

2 Ensure adequate warmth.

3 Stimulate the circulation by vigorous skin massage and by rhythmical movements of the limbs. The new-born puppy in need of resuscitation is limp and shows feeble and intermittent attempts to breathe. Simple resuscitation methods ensure that the respiratory tree is unobstructed and provide the stimulus that is necessary to encourage the new pulmonary circulation and to initiate normal respiration. Providing that there is a regular pulse, resuscitation should be continued until the puppy is

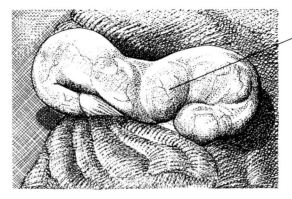

Fig. 4.36. The gravid uterus is lifted outside the abdominal cavity. This relieves respiratory embarrassment due to pressure on the diaphragm, and allows adequate packing off of the abdominal cavity.

Gravid uterus exteriorized and packed off

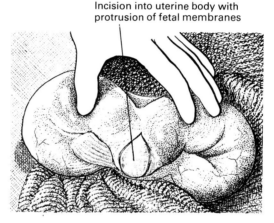

Incision into uterine body with protrusion of fetal membranes

Fig. 4.37. The uterus is opened at the uterine body, and the fetal membranes of the first puppy usually protrude through the incision.

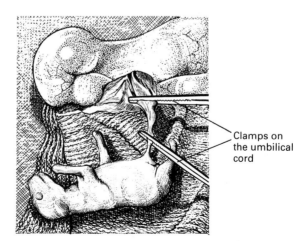

Clamps on the umbilical cord

Fig. 4.38. The membranes are ruptured and the puppy delivered. The umbilical cord is double clamped, and cut between the clamps. The puppy should be handed to an assistant and held head downwards to allow drainage from the pulmonary tree.

crying vigorously, and making purposeful limb movements. An early check should be made to eliminate the presence of common congenital abnormalities, e.g. cleft palate and imperforate anus.

CATTLE

The cow is monotocous, normally carrying one calf to full term, and thus the problem confronting the obstetrician in cattle practice is different from that of the bitch, in which the lives of a whole litter of puppies may be in jeopardy. The large size of the cow makes vaginal manipulation easier than it is in the bitch, and the decision for Caesarean section is only reached after a thorough vaginal examination has eliminated the possibility of vaginal delivery. In addition, fertility following Caesarean section in cattle is considerably reduced compared with that following vaginal delivery so that the operation tends to be performed at a relatively late stage of labour, when more conventional means of delivery have failed.

The operation is frequently carried out in the standing cow under regional analgesia but other operators prefer the animal to be recumbent, in which case it is restrained by sedation which is reinforced by regional analgesia.

The technique for both methods is similar. Laparotomy is carried out through a vertical or oblique left flank incision extending from 15 cm below the external angle of the ilium, down to the level of the fold of the flank (Fig. 4.41). All the muscle layers are incised along the same direction as the initial skin incision.

If possible, the uterus should be drawn up to the incision before it is opened, but in many instances the weight of the gravid uterus will make this impossible and it must be incised blindly within the abdominal cavity. A Roberts' embryotomy knife is ideal for this purpose in that it can be carried safely in the palm of the hand across the peritoneal cavity without risk of damage to the viscera.

The incision should be made along the greater curvature of the pregnant horn, not too close to the tip of the uterine horn and well away from the body of the uterus. If the calf is in cranial presentation to the vagina, the uterus is incised from the point of the calf's hocks which are readily identifiable, distally to just above the fetlock. Each leg in turn can now be flexed and brought out through the incision.

Once the fetus is delivered, the uterus may be lifted through the abdominal incision to facilitate closure. This is carried out with 4 metric synthetic absorbable suture material using an inversion

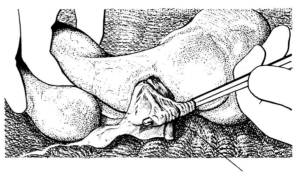

Withdrawing the fetal membranes

Fig. 4.39. The fetal membranes are removed by traction and twisting of the clamp.

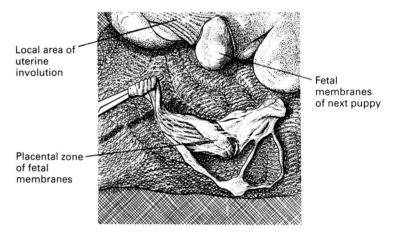

Local area of uterine involution

Fetal membranes of next puppy

Placental zone of fetal membranes

Fig. 4.40. The fetal membranes consist of the thickened zonary placenta, usually stained green, and the thin transparent allanto-chorion and amnion. In a healthy uterus, the uterine wall rapidly retracts in the area from which the puppy has been removed.

suture of the Cushing pattern and, if deemed necessary, oversewn. It is advisable to commence suturing from the cervical end of the incision as this portion tends to retract quite quickly as the uterus involutes. The fetal membranes are frequently impossible to detach during the operation and, if so, should be left to be voided through the vagina.

Special considerations

Monster calves

Schistosoma reflexus is the most common fetal monster encountered in cattle. Although most are smaller than normal calves, the extensor tendon contracture of the limbs can complicate delivery. However, provided each limb in turn is carefully manipulated, taking care to cup the foot in the palm of the hand to avoid damage to the uterine wall, these calves can usually be delivered through a standard-sized incision. An obstetrical hook applied across the vertebral column of the monster is an effective way of applying traction to a Schistosome calf in cephalo-caudal presentation to the vagina.

Irreducible uterine torsion

Owing to the large uterus and oedema of its wall, which makes it unusually friable, it is usually necessary to remove the calf before the torsion is corrected.

Emphysematous fetus

Delivery of a dead, emphysematous calf by Caesarean section frequently results in contamination of the peritoneal cavity with large volumes of highly toxic uterine fluid. Rapid absorption by the peritoneum results in severe toxic shock and death within a few hours of surgery.

Attempts may be made to minimize the contamination by employing a low flank incision (lateral to the mammary vein but below the fold of the flank) which allows access to the smaller, ovarian end of the horn. However, some contamination is inevitable. Lavage of the peritoneal cavity with several litres of warm Hartmann's solution containing antibiotic which are then siphoned off, is often successful in preventing toxaemia. Debridement of the abdominal incision is necessary if the muscle layers are contaminated with fetal hair, placenta, etc.

MARE

A ventral midline incision, commencing just cranial to the udder, is now the standard approach in the mare. Location and delivery of the part of the uterus overlying the foal's hocks usually presents no difficulty. If the placenta is clearly separating, it can be carefully removed, but if it is firmly adher-

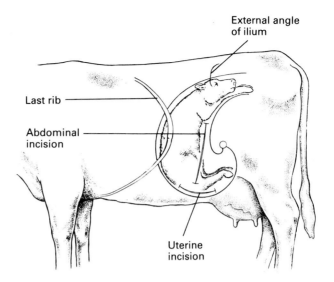

Fig. 4.41. Caesarean section in the cow. Note the relative positions of the abdominal and uterine incisions.

ent, or if haemorrhage occurs as it is being peeled away, it should be left *in situ*. However, it is necessary to detach it for a distance of 3—5 cm to enable a continuous interlocking stitch to be inserted around the margin of the incision. This prevents the mucosa from retracting and any haemorrhage from the numerous submucosal vessels is controlled. The uterine incision is now closed with a double layer of Cushing sutures using 4 metric polyglycolic acid.

EWE

The technique of Caesarean section in the sheep is the same as that described for the cow. The much smaller size of the sheep makes it easy to exteriorize the uterus before opening it to deliver the fetus. Twin pregnancies are common in the sheep, and an incision made in the uterine body will enable both fetuses to be delivered through the same hysterotomy incision.

Cystotomy

DOG

The urinary bladder lies within the abdominal cavity just cranial to the pelvic inlet. Its exact size depends upon the amount of urine that it contains, and in cases of prostatic enlargement, the neck of

the bladder is gradually moved in a cranial direction by the enlarging prostate, so that the complete bladder eventually lies within the abdominal cavity. The bladder is invested in a layer of visceral peritoneum, and is supported by three double folds of peritoneum. The ventral fold or middle umbilical ligament is reflected from the ventral surface of the bladder to the ventral midline of the abdominal wall, and it contains the remnants of the embryonic allantoic stalk or urachus. The two lateral umbilical ligaments are reflected from the lateral walls of the bladder to the lateral pelvic walls and extend cranially to the umbilicus. They contain the remnants of the embryonic umbilical arteries, which were branches of the internal iliac arteries.

The commonest indications for cystotomy are either for the removal of bladder calculi or for the excision of localized tumours of the bladder wall. In the female, the bladder is exposed by a simple caudal laparotomy incision, but in the male, this incision must be made parallel to the prepuce, and of necessity involves transection branches of the external pudendal artery and vein. These are large vessels and must be carefully ligated. The interruption of local venous drainage frequently leads to considerable venous congestion, and swelling of the paraprepuial area during the post-operative period is inevitable.

Following cystotomy (Figs 4.42–4.45) the bladder is washed out with sterile saline, in order to remove the inevitable blood clots.

It is important that the dog should be given the opportunity to empty its bladder at about 6 hours after the operation, and that this should be noted on its case notes. Post-operative retention of urine will lead to leakage and eventual rupture of the suture line, which can be avoided by catheterization if urinary retention develops.

Wound breakdown is also more likely if sutures of polyglycolic acid are used as this material is degraded by the urine.

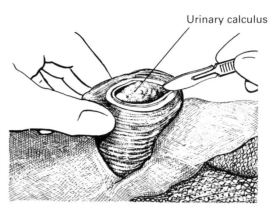

Urinary calculus

Fig. 4.42. The bladder is lifted through the incision and the peritoneal cavity is carefully protected by adequate abdominal packs before the bladder is opened. If possible, the dorsal aspect of the bladder should be chosen for the cystotomy incision.

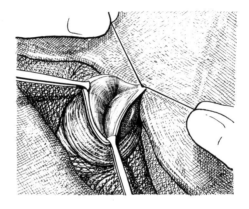

Fig. 4.43. After removal of the calculi or excision of the bladder wall, the thick mucous membrane is closed by a continuous suture of 2 metric synthetic absorbable suture material.

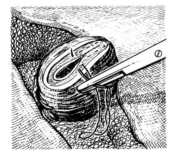

Fig. 4.44. The type of suture employed to close the mucous membrane should be a continuous mattress suture which everts the edges of the mucous membrane away from the lumen of the bladder. This is done to avoid raw edges of the mucous membrane protruding into the bladder lumen, where they can act as a focus for the laying down of further cystic calculi.

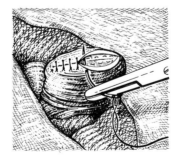

Fig. 4.45. The detrusor muscle of the bladder is closed by a series of simple interrupted sutures using a synthetic absorbable suture other than polyglycolic acid, varying in size from 2 to 3.5 metric depending upon the size of the dog.

HORSE

Cystotomy is sometimes necessary in the male horse to remove a cystic calculus. The calculus which is usually composed of calcium carbonate has a very rough irregular surface which causes intense irritation to the bladder mucosa.

The approach is via a right caudal paramedian incision as close to the pubic brim as possible. The bladder is located within the pelvis and steady traction has to be applied to it for several minutes before it can be brought up to the abdominal incision. Stay sutures of umbilical tape inserted either side of its apex allows further traction to be applied. After packing off the abdominal cavity with swabs, the bladder is incised on its dorsal aspect and carefully peeled away from the surface of the calculus which is then removed. Small fragments of calculus frequently break off during this process and these, and all debris in the bladder, should be removed by lavage and suction to minimize the risk of further calculi forming. Closure of the bladder should be in two layers using 3 or 3.5 metric synthetic absorbable suture material.

The first layer should be a simple continuous pattern; the second, a continuous inverting Cushing or Lembert suture.

REPAIR OF RUPTURED BLADDER — FOAL

Rupture of the bladder is not uncommon in newborn foals and occurs almost exclusively in colt foals. The cause of the condition is unknown, although it is believed that strong forceful abdominal contractions at the time of parturition are the major contributory factor. Occasionally congenital defects of the bladder wall, rather than traumatic ruptures are seen.

The foal is usually presented for surgery between the 3rd and 5th day of life by which time the peritoneal cavity contains several gallons of urine. There is a moderately severe metabolic acidosis, a marked hyponatraemia and hypochloraemia and, most significantly, a marked hyperkalaemia.

As much as possible of the urine should be removed by paracentesis prior to induction of anaesthesia using halothane/oxygen administered via an intranasal tube. Following endotracheal intubation anaesthesia is maintained on a semi-closed circuit. A solution of 0.9 per cent NaCl is administered by intravenous drip to correct the electrolyte imbalance. A catheter is introduced into the urethra and advanced to the level of the ischial arch.

The surgical approach is via a suprapubic paramedial incision as previously described. As much as possible of the remaining urine is removed by suction to facilitate close examination of the bladder which is brought to the abdominal incision without difficulty. Close scrutiny is necessary to determine the extent of the tear which is usually on the dorsal aspect of the bladder, particularly when it extends caudally along the body. The catheter is now advanced into the bladder but not far enough to impinge on its apex before the tear is closed with a double inverting Cushing suture of 3 metric synthetic absorbable suture material. The peritoneal cavity is lavaged with warm saline solution prior to closure of the abdominal incision. The catheter is sutured to the penis near the urethral orifice and a finger of a surgical glove, with a small hole at its apex, is taped to the end of the catheter to act as a one-way valve. The catheter is removed 48 hours later.

....

Urethral obstruction

The urethra in all species of male animals undergoes a sharp change of direction at the ischial arch, where it emerges from the caudal floor of the pelvis and runs forward under the abdominal wall. At the ischial arch, the urethra becomes invested in the ischiocavernosus and bulbocavernosus muscles. This combination of a change in direction together with the muscular reinforcement predisposes the ischial arch as a site for obstruction by small calculi that are washed out of the bladder.

In the dog, the terminal portion of the urethra runs beneath a longitudinal groove in the os penis, and this is the commonest site at which urethral obstruction occurs in this species (Fig. 4.46).

The urethra at the ischial arch is relatively deeply buried in tissue, whereas behind the os penis it is quite superficial. Note the relationship of the low urethrotomy incision to the scrotum and testicles.

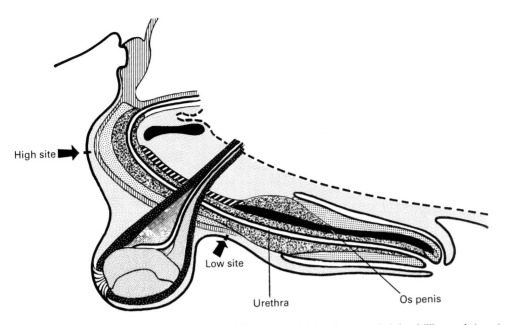

High site

Low site

Urethra

Os penis

Fig. 4.46. The sites of obstruction in the dog at the ischial arch and behind the os penis (after Miller *et al.* (1979) *Anatomy of the Dog*, W.B. Saunders, Philadelphia).

DOG

Low urethrotomy

The symptoms of acute urethral obstruction in the dog soon become obvious. Numerous unsuccessful attempts at urination are followed by signs of discomfort and vomiting. Abdominal palpation will reveal a grossly distended rock-hard bladder. The common site of obstruction is behind the os penis, and this can readily be confirmed by passing a metal sound down the urethra. This will meet resistance at the site of obstruction, and give a very real impression of metal striking against stone. In the majority of cases the obstruction can be removed by a low urethrotomy, which involves opening the urethra between the caudal aspect of the os penis and the scrotum (Figs 4.47−4.48). It must be remembered that urethral obstruction quickly leads to uraemia, and although this is normally reversible once the obstruction is removed, at the time of operation the dog is highly susceptible to the effect of barbiturate narcosis. These drugs should be used with care, and at minimal dose rate, in uraemic animals.

Releasing the grip of the left hand will result in considerable haemorrhage from the edges of the cut urethra, and once all the calculi are removed, there may be a rush of blood-stained urine from the bladder. A catheter should be passed into the bladder to ensure that no more calculi are present,

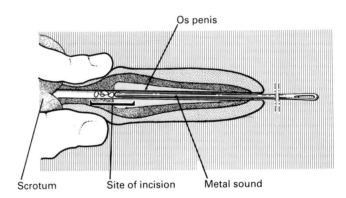

Os penis

Scrotum   Site of incision   Metal sound

Fig. 4.47. Under general anaesthesia, the dog is positioned on its back, and a probe is inserted into the urethra as far as possible. The base of the penis is gripped with the left hand, and an incision is made through the skin and the underlying urethra, to expose the calculi.

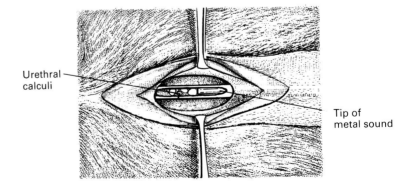

Urethral calculi

Tip of metal sound

Fig. 4.48. The edges of the wound are held with tissue forceps and the calculi are removed under direct vision.

and the bladder should be washed out with sterile saline until the washings are no longer blood-stained.

The urethrotomy incision is not sutured. For up to 7 days post operation there is invariably haemorrhage from the incision each time the dog urinates, or even if it becomes excited. This will cease as the wound slowly heals, which is normally complete in 3–4 weeks. The proximity of the low urethrotomy incision to the scrotum predisposes to scrotal infection, and care must be taken to avoid contamination of the scrotal sac with urine, giving rise to orchitis.

High urethrotomy

If the urethra is obstructed by a calculus that cannot be removed through a low urethrotomy incision, then it is necessary to open the urethra just below the ischial arch by carrying out a high urethrotomy. At this point, the urethra is not a superficial structure, but is invested in the insertions of the bulbo- and ischiocavernosus muscles. In addition the urethra lies embedded in the highly vascular corpus cavernosum of the penis. This contains numerous vascular sinuses supplied by the internal pudendal artery and these have to be incised before the urethra can be exposed and opened. In cases where it is possible to introduce a catheter into the urethra, the lumen of the urethra may be identified by palpation. However, in cases where the urethra is obstructed and will not permit the passage of a catheter then it is often extremely difficult to locate the urethral lumen due to the intensity of the haemorrhage from the corpus cavernosum.

Once the urethra is located and opened, and the obstructing calculus removed, a catheter should be passed into the bladder in order to ensure the free passage of urine, and the bladder should be washed out with sterile saline. It is not usual to suture the urethrotomy incision, which will gradually heal over a period of 3–4 weeks.

Urethrostomy

In dogs which show a tendency to repeated attacks of urethral obstruction, urethrostomy offers the best chance of relief. Two urethrostomy sites are possible.

A high urethrostomy is in essence the same operation as a high urethrotomy, but having opened the urethra longitudinally, its cut edges are sutured to the skin edges, so that after healing a permanent stoma is created in the urethra at the ischial arch (Fig. 4.49). By this means, a by-pass is established which avoids the two areas where obstruction

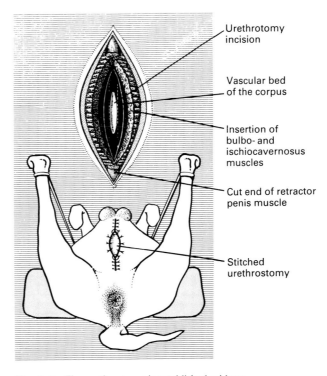

Urethrotomy incision

Vascular bed of the corpus

Insertion of bulbo- and ischiocavernosus muscles

Cut end of retractor penis muscle

Stitched urethrostomy

Fig. 4.49. The urethrostomy is established midway between the anus and the scrotum.

is most likely to occur, namely, the ischial arch and the area just proximal to the os penis. In addition, the pelvic urethra proximal to the urethrostomy is widely dilatable and will allow the passage of small stones which may subsequently be washed out of the bladder. The operation does not render the animal incontinent, but urine scalding of the perineum or scrotum is a potential complication.

The sutures should either be of 2 metric synthetic absorbable material or preferably 1.5 metric blood-vessel silk. Although in many cases a direct suture can be made between the edges of the urethra and the skin, the procedure is simplified by removing a wedge of the ischio- and bulbocavernosus muscles from either side of the urethral incision. This reduces the bulk of tissue and facilitates suturing urethra to the skin, but it does, of necessity, increase the problem of haemostasis, as both of these muscle masses are well supplied with blood.

The preferred urethrostomy site is at the scrotum. This has the advantage of permitting relatively easy access to the urethra since it is superficial at this point. It also has a wide diameter at this level and there is less risk of stenosis. However, castration and scrotal ablation must be performed prior to suturing the urethral mucosa to the skin.

CAT

Urethral obstruction in the cat is complicated both by the nature of the obstructing material which commonly consists of magnesium ammonium phosphate crystals held together in a colloidal 'matrix plug', and also by the length and narrow lumen of the male cat urethra. Many cases can be managed medically, but in cases of recurrent obstruction long-term relief can only be achieved by the surgical elimination of the narrow penile urethra and the construction of an ischial urethrostomy (Figs 4.50–4.55).

The use of a catheter in the new stoma should be avoided as it may promote stricture formation, and the cat should be given shredded newspaper rather than litter in its litter tray in the immediate postoperative period.

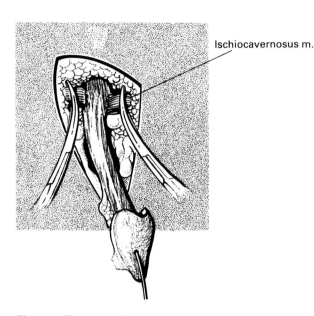

Fig. 4.51. The penis is dissected free of the subcutaneous fat and connective tissue down to its attachment to the ischial arch. Each ischiocavernosus muscle is isolated and clamped for a short period before it is divided.

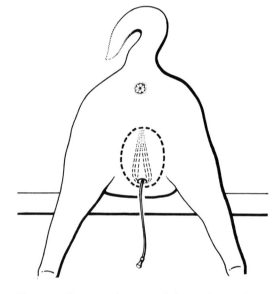

Fig. 4.50. A purse-string suture is inserted around the anus, and the urethra is catheterized. The cat is positioned in ventral recumbency with its hind legs tied over the end of the table and the tail pulled upward and forward. The skin incision encircles the prepuce and scrotum.

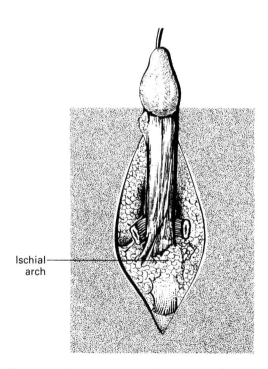

Fig. 4.52. After severing the ischiocavernosus muscles, the penis is completely freed from its attachments to the ischial arch.

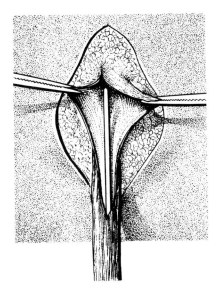

Fig. 4.53. The urethra is split longitudinally to expose the urethral catheter.

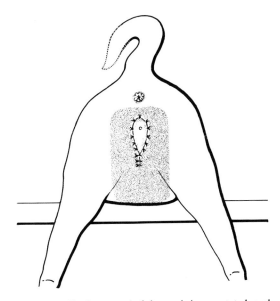

Fig. 4.55. The lower end of the penis is amputated, and the remaining severed edge of the urethra is sutured to the skin.

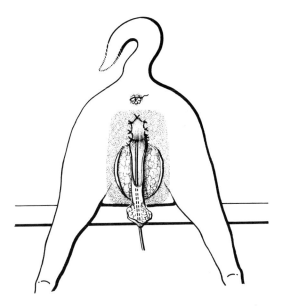

Fig. 4.54. The upper cut urethral margins are sutured to the skin, using 2 metric synthetic absorbable suture material or blood-vessel silk with a cutting atraumatic needle.

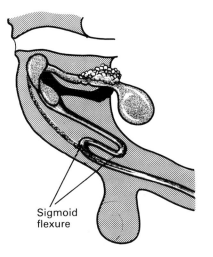

Fig. 4.56. In cattle and sheep and to a lesser extent the goat, urethral obstruction occurs at the sigmoid flexure of the penis. The sigmoid flexure may also be damaged during bloodless castration, giving rise to acute urethral obstruction. (After Oehme & Tillman (1965) *J. Am. Vet. Med. Assoc.* **147**, 1331.)

OTHER DOMESTIC SPECIES

The relatively long narrow urethra in those species with a sigmoid flexure (Fig. 4.56) makes catheterization extremely difficult. In the ram or wether, obstruction to the vermiform urethral extension (Fig. 4.57) can often be cleared by manually 'milking' the appendage, or if this fails by amputation of the urethral appendage.

Obstruction at the sigmoid flexure is normally treated either by a high urethrotomy or urethrostomy, or by amputation of the penis above the sigmoid flexure. It must, of course, be emphasized that these are life-saving procedures and are normally carried out merely to allow the animals to recover sufficiently from the effects of obstructive uraemia so that they may be sent for casualty slaughter. Urethral obstruction in the breeding male animal is a most serious condition, and urethrotomy or amputation will curtail the animal's ability for natural service.

Urethrostomy

Urethrostomy is most commonly performed in steers because of obstruction by urethral calculi or much more rarely due to accidental inclusion of the urethra in the jaws of a Burdizzo during castration. Rupture of the urethra leading to subcutaneous infiltration of urine along the ventral abdomen, or less frequently rupture of the bladder, may have occurred due to delay in diagnosis of the obstruction.

Urethrostomy is performed as a salvage operation to provide an alternative outlet for urine until the animal is fit for slaughter.

Anaesthesia

The surgical procedure is performed under caudal epidural anaesthesia with the animal standing or cast in dorsal recumbency. Although the urethrostomy can be performed at several sites a distal approach at the level of the distal sigmoid flexure has much to commend it in that it allows easy identification of the penis and allows the urethrostomy to be sited in such a way that urine is directed away from the medial aspect of the limbs reducing the risk of scalding.

A 10-cm vertical incision is made over the sigmoid flexure of the penis where it can be palpated immediately caudal to the remnants of the scrotum (Fig. 4.58).

The penis is deeper than one would anticipate and blunt dissection has to extend through subcutaneous adipose tissue and between the paired retractor penis muscle before the firm fibrous penis is located. Gentle traction will allow part of the penis to be withdrawn through the skin incision (Fig. 4.59). It may be possible to palpate the calculus and remove it through a small incision on the ventral aspect of the penis. If there is no urethral necrosis the urethra may be sutured after checking, by passing a catheter proximally and distally, that the urethra is patent. However, in most cases there is usually extensive damage at the site.

The penis is transected to leave an 8–12-cm stump protruding from the dorsal commissure of the skin incision (Fig. 4.60). The dorsal arteries and vein are ligated. The urethra is readily identified and is opened for a distance of 4–5 cm (Fig. 4.61). The stump of the penis is directed caudoventral so that it projects slightly from the skin incision to which it is anchored with a suture which passes through the tunica albuginea and the corpus cavernosus. It is important that the stump should be of sufficient length so that there is no

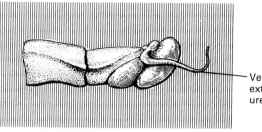

Fig. 4.57. In the ram, the vermiform extension of the urethra is a very common site of urethral obstruction (after Sisson & Grossman (1975) *The Anatomy of the Domestic Animal*, 5th edn, W.B. Saunders, Philadelphia).

Vermiform extension of urethra

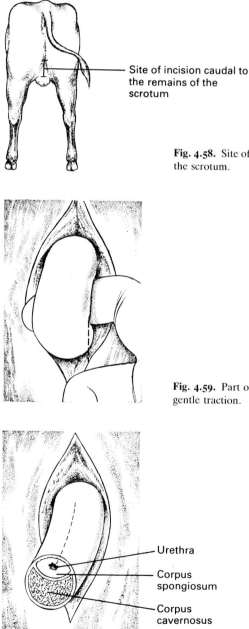

Site of incision caudal to the remains of the scrotum

Fig. 4.58. Site of incision caudal to the remains of the scrotum.

Fig. 4.59. Part of the penis is withdrawn by gentle traction.

Urethra

Corpus spongiosum

Corpus cavernosus

Fig. 4.60. The penis is transected and spatulated.

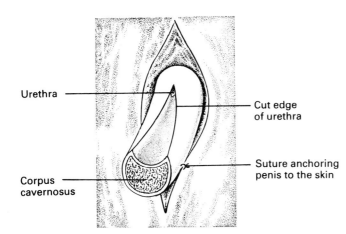

Fig. 4.61. The stump of the penis is anchored to the skin on either side in such a way that it protrudes slightly.

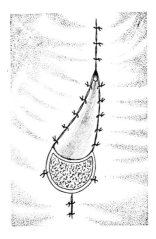

Fig. 4.62. The urethral mucosa and the edge of the corpus spongiosus are sutured to the skin on both sides.

infolding of skin because of excessive tension. The cut edge of the urethra is now sutured to the edge of the skin incisions on each side (Fig. 4.62).

Urethral obstruction in the breeding male animal is a very serious condition and unless diagnosed and treated very early, will curtail the animal's ability for natural service.

Amputation of the penis

Amputation of the penis in any species presents two major problems:
1 The control of haemorrhage.
2 The prevention of subsequent urethral stenosis.

HORSE

Malignant growths of the penis are not uncommon in the ageing gelding. These growths are mostly carcinomas affecting the glans penis. Many of these animals are kept purely as pets, and as the tumour rarely metastasizes, amputation of the penis (Figs 4.63–4.65) is a justifiable and successful means of removing the growth and the associated objectionable preputial discharges.

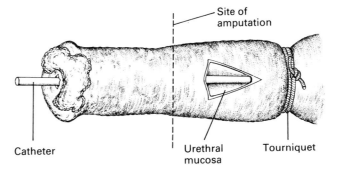

Fig. 4.63. A tourniquet is applied to the penis after the insertion of a urethral catheter. An incision is made in the lower midline of the penis, through the corpus cavernosum to expose the catheter and a length of urethra.

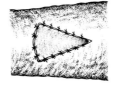

Fig. 4.64. The edge of the urethral mucous membrane is sutured to the integument of the penis, commencing on the cranio-lateral aspect of the incision, and continuing back to the caudal commissure and then forward again on the contralateral side.

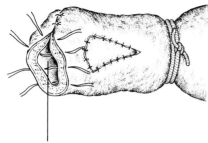

Corpus cavernosus

Fig. 4.65. The penis is amputated through the corpus spongiosum, and the amputated portion is slipped forward along the catheter. The tourniquet is carefully loosened and major bleeding vessels are picked up and ligated. The cranial urethral mucous membrane is sutured to the remainder of the integument, the sutures penetrating the corpus spongiosum so that additionally they are haemostatic in effect. The tourniquet is removed gradually in order to check any uncontrolled bleeding.

Reefing procedure

It is not uncommon for further neoplasms to be present on the preputial ring. These can be removed successfully by employing a reefing procedure.

Parallel circumferential incisions are made through the integument distally and proximally to the lesions (Fig. 4.66). The integument between the incisions is carefully dissected away avoiding damage to the large vessels which lie outside the tunica albuginea of the penis (Fig. 4.67). Bleeding points are identified and ligated after release of the tourniquet. The cut edges of the integument are approximated with interrupted sutures of synthetic absorbable suture material (Fig. 4.68).

DOG

Amputation of the penis in the dog (Figs 4.69–4.74) is indicated as a treatment for neoplasia. It may also be necessary in cases of trauma which have caused irrevocable damage to the penis, particularly when the os penis is involved. The presence of the os penis complicates the technique of amputation, particularly as the urethra lies in a groove on the ventral aspect of the bone. It is also important to guard against urethral stenosis.

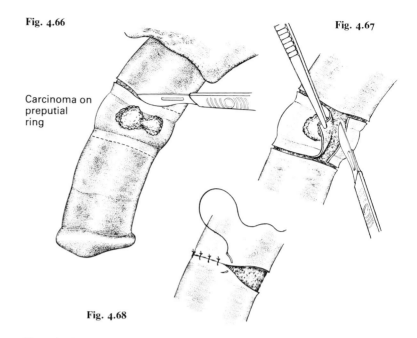

Fig. 4.66

Carcinoma on preputial ring

Fig. 4.67

Fig. 4.68

Fig. 4.66. Two circumferential incisions, proximal and distal to the lesion.
Fig. 4.67. A third longitudinal incision connects the two. The integument is dissected away from the underlying tissues.
Fig. 4.68. The two cut edges are apposed with sutures.

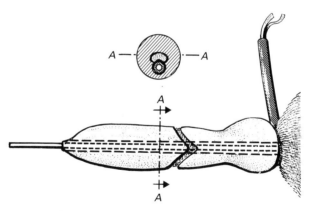

Fig. 4.69. The urethra is catheterized and the penis is snared with a tourniquet. With the patient in dorsal recumbency the os penis is palpated. A pointed knife blade is thrust through the soft tissue of the penis keeping the blade in contact with the edge of the os penis. An incision is then made in an cranio-lateral direction on both sides of the penis in order to create two flaps of corpus spongiosum, and to expose the urethra.

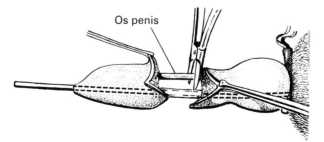

Os penis

Fig. 4.70. The soft tissue of the corpus spongiosum is dissected free from the os penis, and the catheterized urethra is carefully dissected from the groove in the os penis. The os penis is then severed with bone forceps as far back as possible.

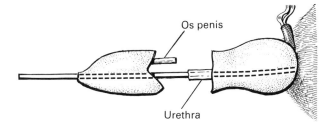

Fig. 4.71. The urethra is transected as far forward as possible, in order to leave a length of urethra still containing the urinary catheter.

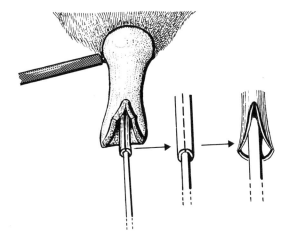

Fig. 4.72. The urethral remnant is split longitudinally on its ventral surface in order to produce a splayed end.

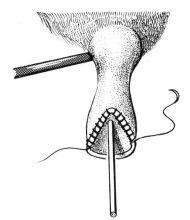

Fig. 4.73. The edges of the split urethra are sutured to the ventral edges of the flaps of the corpus spongiosum.

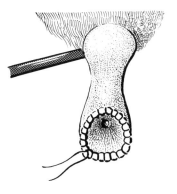

Fig. 4.74. The tourniquet is partially released in order to pick up any major bleeding vessels. The cranial edge of the urethra is then sutured to the remainder of the corpus spongiosum.

RAM

An incision is made through the skin in the midline below the anus. The penis is located by blunt dissection, freed from the surrounding connective tissue, and is then transected above the sigmoid flexure (Fig. 4.75). The dorsal artery of the penis is ligated with a single suture (Fig. 4.76).

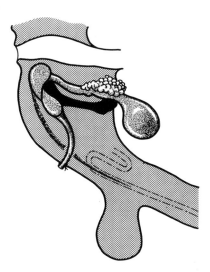

Fig. 4.75. The transected stump of the penis is sutured to the skin, allowing 3 cm to protrude (after Oehme & Tillman (1965) *J. Am. Vet. Med. Assoc.* **147**, 1331).

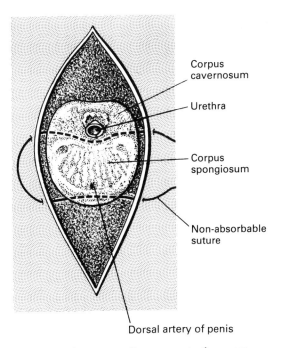

Fig. 4.76. The suture applies pressure to the corpus spongiosum and so controls haemorrhage without interfering with urination (after Oehme & Tillman (1965) *J. Am. Vet. Med. Assoc.* **147**, 1331).

Ureteral ectopia

Ureteral ectopia is a congenital anomaly which results in urinary incontinence. Clinical signs are usually seen in bitches and the incontinence may be continual or intermittent. The diagnosis is confirmed by intravenous excretory urography, combined with pneumocystography.

The ectopic ureters generally enter the neck of the bladder, urethra, uterus or vagina and the ectopia may be unilateral or bilateral. On occasions the ureter may empty into the bladder, yet continue to run within the bladder wall and drain distally beyond the trigone. Hydro-ureter, with or without hydronephrosis, frequently occurs and may be associated with urinary tract infection. The ectopic ureter is usually amenable to surgical re-implantation into the bladder.

The bladder is exposed by a posterior laparotomy incision and the course of the ureters is traced distally from the kidneys. The ectopic ureter may be re-implanted by one of three techniques, depending upon its position.

Intravesical technique

1 An incision is made in the ventral bladder wall and continued to the trigone area (Fig. 4.77a–c). The stoma of each ureter is examined. If the ureter enters the serosal surface of the bladder in the normal position, but then runs intramurally beyond the trigone, a new stoma is created and the distal portion of the ureter is ligated.
2 If the ureter by-passes the bladder it is tran-

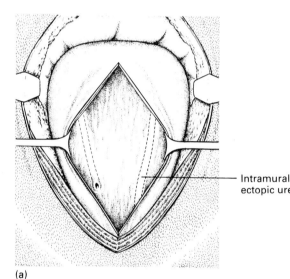

Intramural ectopic ureter

(a)

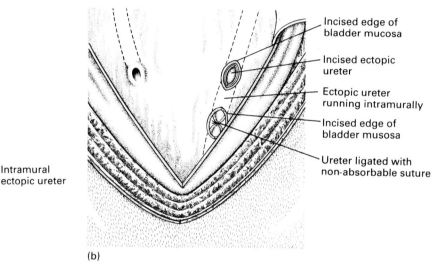

Incised edge of bladder mucosa

Incised ectopic ureter

Ectopic ureter running intramurally

Incised edge of bladder musosa

Ureter ligated with non-absorbable suture

(b)

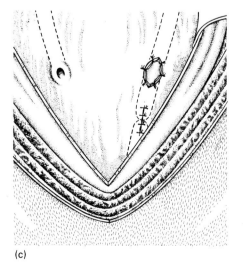

(c)

Fig. 4.77. (a) A ventral cystotomy is performed and the ectopic ureter is identified running within the bladder wall. (b) A small ellipse of mucosa overlying the ectopic ureter is removed and the ureter is incised longitudinally. A second mucosal incision is made just distal to the first, through which the ureter is ligated with a non-absorbable suture. Care should be taken to ensure that the entire ureter is included in this ligature. (c) The new stoma is completed by suturing the edges of the ureter and bladder mucosa with a series of interrupted sutures of 1.5 metric synthetic absorbable suture material. The distal mucosal incision is closed with similar sutures.

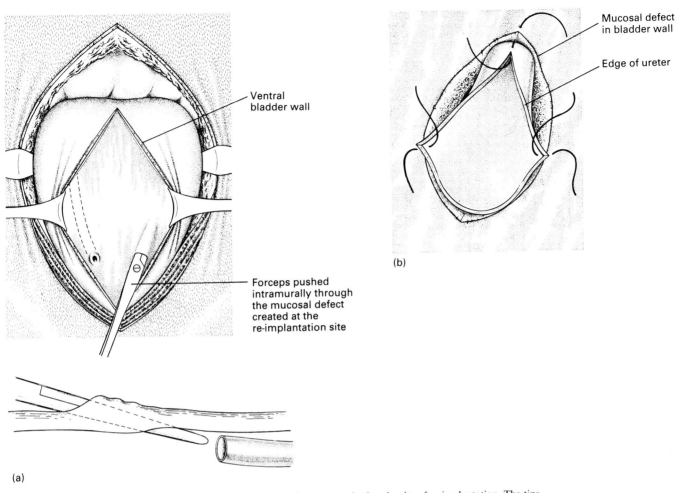

Ventral
bladder wall

Forceps pushed
intramurally through
the mucosal defect
created at the
re-implantation site

Mucosal defect
in bladder wall

Edge of ureter

(b)

(a)

Fig. 4.78. (a) A ventral cystotomy is performed and an ellipse of mucosa excised at the site of re-implantation. The tips of a pair of mosquito forceps are pushed intramurally for a distance approximately three times the diameter of the ureter which is to be transplanted. The serosa of the bladder is incised over the point of the forceps' exit and the end of the ureter is pulled through the tunnel. The end of the ureter is then spatulated. (b) The implantation is completed by suturing the edges of the ureter to the edges of the mucosal defect with interrupted sutures of 1.5 metric synthetic absorbable suture material. The three corners of the ureter are sutured initially to ensure a reasonable fit.

sected, the distal portion ligated and the free end re-implanted (Fig. 4.78). A small ellipse of mucosa is first excised at the proposed re-implantation site on the dorsal wall of the bladder. The tips of a pair of mosquito forceps are then passed through this defect and tunnelled intramurally for a distance approximately three times the diameter of the ectopic ureter. A serosal incision is made over the point of the forceps' exit and the ureter is pulled through the tunnel. The splayed end of the ureter is sutured to the edges of the mucosal defect with interrupted sutures of 1.5 metric synthetic absorbable suture material.

A Foley catheter is inserted in the bladder before the cystotomy incision is closed. Urinary output is monitored post-operatively and a mild diuresis is established for the first few hours following surgery.

Extravesical technique

The transected end of the ureter is spatulated as before but the submucosal tunnel is created through two serosal incisions, thereby obviating the need for a cystotomy (Fig. 4.79). A mucosal ellipse is excised at the site of re-implantation and the splayed end of the ureter sutured to its edges with interrupted sutures of 1.5 metric synthetic absorbable suture material. Finally, the serosal defect is closed with similar sutures.

The bladder is catheterized post-operatively and the remaining management is similar to the intravesical techniques.

If one of the kidneys is severely diseased it is advisable to perform a ureteronephrectomy. It is vital to first establish the presence of a second kidney and that it is functioning adequately.

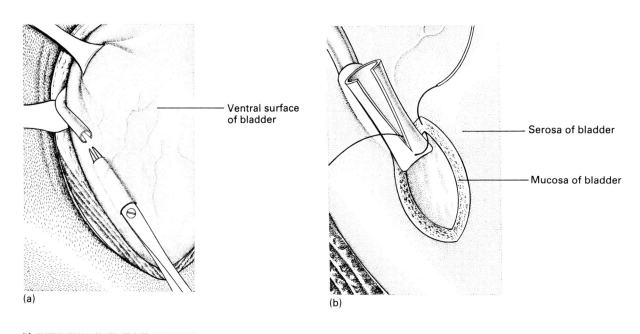

Ventral surface of bladder

Serosa of bladder

Mucosa of bladder

(a)

(b)

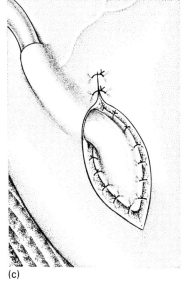

(c)

Fig. 4.79. (a) An incision is made in the bladder serosa at the proposed re-implantation site. The tips of a pair of mosquito forceps are passed through the serosal defect and pushed submucosally for a distance approximately three times the diameter of the ureter. The serosa is incised over the point of the forceps' exit and the splayed end of the ureter is grasped. (b) An ellipse of bladder mucosa is excised, corresponding in size to the splayed end of the ureter. The edges of the ureter and the vesical mucosa are sutured with interrupted sutures of 1.5 metric synthetic absorbable suture material. Care should be taken not to twist or kink the ureter. (c) The serosal defect is closed with interrupted sutures taking care not to occlude the ureter.

Section 5
Surgery of the Mammary Gland and Teat

Mammary neoplasia

Neoplasia of the mammary tissue is the commonest neoplasm in the bitch. In many cases the condition is present for several years as a small, pea-like nodule which tends to be overlooked by both owner and veterinarian until it suddenly increases rapidly in size. This increase is often associated with the stimulus of oestrus, and the rapid growth of the neoplasm often coincides with the development of metastatic lesions which spread via the lymphatics to the local lymph nodes, or by the cardiovascular system to the liver and lungs. Surgical excision is the treatment of choice although the optimal amount of tissue to be removed is still debatable.

Regional mastectomies are based upon the anatomical distribution of the lymphatic and venous drainage. The lymphatic drainage of the three pectoral glands is towards the axillary lymph node while the drainage of the two inguinal glands is towards the inguinal lymph node (Fig. 5.1). It is probable that an indefinite lymphatic link exists between the third pectoral and the first inguinal gland. It is also probable that the third pectoral gland drains forwards through the second and first pectoral glands, and that the first inguinal mammary gland drains through the second one.

Regional mastectomies may either be radical or modified radical procedures (Table 5.1). Both entail elliptical incisions around the relevant mammary tissue down to the body wall (Fig. 5.2).

In both procedures the inguinal lymph node is generally removed while the axillary node is left *in situ*. The importance of removing or leaving the lymph nodes is unclear and the reason for leaving the axillary node is that it is difficult surgically to remove. In contrast, it is difficult to excise the fifth inguinal mammary gland without removing part or all of the inguinal lymph node.

If inguinal glands are affected on both sides, then all the inguinal mammary tissue is removed, including the intervening skin in the midline. If this intervening skin is left, it will frequently slough as it is almost certainly deprived of the majority of its blood supply in a bilateral mastectomy. However, in cases of bilateral neoplasia involving the pectoral mammary glands, it is neither necessary nor desirable to remove the intervening skin.

Radical mastectomies of necessity involve the removal of large quantities of skin, and this frequently leads to undesirable tension on the skin edges in order to co-apt them. It is important that the tension of mastectomy wounds is taken by the subcuticular fascia, and to this end it is necessary to insert a series of interrupted subcuticular absorbable sutures, before the skin is closed with monofilament nylon. The post-operative congestion that is inevitable may be dispersed more rapidly if the bitch is given regular controlled exercise during the immediate post-operative period.

Radical mastectomies are necessary when there are tumours of multiple glands or they may be performed prophylactically in the younger, relatively fit, bitch. The more mammary tissue that is removed, the less there is in which new tumours can develop. There is no value in performing an ovariohysterectomy to reduce the incidence of recurrence.

A local mastectomy can be used to remove tumours of a single breast rather than performing a regional procedure. An elliptical incision is made around the affected gland and the mammary tissue of that gland is removed down to the body wall. Alternatively, lumpectomy, removal of just the

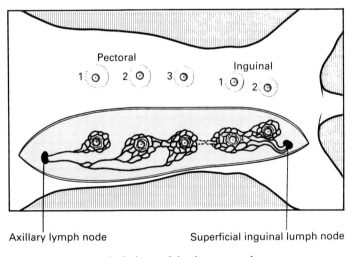

Fig. 5.1. The lymphatic drainage of the three mammary glands is towards the axillary lymph node. The drainage of the two inguinal mammary glands is toward the inguinal lymph node.

Table 5.1. Glands removed in radical and modified radical mastectomies

Tumour	Modified radical	Radical
Gland 1	Remove gland 1	Remove gland 1, 2, 3
2	1, 2	1, 2, 3
3	1, 2, 3	1, 2, 3, 4, 5
4	4, 5	3, 4, 5
5	4, 5	3, 4, 5

tumour tissue, can be performed. This approach may be preferable in older bitches, especially when the volume of the tumour is small.

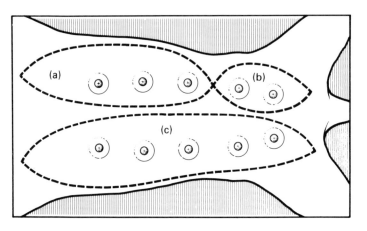

Fig. 5.2. (a) Modified regional mastectomy for neoplasia in the third pectoral gland. (b) Modified regional mastectomy for neoplasia in inguinal glands 4 or 5. (c) Radical mastectomy for neoplasia in pectoral gland 3.

Teats

TEAT OBSTRUCTIONS

Apart from uncommon congenital teat obstructions in the cow, most forms of obstruction are acquired, and many are related to chronic trauma inflicted at milking time due to faulty milking technique. This trauma predisposes to chronic localized infection, and it is therefore important that in addition to dealing with the obstructive lesion, the milking technique should be checked and steps taken to control chronic infection in order to prevent recurrence of the condition.

Basal obstruction

This condition is usually acquired during the dry period, and is predisposed by chronic inflammation and infection of the annular fold of mucous membrane, which separates the mucous membrane of the milk sinus from that of the teat canal. The annular fold is normally kept patent during lactation by the daily passage of milk, but chronic inflammation of the annular fold leads to adhesions developing during the dry period, so that after calving, the affected teat canal cannot fill with milk from the milk sinus. A Hudson's teat probe and spiral can be used to clear the annular fold (Figs 5.3–5.4).

Post-operative antibiotic therapy of the teat canal is essential, bearing in mind that the adhesions in the annular fold are probably predisposed by chronic infection.

Mid-teat obstructions

Localized mid-teat obstructions, or 'peas' are occasionally the result of localized neoplasia, but more commonly arise from localized areas of chronic inflammation, possibly involving the accessory glands which underlie the mucous membrane lining the teat canal. Large lesions may require open teat surgery during the dry period in order to remove them, but many are amenable to surgery through the streak canal, and may be removed by a papillotome (Figs 5.5–5.6).

Apical obstruction

Chronic inflammatory conditions involving the apex of the teat and the streak canal frequently lead to fibrosis and stenosis of the streak canal.

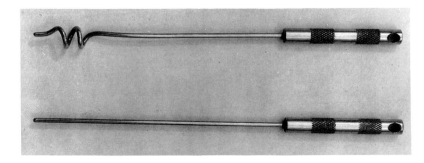

Fig. 5.3. Hudson's teat spiral and probe.

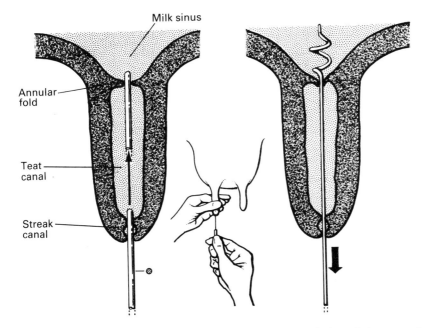

Milk sinus

Annular fold

Teat canal

Streak canal

Fig. 5.4. The probe is carefully inserted into the teat canal and a small hole is made through the centre of the adherent annular fold. The probe is withdrawn, and the teat spiral carefully inserted into the teat canal and insinuated through the hole in the annular fold and up into the milk sinus. The end of the teat is grasped, and the adhesions in the annular fold are broken down by a sharp downward pull on the spiral.

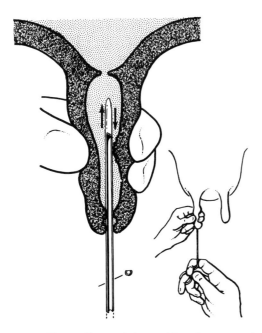

Fig. 5.5. The papillotome is inserted into the teat canal. The cutting surface of the papillotome is pressed against the lesion by pressure of the fingers through the teat wall. Small pieces of the lesion are then 'eroded' by a rhythmical up and down movement of the cutting edge.

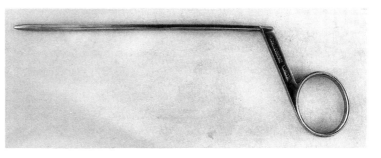

Fig. 5.6. Barrett's papillotome.

Affected animals become very difficult to milk due to the stenosis, and are aptly named 'hard milkers'. The condition may be relieved by longitudinal incision of the fibrosed canal. This treatment tends to be only palliative as the incision eventually heals, accompanied by an insidious recurrence of the stenosis.

The beneficial effect of this procedure will be prolonged if a teat dilator is inserted into the streak canal after milking for 7 days, during which period it is advisable to administer prophylactic intramammary antibiotics. McLean's knife may be used to open the end of a teat which has been severely crushed by a 'tread' injury (Figs 5.7–5.8). It is also useful in some cases of udder injury in which large blood clots collect in the teat canal, and which may prove impossible to milk out until the streak canal has been enlarged.

TEAT LACERATIONS

These fall into three main categories.

1 Flap wounds involving a V-shaped superficial layer of the teat skin, and usually associated with a self-inflicted 'tread' injury. The thin layer of detached skin is deprived of its blood supply and undergoes rapid necrosis, leaving a large raw area which heals only slowly. In these cases the area should be protected by a bactericidal emollient cream, and covered with a non-stick, self-adhesive dressing between milking.

2 Deep lacerations of the teat wall which do not penetrate into the teat canal. These will invariably heal if left unsutured, but in all cases the healing is greatly accelerated if the edges of the wound are cleaned and any bruised and devitalized tissue is removed before co-apting the edges with simple interrupted sutures of fine monofilament nylon.

3 Deep penetrating wounds into the teat canal, through which milk escapes. These lacerations must be sutured, otherwise milk will be lost continuously through the torn wall of the teat canal, and infection may readily become established.

Although in the past it has been customary not to suture the mucosal lining this can now be carried out to advantage using very fine absorbable suture material and an atraumatic needle. The remainder of the teat wall is gently opposed using vertical mattress sutures of fine monofilament nylon (Fig. 5.9).

Many penetrating teat lacerations are extremely irregular in shape, and are not the ideal straight tear as illustrated. In addition, the wound is rarely caused by a sharp instrument and so the wound edges contain bruised and potentially dead tissue which will eventually slough. Although many teat lacerations are successfully repaired by direct suture, others fail to heal completely due either to sloughing of devitalized tissue, or to the interference that is unavoidable each time the cow is milked. These small areas of breakdown rapidly develop an organized lining and form a teat fistula. Once a true fistula has formed it is unlikely to heal until the lining is dissected out and the wound sutured. This is best carried out after the cow is dried off, so that the incision may be left to heal undisturbed before the next lactation commences.

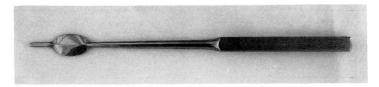

Fig. 5.7. McLean's knife. The blade is designed to cut on insertion and withdrawal.

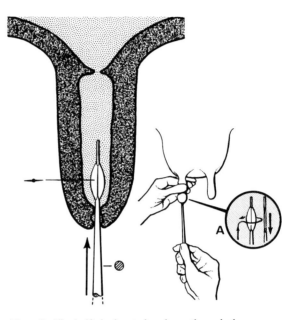

Fig. 5.8. The knife is thrust sharply up through the streak canal, after first cleaning the teat and distending the teat canal with milk. Once in the teat canal, the knife may be rotated through 90° before it is withdrawn to produce a cruciate incision in the streak canal (see insert A).

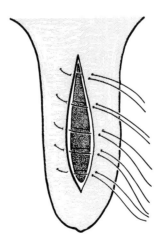

Fig. 5.9. Vertical mattress sutures of fine monofilament nylon are inserted. These sutures are left untied until all have been inserted, making certain that the deep part of the stitch passes through the submucous tissue without penetrating into the teat canal.

Section 6
Hernia and Rupture

A hernia is the protrusion of a viscus through a physiological opening of the abdominal cavity, namely, the umbilical or the inguinal rings. These physiological openings normally close either before or soon after birth, but in certain instances they remain patent, allowing abdominal viscera to pass through the open ring.

In the case of the inguinal canal, in both the male and female it is lined by the tunica vaginalis, which is an outpouching of the peritoneum and thus the protruding viscus is contained within the sac of the tunica vaginalis. In the female this gives rise to a swelling in the inguinal area, but in the male the swelling usually progresses down into the scrotum and is referred to as a scrotal hernia, which is complicated by the presence of the testicle in the tunica vaginalis.

An umbilical hernia arises due to failure of the linea alba to close around the stalk of the umbilical cord, and in many cases this is predisposed by low grade infection of the umbilical remnant. Through this defect a portion of abdominal viscus will protude, pushing with it a pouch of peritoneum. Also attached to the peritoneal sac may be found the vestigial remnants of the umbilical vein (the falciform ligament), umbilical arteries (the round ligaments of the bladder) and the allantoic stalk (the ventral ligament of the bladder).

Surgically, a hernia consists of a ring, which is either the umbilical or inguinal ring; a sac lined with peritoneum, and the contents which may be omentum, broad ligament or a portion of uterus or small intestine. In its simplest terms, therefore, surgical reduction involves returning the herniated contents into the abdominal cavity, obliterating the peritoneal sac and closing the ring with sutures to prevent recurrence of the hernia. All hernias are areas of anatomical weakness and their successful repair depends upon the tissues being permanently co-apted by sutures. It is therefore essential that all hernias are repaired with non-absorbable suture material.

. . . .

Incarcerated hernia

When it is not possible to return the contents to the abdominal cavity, because they are trapped in the hernia sac by the ring, the hernia is said to be incarcerated. If a portion of intestine, or less commonly uterus, becomes incarcerated there is a grave danger that the blood supply to the trapped viscus may be impaired and finally cut off, causing strangulation and necrosis of the trapped viscus, and giving rise to a grave surgical emergency. In dealing with an incarcerated hernia, therefore, it is necessary to enlarge the hernia ring in order to free the trapped contents. The umbilical ring may be enlarged in a cranial or caudal direction, but the inguinal ring can only be enlarged in an craniolateral direction, as its cranio-medial canthus is adjacent to the bony pelvic brim. Having freed the trapped contents, it is then necessary to remove any devitalized tissue, possibly necessitating enterectomy or hysterectomy, before the hernial ring is closed.

. . . .

Umbilical hernia

Figures 6.1—6.3 illustrate the standard procedure for dealing with umbilical hernias.

Figures 6.4—6.6 show an alternative procedure if the peritoneal sac cannot be maintained intact.

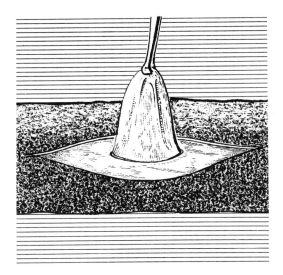

Fig. 6.1. The skin of the hernial sac is freed by an elliptical incision, and the connective tissue is broken down by blunt dissection to expose the glistening peritoneal sac and the ring where it emerges through the abdominal wall. The skin remnant is detached from the peritoneal sac, leaving the sac intact.

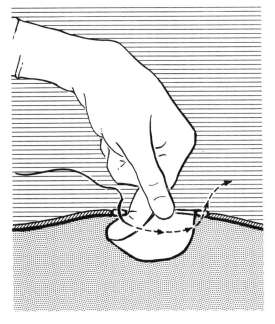

Fig. 6.2. The intact hernial sac is invaginated through the ring, and the edge held between the thumb and forefinger while the stitches are inserted. This ensures that no abdominal viscera are inadvertently damaged by the needle.

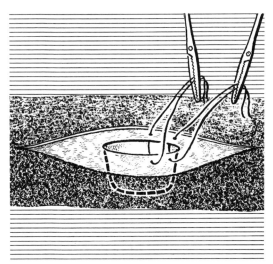

Fig. 6.3. Closure of the hernial ring is simplified if all the sutures are inserted and 'laid' before they are tied.

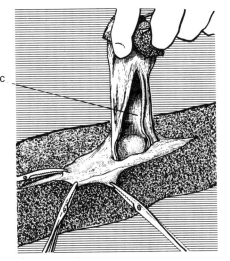

Open hernial sac

Fig. 6.4. The peritoneal sac may be inadvertently opened when attempting to free it from the overlying skin, or purposely opened in order to inspect the contents.

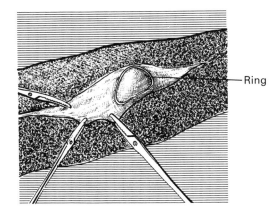

Ring

Fig. 6.5. The peritoneal sac is trimmed off down to the level of the ring.

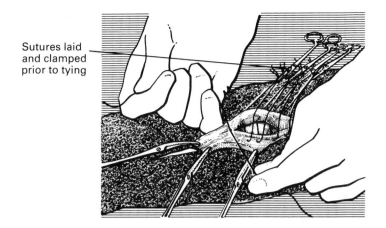

Sutures laid
and clamped
prior to tying

Fig. 6.6. The ring is closed by a series of simple interrupted sutures of non-absorbable suture material. It is easier if the sutures are 'laid', i.e. each suture is inserted but is left untied until all the sutures are in position. This overcomes the danger of accidentally incorporating a loop of intestine in the suture line. It is most important that the sutures are placed well away from the edge of the hernial ring, to ensure that they are co-apting strong tissue. The skin is closed by monofilament nylon.

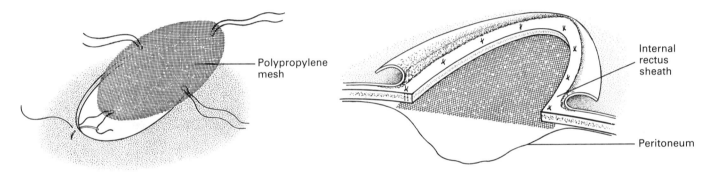

Polypropylene
mesh

Internal
rectus
sheath

Peritoneum

Fig. 6.7. When using polypropylene mesh to repair a hernia it is best to suture it between the peritoneum and the internal rectus sheath.

When the hernial ring is large and its edges thick and rounded, it may be difficult if not impossible to bring them into apposition. In these cases, bridging the defect with a prosthetic material in the form of a mesh provides a simple and very effective alternative method of treatment. Polypropylene mesh has proved to be the most useful of the variety of synthetic materials which have been used for this purpose in animals.

The mesh is best placed in an extraperitoneal position between the internal rectus sheath and the peritoneum where it has a greater mechanical advantage than if it is placed overlying the defect.

The sac is isolated and returned to the abdominal cavity as previously described (Figs 6.1−6.2). The intact peritoneum is reflected peripherally from the deep fascial sheath of the rectus muscle for 1−2 cm. The mesh is cut so that it overlaps the margin of the ring by the same amount. At least eight sutures are preplaced around the margin of the mesh (Fig. 6.7). The two ends of each suture are taken in turn through the margin of the hernial ring from inside outwards and tied, thereby drawing the mesh between the muscle and the peritoneum. The subcutaneous tissue and skin are then carefully apposed over the mesh.

A similar technique can be employed to repair incisional and traumatic flank hernias.

Inguinal hernia

Inguinal hernia in the female

In both the female and the male, an inguinal hernia should be approached by an incision overlying the external inguinal ring (Figs 6.8–6.11). In the female this is best accomplished by an incision medial to the inguinal mammary tissue, whereas in the male the incision should be over the inguinal ring, and parallel to the fold of the flank.

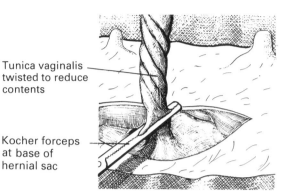

Fig. 6.10. A ligature of non-absorbable material is placed below the Kocher forceps, and is tied into the crushed tissue. The sac above the ligature is cut off.

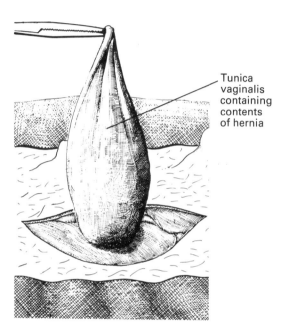

Fig. 6.8. The skin is incised over the inguinal ring. The hernial sac is dissected free by blunt dissection and gripped at its apex by a pair of forceps.

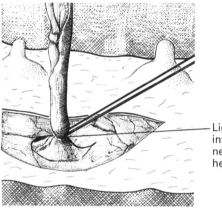

Fig. 6.9. The contents of the sac are returned to the abdominal cavity by twisting the sac, the base of which is then clamped with Kocher forceps.

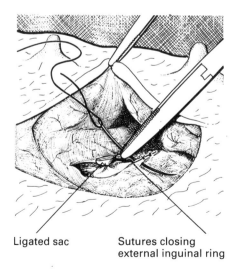

Fig. 6.11. The external inguinal ring is closed by interrupted sutures, burying the ligated pedicle of the hernial sac.

Inguinal (scrotal) hernia in the male

Any hernia is a possible hereditary weakness, and it is not desirable to breed from an animal so affected. It is therefore normal practice to combine castration with scrotal herniotomy (Figs 6.12–6.14), although this is not an essential part of the operation, which, if necessary, can be carried out without sacrificing the testicle.

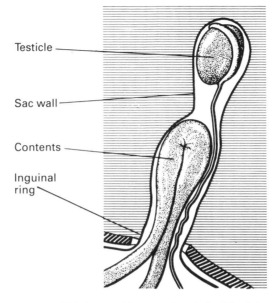

Fig. 6.13. This diagram illustrates the relationship of the testicle and spermatic cord to the hernial contents.

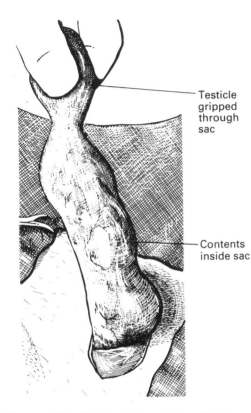

Fig. 6.12. The skin is incised over the inguinal ring, and the hernial sac is dissected free from its attachment to the scrotum. The testicle is held through the wall of the tunica vaginalis.

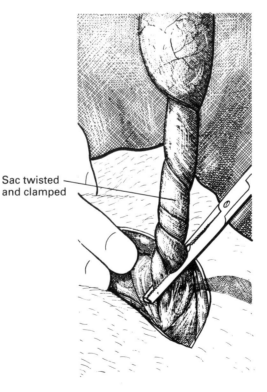

Fig. 6.14. The contents are reduced into the abdominal cavity by twisting the sac, but maintaining a hold on the testicle through the sac wall. Once the contents are reduced, the base of the sac is crushed by Kocher forceps, including the spermatic cord. The sac is then ligated, and cut off above the ligature, so that both the sac and the testicle are removed. The inguinal ring is then oversewn, as shown in Fig. 6.11.

Rupture

A rupture is a tear in the abdominal wall, or in the anatomical boundaries of the abdominal cavity, i.e. the diaphragm and the pelvic diaphragm. It is not related to a physiological opening and is not congenital in origin, but it is always associated with violent trauma or with prolonged subacute trauma. Unlike a hernia, the contents of a rupture are not enclosed within a sac of unbroken peritoneum, and therefore adhesions between the contents and the rupture sac are a common complication and add greatly to the difficulty of repair. It is not proposed to consider the treatment of traumatic tears in the abdominal wall, which are normally repaired by the application of standard surgical principles. Each case is different and requires individual modification.

Rupture of the diaphragm and rupture of the pelvic diaphragm are two conditions which call for rather special skill, and being comparatively common are dealt with in some detail.

RUPTURE OF THE DIAPHRAGM

Any violent trauma, often associated with a car accident or a fall, may lead to rupture of the diaphragm. In the majority of cases the tear occurs in the central membranous portion of the diaphragm, and spreads radially to its attachment with the costal arch, and may then tear this attachment for variable distances. The majority of tears, therefore, tend to be triangular.

In animals which survive this initial trauma, the abdominal contents move forward into the pleural cavity giving rise to lung collapse in direct proportion to the volume of migrating viscera. Dyspnoea is therefore the most common presenting symptom, as respiration is impaired partly by lung collapse and partly by the loss of the diaphragm as an integral part of the mechanics of respiration.

The surgical approach to the repair of the ruptured diaphragm is a matter of controversy, but the authors are in no doubt that this condition is most effectively dealt with through a cranial laparotomy. They justify this approach against repair through a thoracotomy incision for the following reasons.

1 Laparotomy gives a 360° approach to the diaphragm, whereas a thoracotomy only offers a 180° approach unless one is prepared to tear through the mediastinum.

2 Laparotomy is a more familiar technique to the general surgeon than is a thoracotomy.

3 Problems of acute post-operative discomfort do not arise following laparotomy to the same extent as they do following thoracotomy.

4 Intrathoracic adhesions are extremely uncommon. If they do occur, they can usually be safely broken down through an abdominal approach, and only in very exceptional cases is it necessary to resort to thoracotomy to relieve them.

5 Laparotomy allows an examination to be made of the abdominal viscera, which are frequently damaged at the time of the diaphragmatic rupture.

No matter which surgical approach is used, successful repair is in large measure an anaesthetic

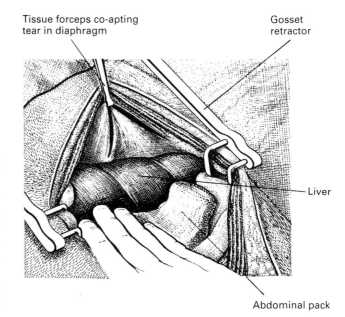

Fig. 6.15. The tear in the diaphragm is located, and the edges are temporarily held together by tissue forceps.

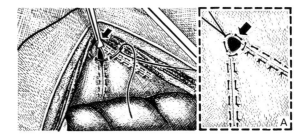

Fig. 6.16. The tear is sutured using either simple interrupted or mattress sutures of a non-absorbable suture material. It is often helpful to lay the last suture and leave it untied until the anaesthetist fully inflates the lungs (A). This tends partially to eliminate the surgical pneumothorax, but it is by no means absolute, as the initial closure of the tear in the diaphragm is rarely completely airtight.

problem, and calls for close co-operation between the surgeon and anaesthetist. An animal with a ruptured diaphragm is suffering from a variable degree of general hypoxia, which may precipitate a cardiac arrest on anaesthetic induction. For this reason we do not induce anaesthesia in cases of ruptured diaphragm until the surgeon is scrubbed for surgery, so that in the event of an emergency arising during induction he or she can rapidly open the abdomen and take whatever remedial steps are necessary.

Following induction, a cranial laparotomy incision is made lateral to the linea alba, avoiding the underlying falciform ligament. The incision should extend from the xiphisternum to beyond the umbilicus. Once the abdomen is opened the incision should be held apart by retractors and the abdominal viscera removed as quickly as possible from the pleural cavity in order to relieve respiratory embarrassment due to lung collapse.

The tear in the diaphragm is located and the edges are temporarily held together by tissue forceps before being sutured (Figs 6.15–6.16).

Following inspection of the abdominal viscera to check for any additional damage, the abdominal wall is closed. It must be emphasized that it is essential to aspirate both pleural cavities by means of a plastic intrapleural catheter connected to a sucker and underwater seal (see pp. 132–3) following abdominal closure. Animals can die following an apparently successful repair due to failure to eliminate the surgical pneumothorax.

PERINEAL RUPTURE — DOG

This arises in the mature male dog due to a degeneration of the muscles of the pelvic diaphragm (Fig. 6.17), which support the lateral walls of the rectum, and seal the pelvic inlet from the abdominal cavity.

The aetiology of this condition is not clear. Many factors have been implicated including tenesmus, congenital weakness, prostatic hypertrophy and hormonal imbalances.

The levator ani and coccygeus muscles tend to overlie and support each other, but there is a weak point between the levator ani and the sphincter ani internus, and it is at this point that the rupture first occurs (Fig. 6.18). This is readily differentiated from a neoplastic enlargement by rectal examination. Neoplasms are space-occupying, whereas in perineal rupture the examining finger readily enters the rectal sacculation.

The accumulation of faecal matter in the sacculation increases the tenesmus, which often forces the prostate gland back into the pelvic inlet, and in extreme cases will cause the bladder to become retroverted into the pelvis, causing acute urinary obstruction. Surgical treatment, therefore, should not be delayed, and is based upon accurate recon-

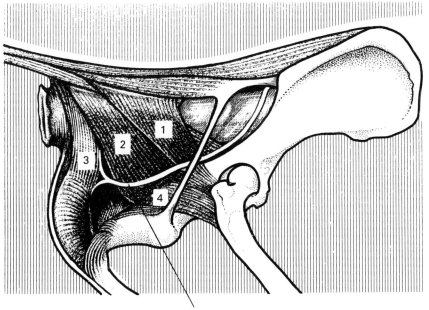

Perineal artery and nerve

Fig. 6.17. The pelvic diaphragm consists of the coccygeus (1) and the levator ani muscles (2). Fibres of the levator ani blend with the sphincter ani internus (3). The floor of the pelvis is covered by the obturator internus muscle (4).

struction of the pelvic diaphragm. The authors consider that castration should be an integral part of the surgical procedure, as it offers the only effective long-term treatment for prostatic hypertrophy.

After anaesthetic induction, the rectum and rectal sacculation should be emptied of faeces, and a purse-string suture inserted around the anus. The dog is then placed in dorsal recumbency and castrated before repairing the perineal rupture. The animal is repositioned in ventral recumbency, with its hind legs strapped over the end of the operating table and the tail pulled upward and forward. The table should have a head-down tilt to enable the pelvic contents to be reduced into the abdomen.

The rupture is approached through an incision starting at the base of the tail, curving around the anus and ending above the scrotum in the midline. The rupture sac contains blood-stained fluid, loose connective tissue and fat, and occasionally the prostate gland and prostatic cysts are found. The contents are pushed forward and the rectum and sphincter ani are recognized medially, whereas the remnants of the pelvic diaphragm may be seen sloping forward laterally, or more frequently are only appreciated by palpation. The floor of the defect is formed by the obturator internus muscle, and the perineal artery and nerve must be recognized as they cross the defect low down in the edge of a fold of connective tissue.

The muscles are sutured together as shown in Fig. 6.19, with a hiatus in the suture line which allows the passage of the perineal artery and nerve, both of which supply the anal ring. This suturing must be accurate, and is made easier if the stitches are first inserted and 'laid' and then finally are all tied in succession. Non-absorbable material is used.

This suture line is then reinforced by dissecting the subcutaneous fascia away from the excess skin flap lateral to the incision, back to the line at which the excess skin is to be cut off, and then stitching the edge of the fascia to the sphincter ani, caudal to the first row of sutures.

The skin is closed and the purse-string suture removed from the anus. If the lesion is bilateral it is normal practice to repair the worst side and to allow 4–6 weeks before repair of the second side. In bilateral cases it is important to avoid damage to the perineal nerve, otherwise faecal incontinence may occur.

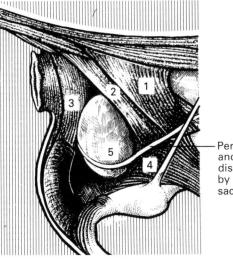

Perineal artery and nerve displaced by rectal sacculation

Fig. 6.18. Once the rectum is deprived of local support due to the rupture, there is a tendency for faecal matter to force the rectum through the muscle defect to produce a rectal sacculation (5) which is clinically recognizable by a swelling in the ischiorectal fossa. The displacement of the perineal artery and nerve makes them liable to damage during the early stages of surgical exposure of the rupture sac. Care must be taken to preserve these structures particularly when a bilateral repair has to be undertaken. (1–4 as in Fig. 6.17.)

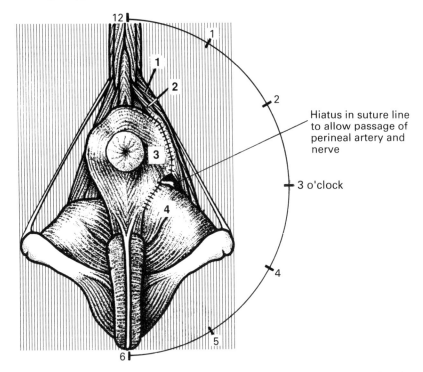

Hiatus in suture line to allow passage of perineal artery and nerve

3 o'clock

Fig. 6.19. Starting at the top of the defect, the levator ani muscle (2) is sutured to the cranial border of the sphincter ani muscle (3), and these sutures are continued round the 'clock face' until at 3 o'clock the forward slope of the levator ani muscle makes it necessary to complete the closure by stitching the obturator internus muscle (4) to the sphincter ani. Alternatively, rather than suturing the obturator internus muscle from 3 o'clock to 6 o'clock, the repair can be strengthened by transecting its tendon of insertion from the ischium, elevating the muscle and suturing into the cranial border of the sphincter ani muscle. Although the coccygeus muscle (1) forms part of the pelvic diaphragm, it is only involved in the closure when the levator ani has become too degenerate to support sutures.

Section 7
Thoracic Surgery

Thoracotomy

LATERAL APPROACH – DOG

A thoracotomy incision is always restricted on either side by the presence of a rib, and this limits the amount of exposure that may be obtained, even with the use of a rib retractor. The incision must therefore be accurately placed in relation to the area of the chest that is to be explored and this can only be decided by an accurate pre-operative assessment of the lesion by radiography. A simple thoracotomy incision may be made by cutting through the intercostal muscles, but this produces a very limited exposure and often proves difficult to close. Better exposure is achieved by the subperiosteal resection of a rib (Figs 7.1–7.5). It is possible to locate the correct rib for resection by first palpating the last rib, and then counting numerically backwards until the correct rib is palpated. If the skin over the rib is then scratched with a scalpel it is easier to identify after the patient is draped.

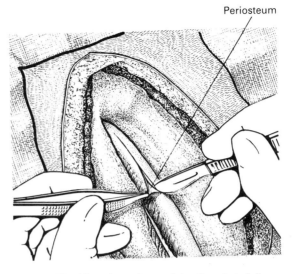

Fig. 7.1. The skin and muscles overlying the selected rib are incised so that the rib is exposed. Haemostasis must be meticulous. The periosteum of the rib is incised along its length, and dissected free from the underlying bone.

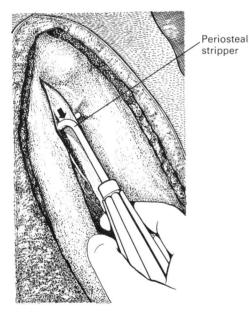

Fig. 7.2. Once a short section of rib has been completely freed from its periosteum a periosteal stripper is inserted below the rib. By carefully running the stripper along the length of the rib it is possible to strip the periosteal covering along its length down to the costochondral junction.

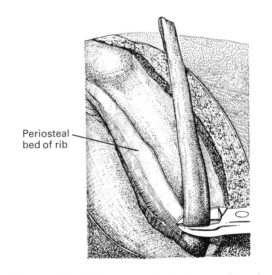

Fig. 7.3. The rib is then severed at each extremity and lifted out of its periosteal bed.

Periosteum and pleura

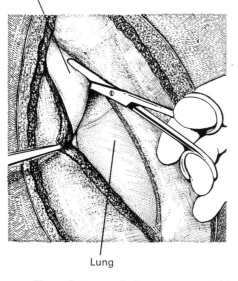

Lung

Fig. 7.4. The periosteum and pleura are opened with scissors, carefully avoiding damage to the underlying lung tissue.

Rib retractor

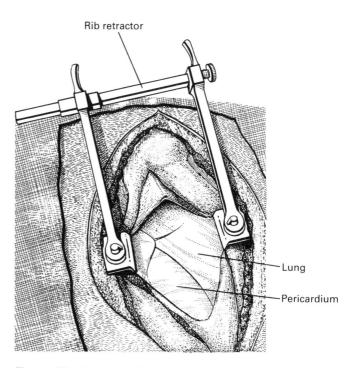

Lung

Pericardium

Fig. 7.5. The thoracotomy incision is then 'spread' and held open by means of a rib retractor.

Surgical closure

Before the thoracotomy incision can be closed it is essential to eliminate the surgical pneumothorax by means of an intrapleural drainage tube connected to an underwater seal (Figs 7.6—7.7).

The pleura and periosteal layer should be closed by a continuous suture to produce an airtight seal. The superficial muscle layers may be closed by either continuous or interrupted sutures.

Management of the chest drain

Once an airtight closure of the chest wall has been achieved, air will be sucked out of the pleural cavity as indicated by a stream of bubbles from the plastic tube beneath the surface of the water, and bubbles will continue to flow until the surgical pneumothorax has been eliminated and the lungs fully re-expanded.

At this stage the water level in the plastic tubing will rise indicating a negative pressure within the pleural cavity, and this level will rise and fall slightly at inspiration and expiration. Once a satisfactory negative pressure has been achieved with minimal respiratory swing the pleural drainage tube is removed by traction, and the small skin incision closed by a simple purse-string suture which in most cases will already have been inserted in the skin but left untied.

If it is considered that further chest aspiration is necessary, the chest drainage tube is disconnected from the underwater seal, having first occluded the tubing by a gate clamp, reinforced by doubling over the tubing and securing it with adhesive plaster. This occlusion must be absolute because if the chest drain is inadvertently opened so that the pleural cavity is in direct contact with the atmosphere, then a massive pneumothorax will result which may well prove fatal. The occluded tube is then lightly bandaged to the patient's body in such a way that it cannot become displaced or be interfered with. If further chest aspiration is necessary, the chest drain must be reconnected to the underwater seal before the gate clamp and adhesive plaster are removed. This method of underwater seal drainage will also remove any fluid which may accumulate within the pleural cavity.

MEDIAN STERNOTOMY — DOG

An alternative thoracotomy approach involves splitting the sternum (Fig. 7.8). This approach provides good exposure of the thoracic contents but has the disadvantage that the heart presses on the great vessels and reduces cardiac output.

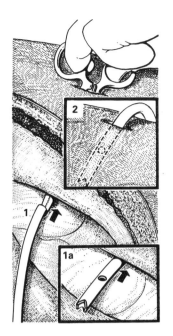

Fig. 7.6. With the chest still open a small skin incision is made high in the chest wall at either one or two intercostal spaces in front or behind the thoracotomy incision. A pair of Kocher forceps is inserted into the skin incision and then thrust through the thickness of the chest wall (1). The jaws of the forceps are opened and the drainage tube is grasped and drawn out through the thickness of the chest wall and skin. The end of the drainage tube which remains in the pleural cavity should have a 'kettle-spout' end and one side hole (1a) and this should be positioned to lie just within the pleural cavity (2). The drainage tube is then anchored to the skin with a suture, avoiding penetrating the tubing or transfixing it in any way as this may give rise to an air leak. A second, purse-string, suture is laid to close the skin incision when the tube is removed.

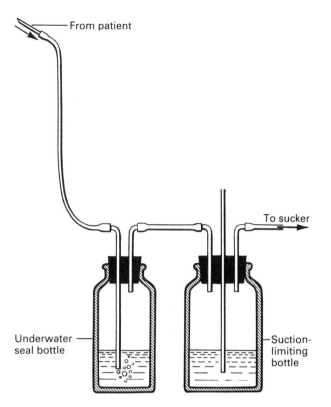

Fig. 7.7. The free end of the drainage tube is attached to the underwater seal which in turn is connected to a mechanical sucker. In order to limit excessive suction, a suction-limiting bottle may be interposed between the water seal and the sucker. The water seal must be at least 1.2 m below the level of the dog.

The dog is placed in dorsal recumbency and the skin is incised from the manubrium to the xiphisternum. The incision is continued through the subcutaneous tissues and fascia down to the sternebrae. Starting at the xiphoid cartilage, the sternebrae are split with an osteotome or oscillating saw, taking care to remain in the midline. If the first one or two sternebrae can be left intact, the ensuing closure will be more stable.

The sternotomy is closed with sutures of monofilament stainless steel wire taken around each split sternebra. The overlying soft tissues and skin are co-apted in the usual manner. A chest drain is inserted before closure.

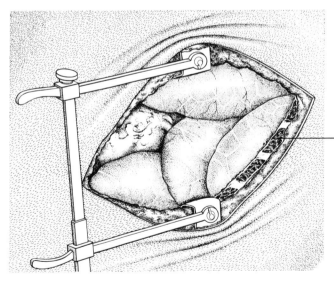

Fig. 7.8. The sternebrae have been split from the xiphoid cartilage to the manubrium. The internal thoracic vessels course on either side of the midline and should be avoided.

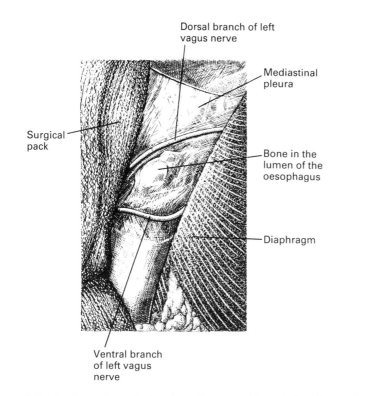

Dorsal branch of left
vagus nerve

Mediastinal
pleura

Surgical
pack

Bone in the
lumen of the
oesophagus

Diaphragm

Ventral branch
of left vagus
nerve

Fig. 7.9. Following thoracotomy the lung is gently retracted towards the hilum and packed away from the operation site. The bone is readily visible through the oesophageal wall, as are the dorsal and ventral branches of the left vagus nerve which run above and below the oesophagus as it penetrates the oesophageal hiatus in the diaphragm.

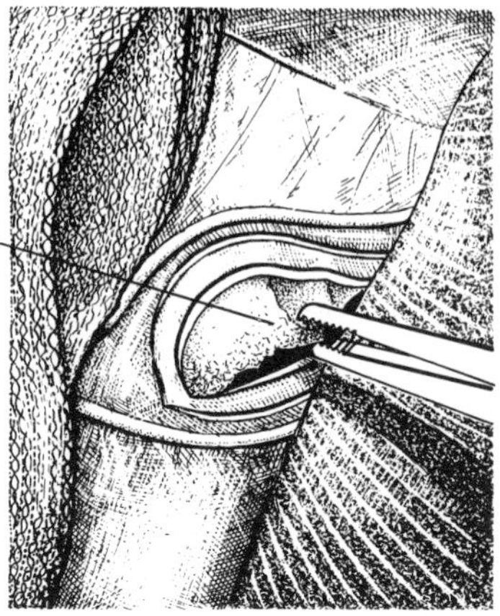

Bone gripped
by forceps

Fig. 7.10. The oesophagus is opened with care to avoid damage to the branches of the vagus and the obstructing bone is removed with forceps.

OESOPHAGEAL OBSTRUCTION – DOG

Oesophageal obstruction in the dog is commonly caused by swallowing an irregular-shaped bone. It then becomes held up either where the oesophagus passes close to the right side of the aortic arch at the base of the heart or, more frequently in the low pressure zone between the heart and the diaphragm. In the majority of cases it is possible to remove the bone by means of an oesophagoscope and crocodile forceps. In cases where the bone has been *in situ* for several days and its sharp projections have eroded into the oesophageal mucous membrane, it may prove very hazardous to attempt a forced extraction by endoscopy due to the danger of tearing the oesophageal wall. In such cases it is usual to remove the bone through a transthoracic oesophagotomy, resecting the left fifth rib to approach the aortic arch and the left eighth rib to approach the oesophagus immediately in front of the diaphragm (Figs 7.9–7.10).

Care must be taken to protect the pleural cavity from contamination by careful packing off, as the bone is frequently in an advanced state of putrefaction and the oesophagus also contains decomposing ingesta. It must be emphasized that bleeding from the oesophageal wall must be controlled before closure is commenced. The oesophagus is liberally supplied by the broncho-oesophageal artery and fatal haemorrhage can occur if a major branch is cut, particularly if this occurs in an area where pressure necrosis has largely destroyed the elastic retractile wall of the artery.

Closure of the oesophagus

Unlike the intestine, the oesophagus is not covered with a layer of serous membrane and therefore surgical closure must be particularly thorough (Figs 7.11–7.12). This is often made difficult by devitalized areas of tissue caused by local pressure necrosis from the sharp edges of the obstructing bone.

A single layer closure using simple interrupted oppositional sutures is a satisfactory alternative. In this case, the sutures should be pre-placed before being tied.

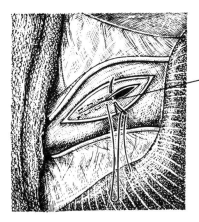

Fig. 7.11. Continuous horizontal mattress suture in mucous membrane using a synthetic absorbable suture material.

Continuous suture in mucous membrane

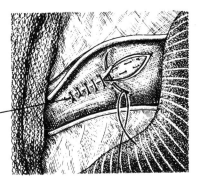

Interrupted sutures in muscle coats

Fig. 7.12. The muscular coats of the oesophagus are closed by a single layer of interrupted sutures. On completion, the pleural cavity is checked to make certain that all packs have been removed, a chest drain is inserted and the routine thoracotomy closure carried out.

VASCULAR RING OBSTRUCTION OF THE OESOPHAGUS — DOG

Oesophageal obstruction can also be caused by a developmental anomaly of the great vessels of the chest (Figs 7.13–7.16). The condition produces clinical symptoms when the affected puppy is weaned onto solid food. This can only pass through the vascular ring with difficulty and so most of it is retained within the oesophagus, cranial to the vascular ring where it causes gross dilatation. Most of this retained food is eventually regurgitated, although this is frequently mistaken for vomiting by the owner of the puppy. The presence of a vascular ring obstruction has a characteristic radiographic appearance and unless oesophageal dilatation is very severe, in the majority of cases the vascular ring is amenable to surgical division (Figs 7.17–7.18).

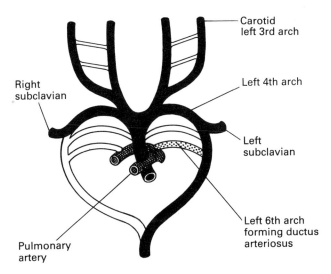

Carotid left 3rd arch

Right subclavian

Left 4th arch

Left subclavian

Left 6th arch forming ductus arteriosus

Pulmonary artery

Fig. 7.13. A simplified diagram of the normal aortic arch complex shows that the arch of the aorta develops from the fourth left embryonic aortic arch, and the pulmonary artery from the sixth embryonic aortic arch, which during intrauterine life maintains a patent connection with the left fourth aortic arch in order to by-pass the lungs. This vessel, the ductus arteriosus, rapidly closes in the neonatal animal but persists throughout life as the fibrous ligamentum arteriosum.

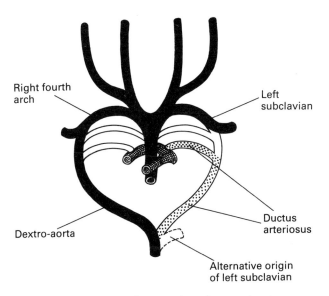

Right fourth arch

Left subclavian

Dextro-aorta

Ductus arteriosus

Alternative origin of left subclavian

Fig. 7.14. The commonest departure from the normal pattern involves the development of the fourth right aortic arch into the definitive aorta, while the ductus arteriosus makes contact with this dextro-aorta by utilizing the remnants of the left fourth arch. Once the ductus arteriosus closes and contracts, the oesophagus is trapped in a vascular ring composed of the base of the heart, the dextro-aorta and the ligamentum arteriosum.

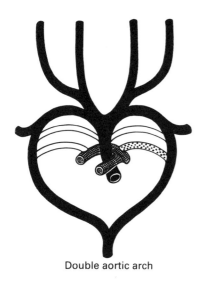

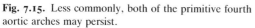

Double aortic arch

Fig. 7.15. Less commonly, both of the primitive fourth aortic arches may persist.

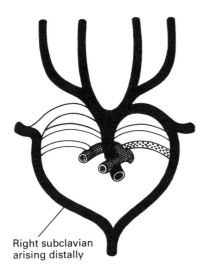

Right subclavian arising distally

Fig. 7.16. The right subclavian artery may arise from the distal instead of the proximal root and gives rise to oesophageal obstruction.

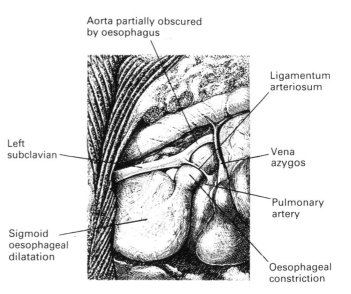

Aorta partially obscured by oesophagus

Ligamentum arteriosum

Left subclavian

Vena azygos

Pulmonary artery

Sigmoid oesophageal dilatation

Oesophageal constriction

Fig. 7.17. A left thoracotomy at the level of the fourth rib will expose the vascular ring (Fig. 7.18). After gently retracting the left apical lung lobe the mediastinal pleura is broken down with care to avoid damage to the adjacent thoracic duct, and the vascular ring may be identified at the caudal end of the oesophageal dilatation. The ligamentum arteriosum is dissected free of the oesophagus by blunt dissection and ligated close to its aortic and pulmonary artery connections before it is divided. The oesophagus should be freed by blunt dissection and then dilated by means of a blunt sound, inserted into the puppy's mouth by an assistant, which is then guided with care through the obstructed area, making certain that the site of obstruction is well dilated.

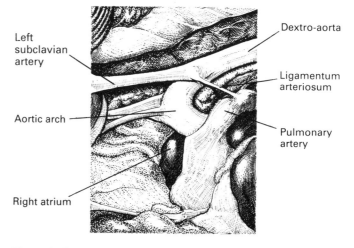

Left subclavian artery

Dextro-aorta

Ligamentum arteriosum

Aortic arch

Pulmonary artery

Right atrium

Fig. 7.18. Oesophagus removed to show the complete vascular ring.

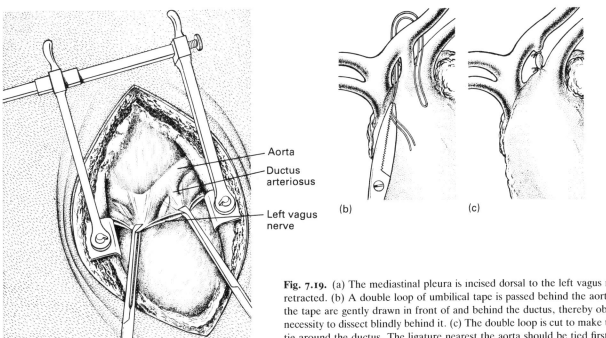

Aorta
Ductus arteriosus
Left vagus nerve

(a)

(b)   (c)

Fig. 7.19. (a) The mediastinal pleura is incised dorsal to the left vagus nerve and retracted. (b) A double loop of umbilical tape is passed behind the aorta. The ends of the tape are gently drawn in front of and behind the ductus, thereby obviating the necessity to dissect blindly behind it. (c) The double loop is cut to make two ligatures to tie around the ductus. The ligature nearest the aorta should be tied first. The ductus should not be divided but the ligatures should be placed as widely apart as possible.

PATENT DUCTUS ARTERIOSUS — DOG

The ductus arteriosus normally closes within the first few days of life and becomes a fibrous band. Failure to close allows blood to pass between the aorta and pulmonary artery. The flow is usually towards the pulmonary artery, thereby causing over-circulation of the lungs. Flow through the ductus in this direction causes turbulence and a typical continuous (machinery) murmur is heard over the left third intercostal space. The increase in the pressure in the pulmonary vessels, left atrium and left ventricle may result in dilatation of these structures and the dog eventually suffers from left-sided congestive heart failure. Ligation of the patent ductus arteriosus should be performed as soon as possible to prevent the above changes (Fig. 7.19).

Occasionally, when the pulmonary pressure is greater than the systemic pressure, the flow within the ductus will reverse and unoxygenated blood enters the aorta. Since the pressure difference between the two sides is much less, and the flow is more laminar, the murmur may be absent. The dog may experience severe exercise intolerance and cyanosis may be noted. Surgery is contra-indicated in these cases since ligation of the ductus will result in unacceptably high pressures in the pulmonary circulation.

The aim of surgery is to ligate the patent ductus and prevent blood flowing from the aorta to the pulmonary artery. Access is achieved by removing the left fourth rib and retracting the cranial and middle lung lobes. The mediastinal pleura is incised parallel and dorsal to the left vagus nerve and both are retracted ventrally to expose the ductus.

Blunt dissection cranial and caudal to a long ductus is relatively easy compared to those cases where the vessel is short and wedge shaped. In some cases dissection is facilitated by elevating the aorta distal to the ductus with a length of umbilical tape. The ductus is occluded with two ligatures of similar material. These are passed behind the aorta and their ends grasped by forceps gently introduced in front of, and behind the ductus. This avoids dissecting behind the fragile ductus and reduces the likelihood of tearing it. The aortic end of the ductus is ligated first and the ends of the ligature are left uncut so that gentle traction can be applied while the second ligature is tightened. The distance between the two ligatures should be as great as possible. The ductus should not be divided since there is always a possibility that the ligatures may slip.

LOBECTOMY — DOG

Lobectomy is indicated for the extirpation of disease conditions which are limited to a discrete area of lung tissue such as early bronchiectasis or a localized primary neoplasm, or to cases of trauma which involve gross laceration of lung tissue. The operation falls into two separate stages. In the first stage the blood supply to the affected lung lobe must be identified and ligated (Figs 7.20–7.21). The second stage involves the excision of the lobe by transection of the bronchus and surgical closure of the bronchial stump (Figs 7.22–7.23).

In the dog, all lobes of the lung are separated by distinct fissures apart from the left cranial and middle lobes which are fused over a transverse

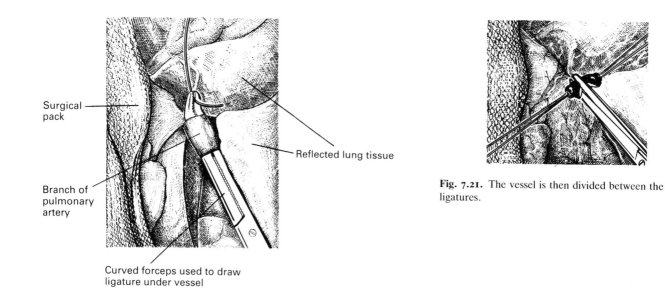

Surgical pack

Reflected lung tissue

Branch of pulmonary artery

Curved forceps used to draw ligature under vessel

Fig. 7.21. The vessel is then divided between the ligatures.

Fig. 7.20. The pulmonary artery and vein are dissected free from the bronchus by careful blunt dissection, remembering that the major vessels of the pulmonary tree are thin walled and easily torn, so they must be handled with considerable care. Two ligatures are passed around each vessel.

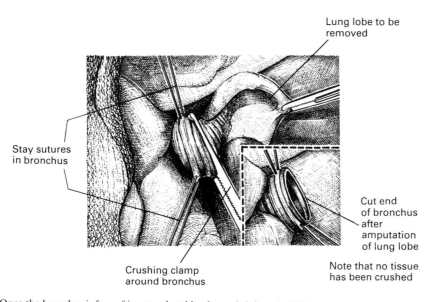

Lung lobe to be removed

Stay sutures in bronchus

Cut end of bronchus after amputation of lung lobe

Crushing clamp around bronchus

Note that no tissue has been crushed

Fig. 7.22. Once the bronchus is free of its attendant blood vessels it is occluded by a crushing clamp placed close to the lung parenchyma and as far as possible from the junction with the main bronchus. Two stay sutures of monofilament nylon are then inserted into the wall of the bronchus as close as possible to the junction with the main bronchus, using a round-bodied needle.

distance of approximately 2.5 cm from the vertebral border to the fissure between the two lobes. The main pulmonary vessels follow the distribution of the bronchial tree and are therefore recognized by first identifying the bronchus supplying the diseased or traumatized lung lobe.

Normal chest closure is carried out, but as most lobectomies are followed by a mild pleural effusion it is usual to blank off the chest drain and to leave it bandaged to the patient's chest, as previously described. Subsequent aspirations may then be carried out and in most cases the chest drain can be removed after 12 hours. It should be remembered that if a breakdown in the bronchial stump is going to occur, the fifth post-operative day is the most critical and any increasing dyspnoea at this time may indicate a bronchial leak. In some cases this will seal spontaneously providing that continuous chest aspiration can be applied, but the majority require a re-suture of the bronchial stump.

The space that is left following lobectomy is obliterated mainly by an expansion of the adjacent lung lobe, often accompanied by an elevation of the diaphragm on the affected side. Providing that adequate lung re-expansion is achieved, the deformity that results will almost be obliterated.

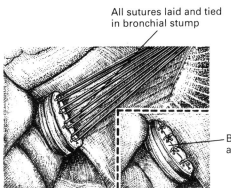

All sutures laid and tied in bronchial stump

Bronchial stump after closure

Fig. 7.23. The lobe is amputated by dividing the bronchus between the stay sutures and the crushing clamp with a scalpel, taking particular care to avoid damaging the bronchial wall, as the cartilage rings are very prone to undergo necrosis which will result in a slough of the bronchial stump and a resultant pneumothorax. The open bronchial stump is aspirated free of blood and mucus and is closed by a series of carefully placed sutures of monofilament nylon, which are all tied but are left uncut until it is certain that there is no air leak from the occluded bronchus.

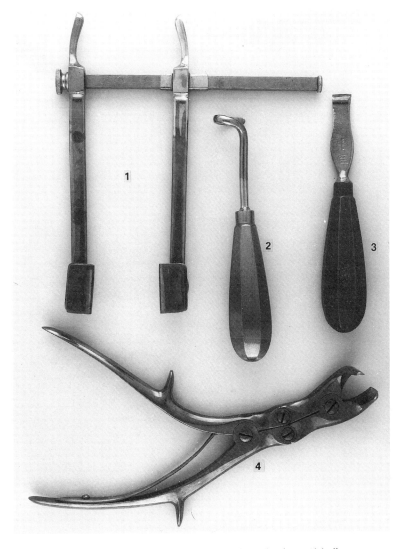

Fig. 7.24. Instruments: (1) rib retractor; (2) rib periosteal stripper; (3) rib raspatory; (4) rib-cutting shears.

Section 8
Ophthalmic Surgery

In all ophthalmic surgery a precise technique and exact suturing are essential. Some special instruments (Figs 8.36–8.43, see pp. 152–4), needles and suture materials are required and without them this branch of surgery should not be attempted. All operations to be described are best performed under general anaesthesia. Pre-operative preparation varies with each individual operation but all procedures require shaving the peri-orbital area, trimming the eyelashes, and applying a 1 per cent aqueous solution of iodine to the skin. Post operation the eye is left uncovered but to prevent self-inflicted injury the ipsilateral front foot is bandaged.

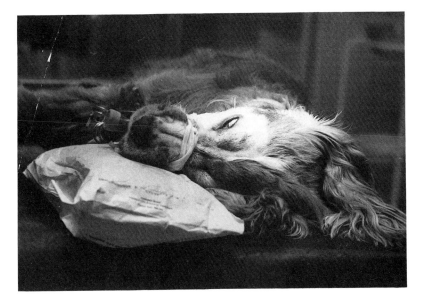

Fig. 8.1. For ophthalmic surgery the patient is positioned in lateral recumbency with a sandbag placed under the nose to keep it and the eye horizontal.

Eyelids

ENTROPION

The simplest and most satisfactory method of treating entropion in the dog is to remove an elliptical piece of skin parallel to the edge of the eyelid together with the underlying orbicularis muscle (Figs 8.2–8.4). The exact amount of skin to be removed varies with each individual and should be assessed prior to anaesthesia.

It must be realized that success in this operation will depend on the degree of out-turning of the eyelid that is achieved and this depends not only on the width of the piece of skin removed but also on the depth of tissue removed and the closeness of the first incision to the margin of the eyelid.

ECTROPION

This condition is the outward turning of the lower eyelid and is the opposite to entropion. It is corrected by shortening the lid either by removing a wedge of eyelid at the outer canthus in a manner similar to that described for removing an eyelid tumour (see Figs 8.6–8.9) or by performing a V-Y plasty (see Section 12, Fig. 12.2b) with the arms of the V embracing the extremities of the out-turning of the lid.

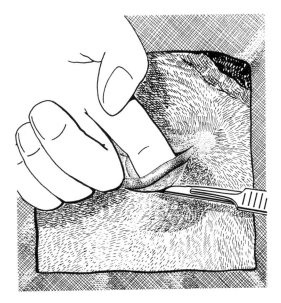

Fig. 8.2. A scalpel is used to make the first incision. Looseness of the eyelid makes this incision difficult but the tissue can be satisfactorily tensed by putting the end of a finger underneath the lid.

143

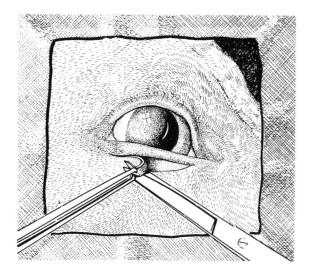

Fig. 8.3. Scissors will be found more satisfactory than a scalpel for removing the piece of skin particularly when it is of irregular shape due to an uneven in-turning of the lid.

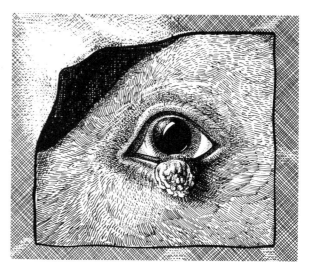

Fig. 8.5. A typical carcinoma of the eyelid which is infiltrating the deeper tissues. The most satisfactory method of removing these neoplasms is by excising a V-shaped wedge of eyelid.

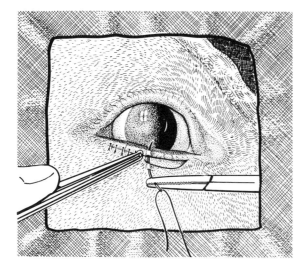

Fig. 8.4. The incision is closed with a series of interrupted sutures using 1 metric braided nylon on a small full-curved needle (Lanes's curved No. 1). The edges of the skin are just brought into apposition, the knot tied tightly and pulled away from the edge of the eyelid. If these simple measures are not practised then, due to constant movement of the eyelid, the sutures become loose and wound breakdown occurs.

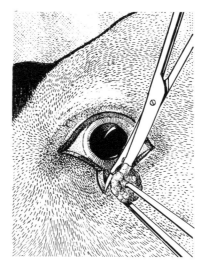

Fig. 8.6. The wedge of eyelid, in which the neoplasm is included, is removed with scissors. The two incisions are made through the whole thickness of normal eyelid and conjunctiva.

EYELID TUMOUR

Neoplasms, such as papillomas and sebaceous adenomas occurring on the margin of the eyelid are removed by simple excision, and haemorrhage is controlled by electrocautery. Neoplasms such as squamous and basal cell carcinomas which infiltrate the deeper tissues must be removed by radical excision (Figs 8.5–8.9). If only the superficial or protruding portion is removed then the growth rapidly recurs.

DISTICHIASIS

The supernumerary eyelashes are treated either by simple removal with cilia forceps or electro-epilation.

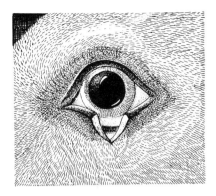

Fig. 8.7. A good deep wedge of tissue is removed from the point where the incisions meet well below the margin of the eyelid. This type of wedge resection ensures that there will be little distortion following repair.

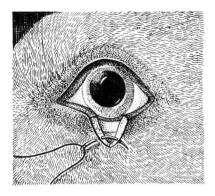

Fig. 8.8. The wound is closed by simple interrupted sutures using 1 metric braided nylon. Each suture is placed deep into the eyelid tissues but not through to the conjunctival surface.

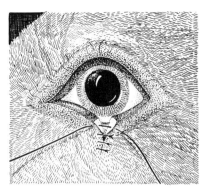

Fig. 8.9. Care must be taken to ensure that the edges of the incision, especially the palpebral margin, are brought into perfect apposition.

Nictitating membrane

REMOVAL OF THE NICTITANS GLAND (HARDERIAN GLAND)

Surgical excision of the nictitans gland is indicated in cases of prolapse or chronic inflammation of the gland (Figs 8.10–8.11). Haemorrhage is controlled either by injection of 0.1 per cent adrenaline solution into the base of the nictitating membrane or instilling a few drops topically.

NICTITATING MEMBRANE USED AS A CONJUNCTIVAL FLAP

The nictitating membrane can be used as a most satisfactory conjunctival flap to protect and support the cornea in cases of wounds and ulcers (Fig. 8.12). There is no tendency for any adhesions to form between it and the corneal lesion.

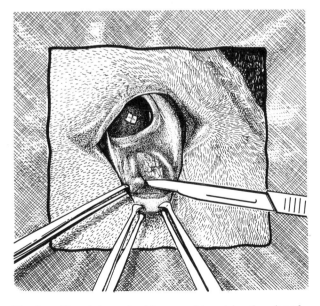

Fig. 8.10. The nictitans gland is exposed by seizing the edge of the nictitating membrane with two pairs of Allis forceps and everting it. The conjunctiva over the gland is then incised.

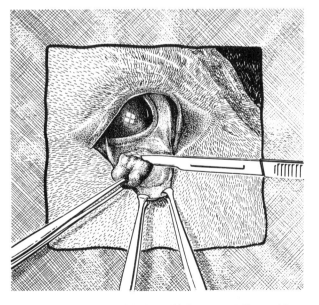

Fig. 8.11. The gland is picked up with forceps and dissected free, starting at the base of the nictitating membrane, taking care not to injure the cartilaginous plate of the nictitating membrane. After removal of the gland, the conjunctiva is just smoothed back into place. No suturing is necessary.

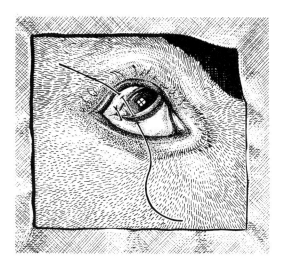

Fig. 8.12. Each suture is first passed through the fleshy ridge of tissue on the free edge of the nictitating membrane and then through a thick piece of bulbar conjunctiva by picking it up and elevating it from the globe with dissecting forceps. Three or four interrupted sutures, using 1 metric braided nylon, are required to pull the nictitating membrane across the cornea and anchor it to the bulbar conjunctiva. Sutures should be left in for about 1 week.

Cornea

PAROTID DUCT TRANSPOSITION

Transposition of the parotid duct is indicated in some instances in dogs suffering from keratoconjunctivitis sicca. Some dogs may be managed medically with the use of artificial tears or pilocarpine, but others require transposition of the parotid duct to enable the secretion of the parotid gland to replace normal tear production.

The parotid gland lies at the base of the ear and its duct runs rostrally under the superficial fascia close to the masseter muscle. It opens at a small papilla on the buccal mucosa opposite the third or fourth upper cheek tooth.

Prior to surgery, the function of the gland and the patency of its duct should be checked by placing a drop of atropine on the tongue, drying the area around the papilla and noting whether it becomes moist again.

A piece of 3 metric monofilament nylon is threaded through the papilla at the commencement of surgery to facilitate identification of the duct (Fig. 8.13). This lies midway between the dorsal and ventral branches of the facial nerve and can be mistaken for either of these structures.

The rest of the procedure is shown in Figs 8.14–8.15.

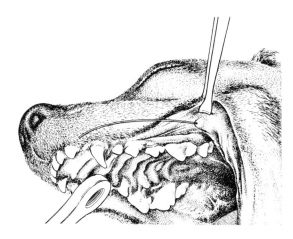

Fig. 8.13. A piece of 3 metric monofilament nylon is threaded through the papilla of the parotid duct opposite the third or fourth upper cheek tooth.

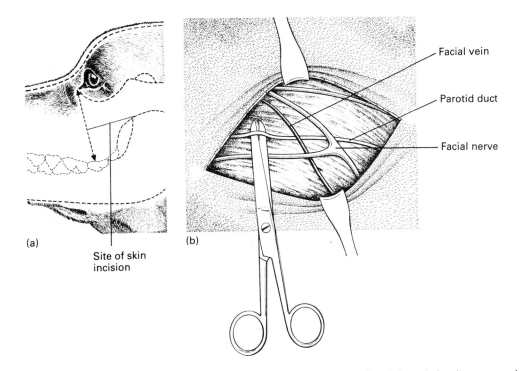

Facial vein

Parotid duct

Facial nerve

(a)

(b)

Site of skin
incision

Fig. 8.14. (a) A skin incision is made over the parotid duct and the dissection continued through the platysma muscle. (b) The duct is freed from the underlying masseter muscle by blunt dissection to the point where it enters the cheek. The dissection is completed by incising a disc of buccal mucosa, 6 or 7 mm in diameter, from around the papilla.

Fig. 8.15. A subcutaneous tunnel is made with a pair of mosquito forceps from the lateral angle of the ventral conjunctival fornix. The forceps are used to grasp the mucosal disc and to pull it through to the conjunctival sac. The disc is secured with six to eight interrupted sutures of 1 metric synthetic absorbable suture material placed around its periphery and the defect in the buccal mucosa is closed with two to three interrupted sutures of 2 metric synthetic absorbable suture material. The subcutaneous tissues are closed with a continuous suture of 3 metric synthetic absorbable suture material and the skin co-apted in the usual manner.

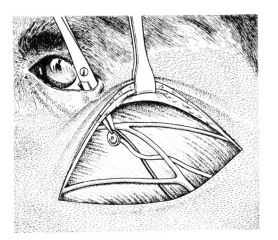

DERMOID REMOVAL

See Figs 8.16–8.19.

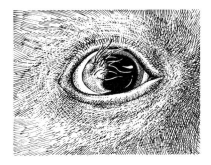

Fig. 8.16. A corneal or conjunctival dermoid is a fleshy, hairy and often pigmented congenital defect. It is usually located on the cornea adjacent to the limbus towards the outer canthus.

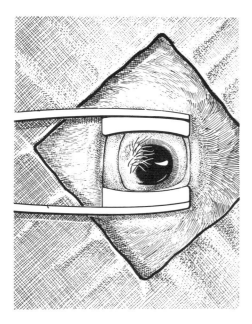

Fig. 8.17. Removal of a corneal dermoid requires a good exposure which is obtained by inserting an eye speculum.

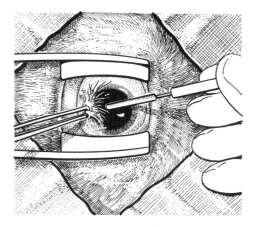

Fig. 8.18. The dermoid is held with dissecting forceps and, starting at the corneal edge, dissected off the cornea back towards the limbus with a Tooke's knife.

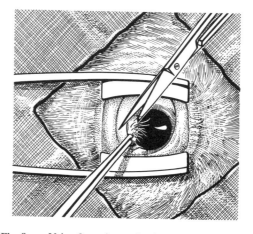

Fig. 8.19. Using fine scissors the dermoid is removed by severing its connection with the conjunctiva just behind the limbus.

Intraocular surgery

A major factor in intraocular surgery is the method by which the eye is entered and repaired. Incising the cornea is a quick and bloodless method but healing is slow and leaves a scar. Entry via a limbal-based conjunctival flap and scleral incision is the method preferred and although it is more complicated, and haemorrhage has to be controlled, healing is satisfactory and no post-operative scar persists.

Extraction of the cataractous lens is made easier when the pupil is dilated and this is obtained by installing 1 per cent atropine into the eye for 2 or 3 days before surgery.

LENS EXTRACTION

Stage I: Opening the eye

See Figs 8.20–8.24.

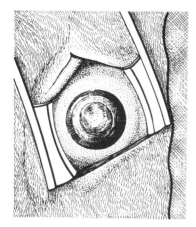

Fig. 8.20. An eye speculum is inserted and a lateral canthotomy performed using straight scissors.

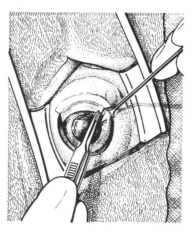

Fig. 8.23. The puncture is made anterior to the iris which is extremely vascular and great care must be taken to ensure that it is not damaged.

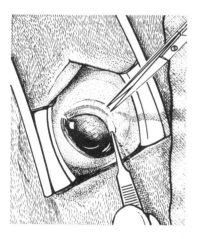

Fig. 8.21. The bulbar conjunctiva is incised, about 4 mm behind the limbus, and then using small sharp pointed scissors is dissected from the underlying sclera to form a conjunctival flap, which is reflected onto the cornea.

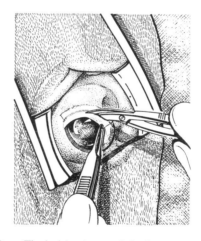

Fig. 8.24. The incision is extended using corneal spring scissors. Care must be taken that the blade of the scissors in the anterior chamber is in front of the iris before each cut is made otherwise there is a grave danger of damage to the iris with considerable haemorrhage.

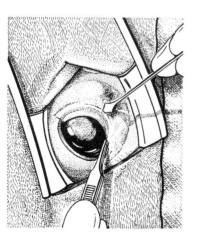

Fig. 8.22. The anterior chamber is entered by puncturing the sclera with a paracentesis needle inserted just behind the limbus.

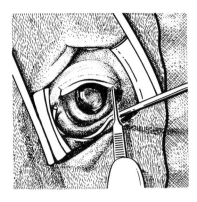

Fig. 8.25. The lens is removed by applying gentle pressure at the inferior limbus using an expressor hook. The luxated lens has a posterior attachment to the vitreous which must be cut with scissors prior to removal to prevent vitreous loss.

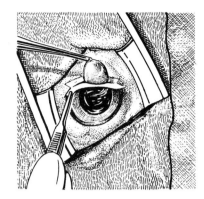

Fig. 8.26. Immediately the lens protrudes through the incision in the sclera it is picked up with fine fixation forceps and extracted.

Stage II: Removing the dislocated lens

For removing a cataractous lens extracapsular extraction is recommended (Figs 8.25–8.26). By this method the zonule and posterior capsule are preserved intact thus preventing the loss of any vitreous. A large circular piece of the anterior capsule is torn away following its rupture with a cystitome and the contents of the lens removed as for a subluxated lens. When the lens substance is soft it is removed with a vectis.

Stage III: Repairing the scleral incision

See Fig. 8.27.

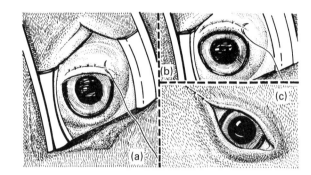

Fig. 8.27. (a) The scleral incision is closed with a series of interrupted sutures using Barraquer virgin silk on a Jameson Evan's 8-mm corneal needle. (b) The conjunctival flap is repositioned covering the sutures in the sclera and sutured to the bulbar conjunctiva with a few interrupted sutures as for the scleral incision. (c) The canthotomy is repaired with interrupted sutures using 1 metric braided nylon.

Surgery of eye trauma

WOUNDS OF THE CORNEA

Lacerations of the cornea with collapse of the anterior chamber require suturing (Fig. 8.28).

The anterior chamber is cleared of all blood clot and foreign material by irrigation with a solution of sterile normal saline. The edges of the cornea are approximated with interrupted sutures using plain collagen 1 metric material with an 8-mm spatulated 1/4 circle needle attached. The sutures must not penetrate the thickness of the cornea. To ensure accurate approximation of the edges any protruding iris is repositioned or excised if infected. To prevent buckling of the cornea care must be taken to place the sutures at right angles to the edges and just far enough apart and tied with just sufficient tension to prevent the escape of aqueous humour.

Reformation of the anterior chamber is rapidly established following suturing but some surgeons practice injecting normal saline solution or an air bubble to ascertain that the suture line is leak proof and to prevent the development of anterior synechia.

Post operation it is necessary to instil atropine solution daily and an antibiotic 4-hourly. The sutures are removed after about 10 days.

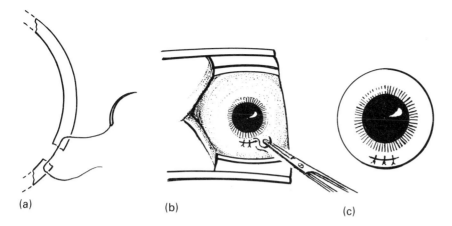

Fig. 8.28. Repair of wounds of the cornea. (a) Sutures must not penetrate the thickness of the cornea. (b) Edges approximated using interrupted sutures of plain collagen 1 metric with 8-mm spatulated needle attached. (c) Completed suturing.

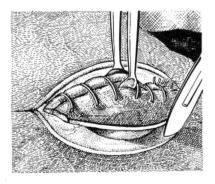

Fig. 8.29. The eyelids are sutured together with a continuous suture of fine braided nylon.

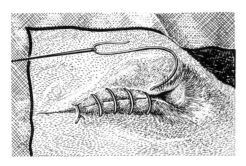

Fig. 8.30. An elliptical incision is made around the margins of the eyelids through the skin and eyelid muscle down to the palpebral conjunctiva.

ENUCLEATION OF THE EYEBALL

Enucleation is indicated in cases of gross injury, panophthalmitis, irreducible prolapse and neoplasia. The operation comprises removing the eyeball together with the bulbar and palpebral conjunctiva and the nictitating membrane (Figs 8.29–8.35).

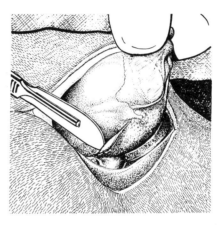

Fig. 8.31. With continual traction on the eyeball and taking care not to incise the conjunctiva the retrobulbar tissues are dissected free and the extraocular muscles are severed as close to the globe as possible. This is continued until the retractor oculi muscle is exposed.

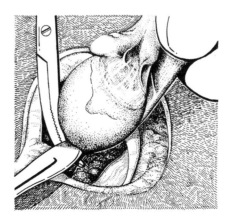

Fig. 8.32. The retractor oculi muscle and the enclosed artery, vein and nerve are clamped with either curved artery or gall bladder forceps. The eye is then removed by severing the tissues above the forceps.

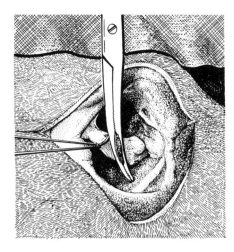

Fig. 8.33. Haemorrhage from the artery and vein is controlled by placing a suture, using 3 metric synthetic absorbable suture material, below the forceps.

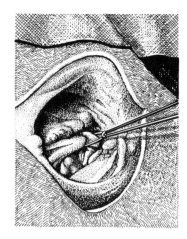

Fig. 8.34. To occlude the dead space in the orbit the retrobulbar tissues and extraocular muscles are drawn together with a few 3 metric synthetic absorbable sutures. This procedure controls haemorrhage and obviates the necessity for packing the cavity.

In the dog this elliptical incision can be made remote from the edge of the eyelids but in the horse the skin is closely adherent to the underlying bone and unless the incision is made close to the eyelid margins it will be difficult to co-apt the skin edges at the end of the operation.

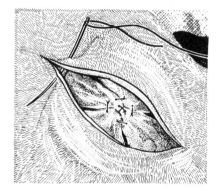

Fig. 8.35. The skin incision is closed with interrupted sutures of monofilament nylon, and protected by oversewing a gauze pad.

Ophthalmic instruments

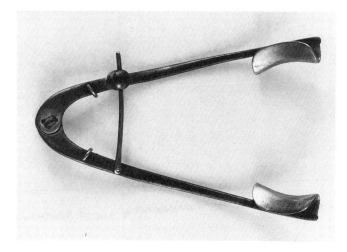

Fig. 8.36. An eye speculum.

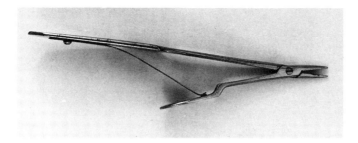

Fig. 8.37. A needle holder.

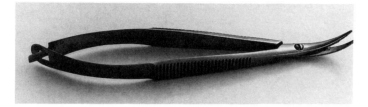

Fig. 8.38. Corneal scissors.

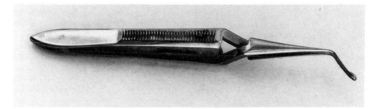

Fig. 8.39. Intracapsular forceps.

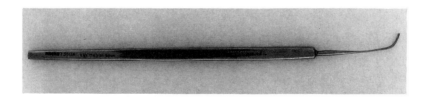

Fig. 8.40. An iris repositor.

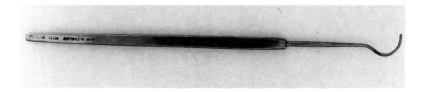

Fig. 8.41. A lens expressor.

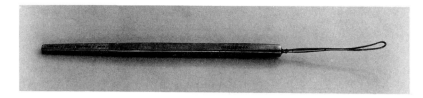

Fig. 8.42. A vectis.

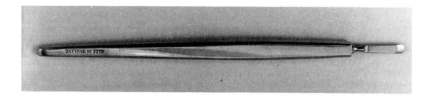

Fig. 8.43. Tooke's knife.

Section 9
Neurosurgery

Nerve suture

Tissues without motor function or sensation are a serious disability and therefore all severed nerves must be repaired by primary suture, even when infection is present (Fig. 9.1).

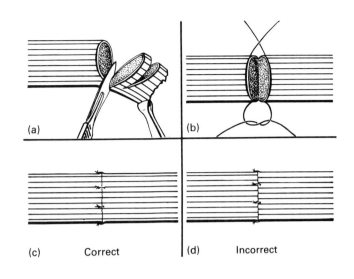

Fig. 9.1. (a) Identify the nerve and remove the cut end, with a sharp scalpel, through normal tissue. (b) Co-apt the neurolemma with a series of interrupted sutures, using 1 metric blood-vessel silk on an atraumatic needle. (c) Correct alignment of the nerve ends. (d) Incorrect alignment of the nerve ends due to axial rotation. This can be reduced by matching the blood vessels in the neurolemma.

Neurectomy — horse

Neurectomy is the excision of a portion of a nerve, and is employed in the horse to treat incurable lameness. Cutting the sensory nerve supply from a painful pathological lesion alleviates pain and enables the horse's working life to be prolonged for a limited period.

Neurectomies can be performed under local analgesia, but it is recommended that these operations should be performed with the horse recumbent and under general anaesthesia.

PALMAR NEURECTOMY

Neurectomy of the medial and lateral palmar nerves deprives all structures below the fetlock of sensation. Midway between the knee and fetlock joint the medial palmar nerve gives off a communicating branch which passes obliquely down over the flexor tendons to join the lateral palmar nerve just above the distal extremity of the fourth metacarpal bone. When performing a neurectomy of the lateral palmar nerve care must be taken to sever it distal to its junction with this communicating branch from the medial palmar nerve. At the fetlock the medial and lateral palmar nerves are called the medial and lateral digital nerves and each divides into two branches, the dorsal branch and the palmar branch of the digital nerves.

With the fetlock joint in extension a skin incision 4 cm long is made along the dorsal edge of the deep digital flexor tendon, extending from just below the level of the distal extremity of the small

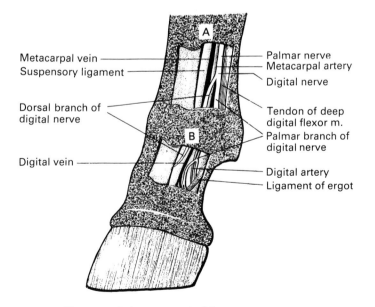

Metacarpal vein
Suspensory ligament
Dorsal branch of digital nerve
Digital vein

Palmar nerve
Metacarpal artery
Digital nerve
Tendon of deep digital flexor m.
Palmar branch of digital nerve
Digital artery
Ligament of ergot

Fig. 9.2. The anatomical arrangement of the nerves, blood vessels, tendons and ligaments of the distal leg of the horse. Site A is used for palmar neurectomy and site B for digital neurectomy.

metacarpal bone to a point level with the apex of the sesamoid bone. A common mistake is to make the incision dorsal to the tendon, i.e. in the depression between the tendon and the suspensory ligament. The deep fascia is incised the length of the incision and the edges separated, when the nerve should be distinctly seen (Fig. 9.3). If not seen the nerve can be brought into view by applying digital pressure to the tendon of the deep digital flexor muscle on the opposite side of the leg.

The skin and fascia are closed together with interrupted sutures, using monofilament nylon. The horse is turned over and palmar neurectomy performed on the opposite side.

DIGITAL NEURECTOMY

Neurectomy of the palmar branch of the medial and lateral digital nerve desensitizes the caudal portion of the foot. The nerve lies immediately palmar to the medial/lateral digital artery and the depression between the deep digital flexor tendon and the palmar border of the first phalanx.

With the fetlock joint in extension draw a finger up the depression between the deep digital flexor tendon and the palmar border of the first phalanx until the base of the sesamoid bone is palpated. From this point make an oblique skin incision 4 cm long directed distally to cross this depression.

Incise the fascia the length of the incision, separate the edges by dissection and isolate the nerve which will be found lying parallel and immediately palmar to the digital artery. The nerve is recognized and neurectomy performed in the manner as described for high palmar neurectomy.

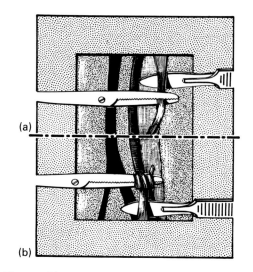

Fig. 9.3. (a) The nerve is identified by its longitudinal striation and dissected free from the surrounding structures. It is then clamped with artery forceps at the proximal extremity of the incision, retracted distally and severed transversely with a scalpel. (b) The distal extremity of the nerve is then twisted up on the artery forceps, retracted proximally and severed in like manner, ensuring that at least 4 cm of nerve are removed.

Near the middle of the first phalanx the nerve is crossed obliquely by the ligament of the ergot, which in appearance is similar to the nerve. It will be seen if the incision is placed too low, but can be differentiated from the nerve because it is more superficially placed, broader, flatter and inelastic, and when clamped with artery forceps does not provoke a reflex movement of the limb.

· ·

Cervical spine

FENESTRATION OF A CERVICAL INTERVERTEBRAL DISC — DOG

This operation consists of making a small hole in the anulus fibrosus which permits the escape of the nucleus pulposus, or enables it to be scooped out (Figs 9.4–9.9). It does not provide access to the spinal cord itself, therefore it is not possible to remove extruded disc material from the vertebral canal. Accordingly, fenestration is not an appropriate procedure for dogs with significant neurological defects, but it may be used where pain is the only clinical sign associated with a prolapsed intervertebral disc.

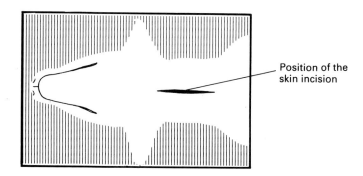

Position of the skin incision

Fig. 9.4. The dog is placed in dorsal recumbency with its head and neck extended. Exposure is improved by placing a sandbag under the neck.

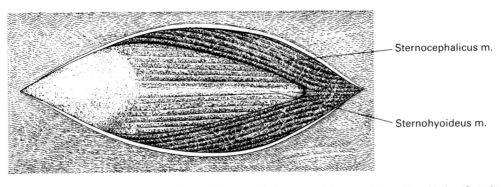

Fig. 9.5. A longitudinal midline skin incision is made between the larynx and the manubrium. The skin is reflected to expose the underlying sternocephalicus and sternohyoideus muscles.

Sternocephalicus m.

Sternohyoideus m.

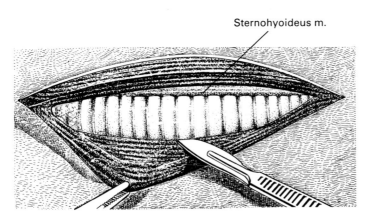

Sternohyoideus m.

Fig. 9.6. The sternohyoideus muscle is incised the length of the skin incision and retracted to expose the trachea.

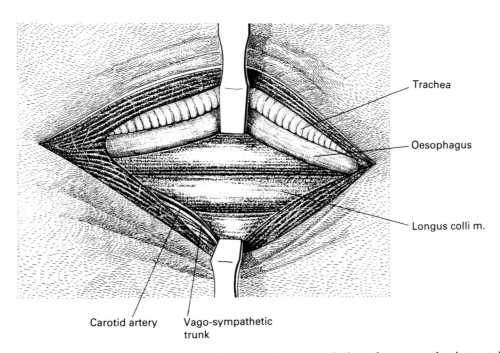

Trachea

Oesophagus

Longus colli m.

Carotid artery   Vago-sympathetic trunk

Fig. 9.7. By blunt dissection the oesophagus, carotid artery and vago-sympathetic trunk are exposed and retracted to reveal the underlying longus colli muscle.

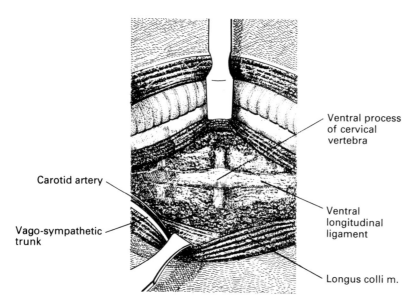

Carotid artery

Vago-sympathetic trunk

Ventral process of cervical vertebra

Ventral longitudinal ligament

Longus colli m.

Fig. 9.8. The longus colli muscle is divided longitudinally, and retracted to expose the ventral longitudinal ligament of the cervical vertebrae. This enables the ventral processes of the cervical vertebrae to be palpated and allows the exact position of any intervertebral disc to be accurately located.

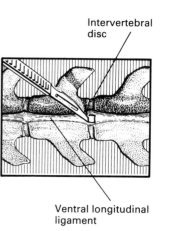

Intervertebral disc

Ventral longitudinal ligament

Fig. 9.9. Fenestration is performed by cutting a hole in the ventral longitudinal ligament and the underlying anulus fibrosus with a sharp pointed scalpel (blade No. 11). The nucleus pulposus either escapes or can be scooped out.

If the nucleus pulposus is completely removed then no further protrusions of the fenestrated disc can occur, but after operation it is not uncommon for a protrusion to develop in the adjacent discs, and therefore it is customary to fenestrate them at the same time as a preventive measure, although they may appear to be quite normal.

The operation is completed by co-apting the longus colli muscle with a synthetic absorbable suture in a simple continuous pattern. The structures of the neck are returned to their normal position and the sternohyoideus and sternocephalicus muscles are sutured separately using a similar suture pattern and material. Subcutaneous dead space is occluded by a subcuticular suture and the skin closed with a continuous suture.

DECOMPRESSION OF THE CERVICAL SPINAL CORD BY A VENTRAL SLOT — DOG

This operation involves cutting a slot in the bodies of two adjacent cervical vertebrae and their associated intervertebral disc. This enables any prolapsed disc material to be retrieved from the vertebral

canal, thereby relieving pressure on the spinal cord.

The surgical approach is similar to that described for a cervical fenestration. Following division and retraction of the longus colli muscle, the relevant intervertebral disc is identified and fenestrated. Bone is then removed from either side of the disc, using a high speed mechanical burr, to create a slot in the midline of the vertebral bodies (Fig. 9.10). The slot is carefully deepened until the spinal cord is exposed. The width of the slot should not exceed one-third of the width of the vertebra. Too wide a slot results in penetration of the vertebral sinuses and severe haemorrhage. The length of the slot should be approximately one-third the length of each vertebral body, although due to the angle of the intervertebral disc the length of the slot in the rostral vertebra should exceed that of the caudal vertebra (Fig. 9.11).

Haemorrhage may either arise from the vertebral sinuses or from the cancellous bone. The former should be controlled by packing the slot with haemostatic gelatin sponge; the latter may be controlled with bone wax.

The closure of the tissues is similar to that described for cervical fenestration.

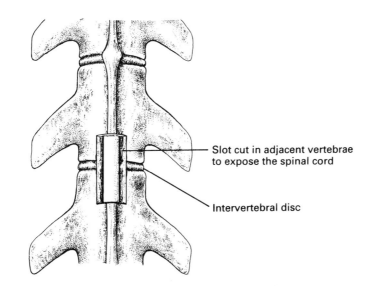

Fig. 9.10. To remove disc material from the cervical vertebral canal it is necessary to perform a ventral slot. The slot is cut with a mechanical burr through the outer cortical bone of the vertebrae and continued through the soft cancellous bone of their bodies. When the inner cortical bone layer is reached, extreme caution is required. The decompression is completed by carefully removing the periosteum of the inner cortical bone and the underlying dorsal longitudinal ligament from the floor of the vertebral canal with a scalpel.

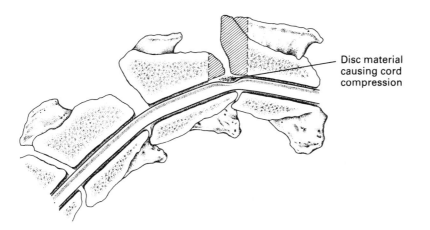

Fig. 9.11. The dog's head is to the left. Due to the slope of the intervertebral disc spaces more bone is removed from the rostral vertebra than the caudal one. The extruded materal may be removed with a small curette or dental scraper.

STABILIZATION OF THE CERVICAL VERTEBRAE — DOG

Instability of the cervical vertebrae, or spondylolithesis, is one cause of the 'Wobbler syndrome'. The fifth, six and seventh vertebrae are generally involved, although the site of compression must be confirmed by myelography. The dynamic compression produced by the abnormal cranial tilting of any or all of these vertebrae results in hindlimb proprioceptive defects. More severe compression may result in forelimb hypermetria, quadriparesis or even quadriplegia.

The condition is treated by arthrodesis of the affected intervertebral joints. The intervertebral disc spaces are fenestrated, the adjacent vertebral endplates are curetted and the vertebrae stabilized by screwing them together (Fig. 9.12). To encourage early arthrodesis, the disc spaces are packed with cancellous bone taken from a suitable site (the proximal humerus is readily accessible and usually used).

The vertebrae are stabilized with 3.5-mm cortical or 4.0-mm cancellous screws. The length of screw is determined by measurements taken from a pre-operative radiograph of the lateral cervical spine.

DISTRACTION-FUSION OF THE CERVICAL VERTEBRAE - DOG

In the older dog, spondylolisthesis may be complicated by disc disease secondary to vertebral instability. In some of these cases it is necessary to decompress the spinal cord by performing a ventral slot (see Figs 9.10 and 9.11).

In other cases, where myelography indicates cord compression can be relieved by traction on the cervical spine, a distraction-fusion technique is indicated. Following a ventral approach the affected disc space is fenestrated and anulus removed from the vertebral end plates. The vertebrae are distracted and held apart with a metal washer (Fig. 9.13), held in place with a screw placed through the adjacent vertebral bodies. The remainder of the disc space is packed with autogenous cancellous bone to promote fusion of the joint.

The washer frequently causes collapse of the adjacent vertebral end plates. If this occurs slowly, it is often of little clinical consequence. However, early collapse frequently results in a marked deterioration in the dog's neurological status.

ATLANTO-AXIAL SUBLUXATION - DOG

Atlanto-axial subluxation is occasionally seen in toy breeds of dogs and is characterized by compression of the cervical spinal cord. Dogs generally have pain and motor dysfunction ranging from fore- or hindlimb paresis to quadriplegia.

The luxation can be reduced and the vertebrae stabilized with a heavy suture of non-absorbable monofilament material passed under the dorsal arch of the atlas and through holes drilled through the dorsal spine of the atlas (Fig. 9.14). Care should be taken not to flex the neck too much during surgery since this may provoke respiratory arrest.

As an alternative to dorsal stabilization, it is possible to stabilize the vertebrae ventrally by placing two screws, one either side of the midline, across the atlanto-axial articulation. This is technically more demanding, but if arthrodesis can be achieved, long-term stability is improved.

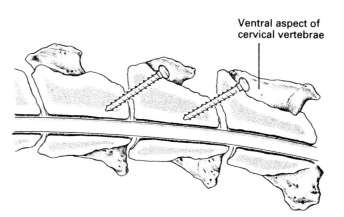

Ventral aspect of cervical vertebrae

Fig. 9.12. Stabilization of the cervical vertebrae with screws through their vertebral bodies. The intervening disc spaces are fenestrated and packed with cancellous bone to encourage arthrodesis.

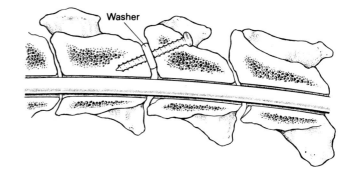

Washer

Fig. 9.13. Distraction-fusion of the cervical spine.

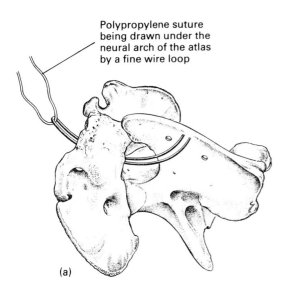

Polypropylene suture being drawn under the neural arch of the atlas by a fine wire loop

(a)

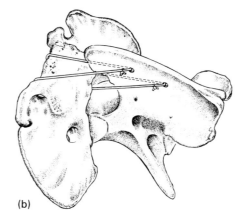

(b)

Fig. 9.14. Dorsal stabilization of an atlanto-axial subluxation. After the loop of suture material has been drawn under the neural arch of the atlas (a), it is cut and the ends threaded through holes drilled in the axis. The suture is knotted as in (b).

Thoracolumbar spine

HEMILAMINECTOMY OF THE THORACOLUMBAR VERTEBRAE – DOG

This operation (Figs 9.15–9.20) consists of removing the articular facets of two adjacent vertebrae, together with a portion of their ipsilateral wall, to expose the spinal cord. This decompresses the spinal cord and enables any extruded disc material to be removed from the vertebral canal.

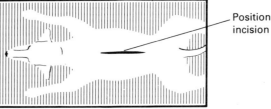

Position of skin incision

Fig. 9.15. The dog is placed in sternal recumbency with a sandbag under its abdomen to obtain a degree of kyphosis. To permit sufficient muscle retraction the dorsal midline skin incision must extend at least two vertebrae cranial and caudal to the intervertebral disc to be exposed.

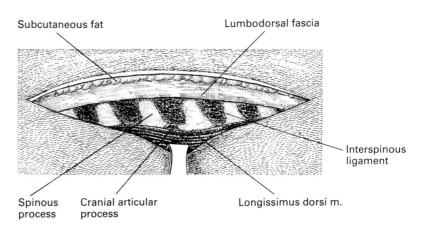

Subcutaneous fat | Lumbodorsal fascia

Interspinous ligament

Spinous process | Cranial articular process | Longissimus dorsi m.

Fig. 9.16. The subcutaneous fat is incised and dissected free from the underlying lumbodorsal fascia, which is incised the length of the skin incision. The supraspinous ligament is incised around and between the apices of the spinous processes and the longissimus dorsi muscle is separated from them by blunt dissection.

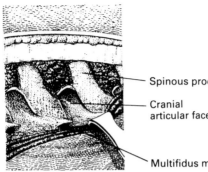

Spinous process

Cranial articular facet

Multifidus m.

Fig. 9.17. The cranial articular facets are exposed by dissecting them free of and retracting the multifidus muscle.

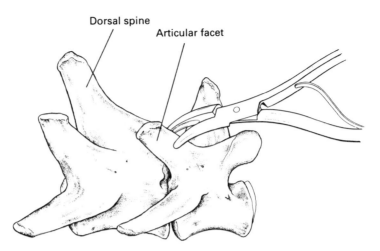

Dorsal spine

Articular facet

Fig. 9.18. Hemilaminectomy is performed by cutting off the articular facets with bone ronguers.

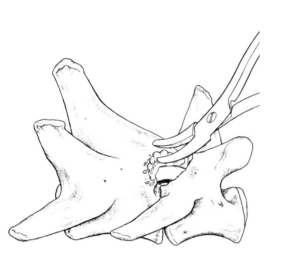

Fig. 9.19. The base of the articular facets is removed and the intervertebral foramen is enlarged with ronguers. The foramen can be opened a little by lifting the caudal vertebrae with a towel clip attached to its dorsal spine.

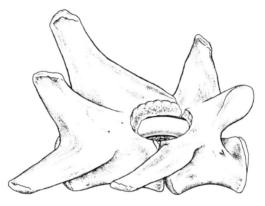

Fig. 9.20. Completion of the hemilaminectomy. The epidural fat is carefully removed, the underlying spinal cord is carefully elevated and any extruded disc material is removed. The disc may be fenestrated if considered necessary.

Tibial neurectomy — calves

Spastic paresis is a progressive condition characterized by contraction of the gastrocnemius and related tendons and muscle bellies leading to severe overextension of the hock.

Tibial neurectomy is carried out under general anaesthesia. The site of the 15–20-cm incision is on the lateral aspect of the thigh in the groove between the two heads of the biceps femoris muscle (Fig. 9.21a). This can be seen clearly in the standing animal but is much less obvious in the recumbent patient. The incision is made so that its distal one-

third overlies the lateral head of the gastrocnemius muscle.

After incising the skin and underlying gluteal fascia, the groove in the biceps femoris is identified and the heads (Fig. 9.21b) are exposed by blunt dissection and separated with a wound retractor. The peroneal nerve which is approximately 8 mm wide can be seen on the lateral surface of the lateral head of the gastronemius muscle. The tibial nerve lies in the adipose tissue associated with the popliteal lymph node. Careful blunt dissection will enable the nerve to be located without damaging the blood vessels in this area. The nerve, which is as broad as the peroneal nerve, will be seen passing between the medial and lateral heads of the gastrocnemius muscle. Its identity can be confirmed by observing a sharp contraction of the muscle when gentle pressure is applied to the nerve with a pair of haemostats.

A 3-cm segment of the nerve is removed (Fig. 9.21c). The incisions in the biceps femoris and gluteal fascia are closed with interrupted and continuous sutures, respectively, and the skin with interrupted sutures. Limited exercise is encouraged for the first few weeks after surgery.

The operation is usually free from complications in animals of relatively low weight but rupture of the gastrocnemius can occur 1–5 days postoperatively in heavy cattle. In these larger animals partial neurectomy is advocated in which only the bundles of the tibial nerve which supply the gastrocnemius muscle (identified by electric stimulation) are cut.

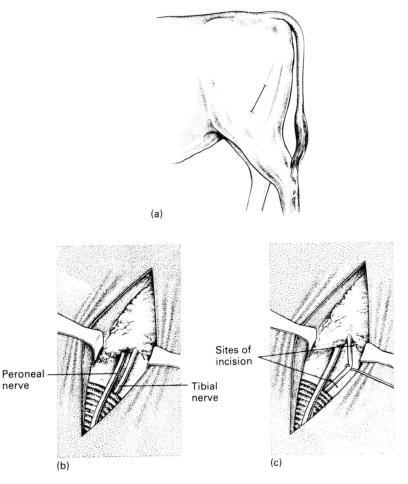

Fig. 9.21. Site of tibial neurectomy (for details see text).

Section 10
Orthopaedic Surgery

Arthrotomy and the internal fixation of fractures have become safe and established practices due to the control of infection by antibiotics and a better understanding of the reaction of tissue to the metals implanted. However, it must still be remembered that operations involving bone and joints require a more precise aseptic technique than similar operations upon soft tissues. The use of inert metals and antibiotics in no way reduces the necessity for sound surgical techniques but rather provides an additional safeguard and a means of supplementing the natural resistance of the patient.

It is the authors' practice in all operations below the elbow and stifle joints in the horse and in selected cases in the dog to obtain a bloodless field by forcing the blood from the limb with a rubber bandage and then applying a tourniquet. At the completion of the operation rather than releasing the tourniquet and ligating the bleeding vessels, a pressure pad and bandage are applied before the tourniquet is removed. The pressure bandage is left on for 24–48 hours.

In order to minimize such complications as muscle atrophy, joint stiffness and disuse osteoporosis following fracture repair, it is important to achieve early weight bearing on the injured limb. This requires accurate reduction and rigid internal fixation of the fractured bones.

To achieve an early return to function of an injured limb following a fracture, the Association for the Study of Internal Fixation (ASIF) advocates rigid internal fixation using compression and has designed bone screws and plates for this purpose. Compression, *per se*, does not stimulate osteogenesis, but by eliminating micromovement, callus formation is reduced to a minimum and healing occurs by creeping substitution. This is called primary bone union.

The ASIF system permits repair of a much wider range of fractures than was previously possible, due in part to an improved understanding of the biomechanics of fracture repair and in part to a greater variety of specially designed implants.

A number of techniques have been devised to create compression at a fracture site and the reader is encouraged to consult G.E. Fackelman and D.M. Nunamaker (1982) *Manual of Internal Fixation in the Horse* and W.O. Brinker *et al.* (1984) *Manual of Internal Fixation in Small Animals* for further details (see Bibliography). Some of these techniques can be applied using 'conventional' implants, such as interfragmentary compression using a lag screw and the application of a tension band wire.

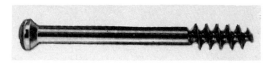

Fig. 10.1. 6.5-mm cancellous bone screw. Diameter of thread 6.5 mm; diameter of core 3.2 mm; diameter of shaft 4.5 mm.

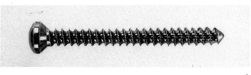

Fig. 10.2. Cortical screw. Diameter of thread 4.5 mm; diameter of core 3.2 mm.

ASIF screws are available in two types: cortical screws for use in cortical bone and cancellous screws for use in the less dense cancellous bone (Figs 10.1–10.2). The cancellous screw has a deeper, more open thread which is designed to have better purchase in the softer trabecular bone of the metaphyses and epiphyses. Both types of screw have a rounded end and therefore a thread has to be cut with a bone tap before they are inserted. The advantage of pre-cutting the thread is that the full depth of the threads of the screw grip the bone. In contrast, self-tapping screws impact bone chips as they are driven into the bone and only the tips of their threads provide purchase on the bone. They are, therefore, more likely to pull out.

When using cortical screws, the size of the bone tap corresponds to the outside diameter of the screw. These are available with diameters of 5.5, 4.5, 3.5, 2.7, 2.0, or 1.5 mm. The corresponding drill bit sizes are 4.0, 3.2, 2.5, 2.0, 1.5 and 1.1 mm respectively.

Cancellous screws may be fully threaded or partially threaded. They are available as 3.5, 4.0 and 6.5-mm diameter screws. The drill bit size for the threaded hole corresponds to the core diameter of the screw and is 2.0 mm for the 3.5-mm screw, 2.5 mm for the 4.0-mm and 3.2 mm for the 6.5-mm screw.

A partially threaded cancellous screw may be used as a lag screw provided the non-threaded shaft crosses the fracture line. These screws are recommended for fractures of trabecular bone.

INTERFRAGMENTARY COMPRESSION USING LAG SCREWS

The principle of the lag screw is that the threads only bite in the distal fragment so that the fragments are pulled together. This effect can be achieved by using a partially threaded cancellous screw or a fully threaded cortical screw where the proximal fragment is overdrilled. In each case static interfragmentary compression is produced.

Using a cancellous bone screw

See Fig. 10.3.

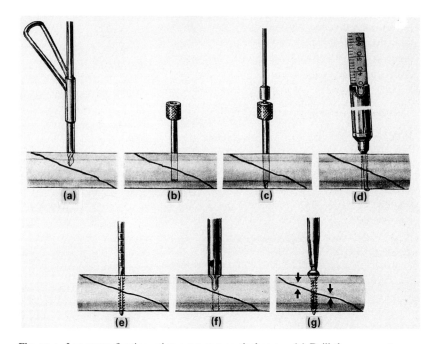

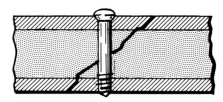

Fig. 10.3. The lag effect obtained with a partially threaded cancellous bone screw. Note that the shaft crosses the fracture line and only the thread takes hold in the far fragment.

Using a cortical screw

This screw has a full length thread and will act as a lag screw provided it can obtain a hold in the far cortex. This requires a larger hole to be drilled in the near cortex than the far cortex, which has to be tapped. The large hole is called the 'gliding hole' and the small hole the 'pilot hole'.

The gliding hole must be the same diameter as the outside diameter of the screw and the pilot hole is tapped with a bone tap of equal size (Fig. 10.4).

A single cortical screw inserted at right angles to the axis of the long bone prevents the fragments moving under *axial* compression (Fig. 10.5). To create maximum *interfragmentary* compression, the screw should be placed at right angles to the fracture. In practice, the screw is often inserted along the line that bisects these two angles.

INTERFRAGMENTARY COMPRESSION USING THE TENSION BAND PRINCIPLE

Tensile forces acting at a fracture site can be counteracted and converted into compressive

Fig. 10.4. Lag screw fixation using a 4.5-mm cortical screw. (a) Drill the near cortex with a 4.5-mm drill using a 4.5-mm tap sleeve. (b) Insert a drill sleeve, with an external diameter of 4.5 mm and an internal diameter of 3.2 mm, into the hole until it meets the opposite cortex. (c) The far cortex is drilled using a 3.2-mm drill bit. (d) The length of screw required is measured with a depth gauge. (e) The far cortex is tapped out using a 4.5-mm cortical tap. (f) A countersink is cut in the near cortex for the head of the screw. (g) Drive in a cortical screw.

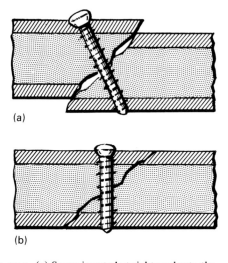

Fig. 10.5. (a) Screw inserted at right angles to the fracture line. Under axial compression, movement may occur. (b) Screw inserted at right angles to the axis of the long bone. Under axial compression there is greater resistance to movement.

forces by using the tension band principle. This type of compression is termed dynamic compression since it relies upon muscular forces to create the compressive effect. A tension band may either be a bone plate (Fig. 10.6) or a figure-of-eight wire. In both cases they must be applied to the tensile side of the bone.

AXIAL COMPRESSION USING A BONE PLATE

A plate with round holes can be used as a compression plate by employing a tension device (Fig. 10.7). This round hole plate has now been largely superceded by the dynamic compression plate which has oval holes. By inserting the screw at one end of the oval hole, i.e. eccentrically, the plate is placed under tension as the conical head of the screw engages the plate (Fig. 10.8). This obviates the need for the tension device.

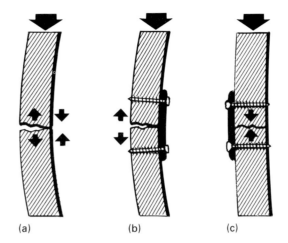

(a)　　　　　(b)　　　　　(c)

Fig. 10.6. The principle of a tension band plate. (a) Transverse fracture of a long bone under axial compression. Note the effect of the tension forces on the convex side. (b) A plate applied to the concave side does not overcome the tension as the plate is under bending stresses, this results in metal fatigue and the plate breaking. (c) A plate applied to the convex side counteracts all tension forces and provides rigid internal fixation.

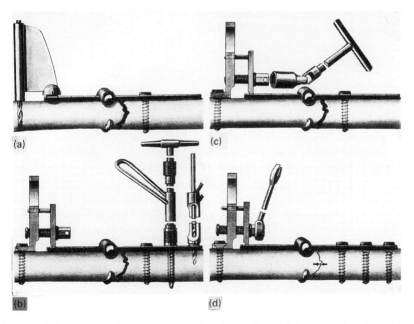

Fig. 10.7. Using the tension device and a 4.5-mm round hole bone plate. (a) A 3.2-mm hole is drilled 1 cm from the fracture line. The 4.5-mm thread is tapped, the fracture reduced, a bone plate applied and held in position with a 4.5-mm screw. While retaining the reduction with the bone-holding forceps a hole is drilled 18 mm from the end of the plate using the special drill sleeve, a 3.2-mm drill bit and the 4.5-mm thread tapped out.

(b) The hook of the tension device is inserted and engaged in the horizontal slot in the end hole of the plate and the tension device fixed to the bone with a 4.5-mm screw. The nut on the tension device is now tightened until a satisfactory reduction is attained.

(c) The remaining screws are driven into the first fragment using the drill guide, a 3.2-mm drill bit and tapping the 4.5-mm thread.

(d) The tension device is now tightened, using an open-ended wrench, until full compression and rigid fixation is attained. The reduction is checked and the remaining screws inserted. Finally the tension device is removed and the last 4.5-mm screw inserted in the hole of the plate occupied by the screw fixing the tension device.

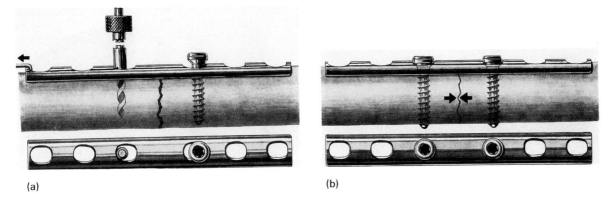

(a)   (b)

Fig. 10.8. Using a 4.5-mm dynamic compression plate. (a) A 3.2-mm hole is drilled 1 cm from the fracture line. The 4.5-mm thread is tapped, the plate applied and the first cortical screw driven until its head just touches the plate. The fracture is reduced and an assistant pulls on the plate with a hook to engage the oval hole firmly against the screw. The second hole is now drilled eccentrically on the opposite side of the fracture and the thread tapped.

(b) The second screw is now driven and tightened, followed by tightening the first screw. Because the screws are placed eccentrically, tightening will press the conical head of the screw down against the edge of the oval hole thus forcing the fragments together and compressing them. The remaining screws are inserted in the centre of each oval hole.

Thoracic limb — horse

Elbow

FRACTURE OF THE OLECRANON

In most fractures of the olecranon the attachment of the triceps brachii to the summit of the bone causes separation of the fragments.

These fractures should be treated by open reduction and fixation using a tension-band plate applied to the caudal aspect of the bone (Fig. 10.9).

Surgery is performed with the horse in lateral recumbency with the affected leg uppermost. The fracture is approached by a curved skin incision over the caudo-lateral aspect of the point of the elbow and extending to the lower third of the ulna. The common digital extensor and the ulnaris lateralis muscles are separated by blunt dissection to expose the fracture site.

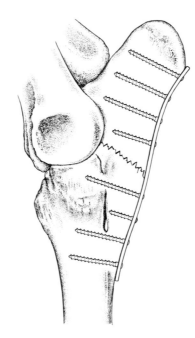

Fig. 10.9. Fracture of the ulna repaired with a 3.5-mm dynamic compression plate applied as a tension-band plate.

Carpus

ANGULAR DEFORMITIES OF THE CARPUS — FOAL

Angular limb deformities resulting from unequal physeal growth are quite common in foals. The most frequent location is the carpal joint where valgus deformity — outward deviation of the distal limb — predominates. Varus deformity, in which the distal limb is deviated towards the midline, is much less common as are fetlock varus and tarsal valgus deformities.

Conservative therapy is successful in correcting most of the angular deformities. This should include trimming the hooves to remove the fulcrum effect caused by a long toe and reduction of con-cussive forces by confining the foal to a large pen. If very definite improvement is not apparent within 4–6 weeks, surgery is advisable. This may be directed at retarding maturation and calcification of endochondral ossification on the more active side of the physis by temporarily bridging it with staples, or screws and a figure-of-eight tension band wire. Alternatively, growth may be stimulated on the less active side by horizontal transection of the periosteum and periosteal stripping.

Transphyseal bridging

See Figs 10.10–10.11.

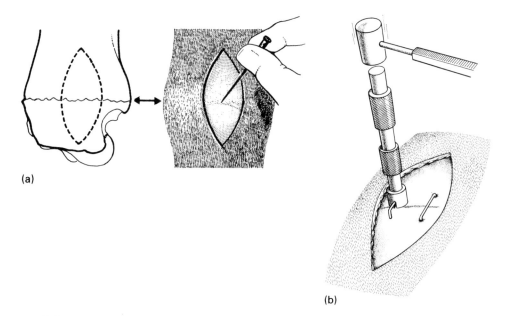

(a)

(b)

Fig. 10.10. (a) In cases of valgus deformity affecting the carpus, the distal growth plate of the radius is exposed by a 6–8-cm curvilinear skin incision over the point of maximum convexity on the medial aspect and its exact location delineated using a hypodermic needle.

(b) Using staples: the size of staple selected varies with individual foals and is determined by reference to the preoperative radiographs. The staples are held in a special staple inserter, centred on the hypodermic needle and inserted at right angles to the growth plate. They are driven into the bone using an orthopaedic hammer until the body of the staple lies flat against the periosteum. Two staples are sufficient, one placed medially and the other cranio-medially. Their position should be checked by radiography before skin closure. Removal of the staples once the leg is straight is achieved by incising the skin and overlying fibrous tissue and prising them out using a staple elevator or old orthopaedic chisel.

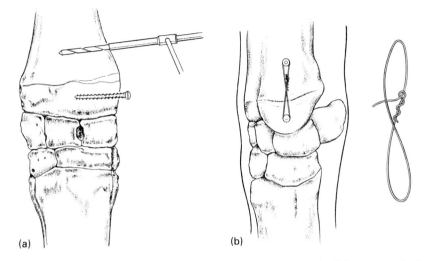

(a)   (b)

Fig. 10.11. Using screws and cerclage wire: (a) A 3.2-mm hole is drilled to a depth of about 40 mm in the distal radial epiphysis parallel to the plane of the growth plate and radiocarpal joint. An intra-operative radiograph should be taken at this point to ensure that the drill does not endanger the physis or radiocarpal joint. The hole is then tapped using an ASIF 4.5-mm tap. A 4.5-mm cortical screw 32−38 mm in length is inserted and tightened to a point where the head still protrudes from the collateral ligament. A second screw is inserted in the metaphyseal region in a similar manner to the first.

(b) A figure-of-eight (1.2 mm) wire loop is placed around the heads of the screws. Additional tension is then brought about in the wire by alternatively tightening the screws. The subcutaneous tissues are carefully opposed to ensure that the implants are covered before closing the skin.

This technique has the advantages of applying more immediate compression at the growth plate, producing less fibrous reaction at the site and allowing easier removal of the implant. However, there does not appear to be any significant reduction in the time taken for the limb to straighten compared to that when staples are used.

Hemicircumferential transection of the periosteum

Stimulating growth on the concave side of the growth plate by hemicircumferential transection and elevation of the periosteum offers a much simpler but equally effective method of correcting angular deformities.

The growth plate is identified with a needle. A curvilinear incision 6 cm long is made commencing just below the physis and extending proximally. The subcutaneous connective tissue is incised and reflected exposing the periosteum which is incised parallel to, and approximately 1−2 cm proximal to the growth plate extending to the cranial and caudal borders of the radius. A vertical incision 4−5 cm long is made creating an inverted T (Fig. 10.12a). The triangular portion of periosteum on either side is elevated from the underlying bone with a

chisel, allowed to fall back into place and is left unsutured (Fig. 10.12b). The operation is completed by closing the subcutaneous connective tissue with a continuous suture of 3 metric synthetic absorbable suture material and the skin with a subcuticular suture of the same material (Fig. 10.12c).

In foals with very severe angulations, simultaneous transphyseal bridging on the convex side, and periosteal elevation on the concave side, will bring about a more rapid correction of the deformity. This is of particular importance in varus deformity of the fetlock joint which carries a much less favourable prognosis than angular deformities of the carpus because of early closure of the distal metacarpal or metatarsal growth plate. Clinical experience has shown that to be successful, corrective surgery must be carried out in these cases before the foal is 2 months of age.

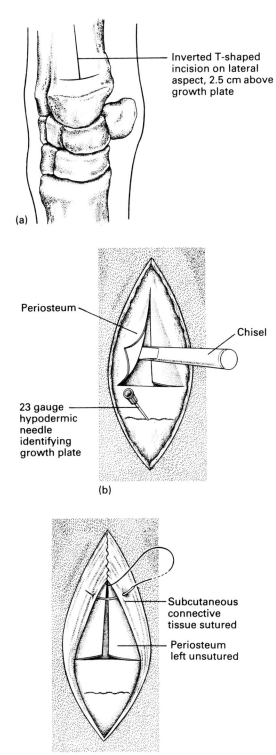

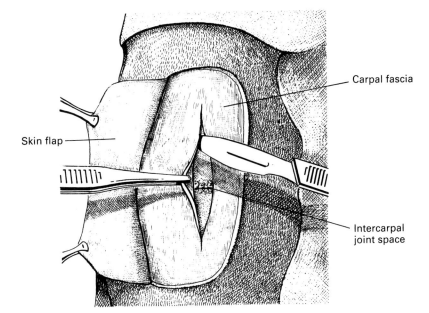

FRACTURE OF THE CARPAL BONES

The bones most frequently fractured are the radial, intermediate and third carpal bones. Slab fractures must be immobilized by a lag screw, whereas in smaller chip fractures the bone fragment(s) must be removed. This can be effected through an arthotomy incision or via arthroscopy. In either case the subchondral bone defect should be curetted to make a smooth surface. In chronic cases excrescences of cartilage and bone may develop along the joint edges and these also must be removed with rongeurs.

Carpal arthrotomy

The horse is restrained in lateral recumbency with the affected leg ventral so that the carpus can be exposed from the medial aspect.

Figures 10.13—10.15 show the procedure for removing a chip fracture from the proximal border of the third carpal bone.

Slab fractures of the carpus are most commonly associated with the third carpal bone. Thin slabs of bone which only involve the dorsal edge of the joint surface are best removed as the area of weight bearing surface that is lost is minimal and of little consequence.

Fig. 10.12. Hemicircumferential transection of the periosteum (for details see text).

Fig. 10.13. Removal of a chip fracture from the proximal border of the third carpal bone. On the dorso-medial aspect of the carpus the skin is incised to form a flap between the tendons of extensor carpii radialis and the common digital extensor muscles. The underlying fascia and joint capsule are incised longitudinally between these tendons to expose the radial and third carpal bones. A medial view of the right carpus is shown.

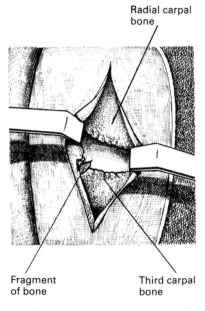

Radial carpal bone

Fragment of bone

Third carpal bone

Fig. 10.14. The carpus is flexed which opens the intercarpal articulation. The fascia and joint capsule are retracted. This permits the edges of the intercarpal articulations to be examined and enables the fragment to be dissected free. Any excrescences are removed with rongeurs and the area is curetted to create a smooth surface.

On the other hand thick slabs of bone must be accurately replaced, repositioned and immobilized with a lag screw if the normal weight bearing area of the joint is to be maintained (Figs 10.16–10.17). It is essential that the slab of bone is accurately positioned and the joint surface is congruent. To

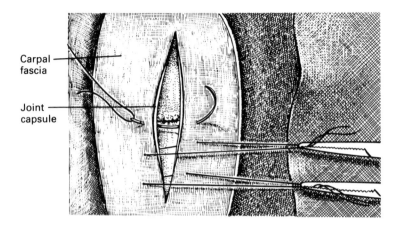

Carpal fascia

Joint capsule

Fig. 10.15. The carpus is extended and the incision closed by co-apting the fascia and joint capsule together with a series of interrupted synthetic absorbable sutures. It is an advantage to lay the sutures individually before tying them. The skin flap is replaced and retained in position with mattress sutures using monofilament nylon.

attain this the following points require attention:

1 The operation must not be delayed more than 5–7 days because new tissue growth will prevent accurate reduction and result in an articular defect.

2 The slab of bone moves proximally and it cannot be accurately replaced unless the carpus is flexed.

3 The slab of bone must be immobilized with a lag screw to obtain compression of the fracture. The screw should be inserted in the centre of the slab and at right angles to the fracture plane. Countersinking the screw head reduces the chances of splitting the slab during tightening but care must be taken not to overtighten the screw.

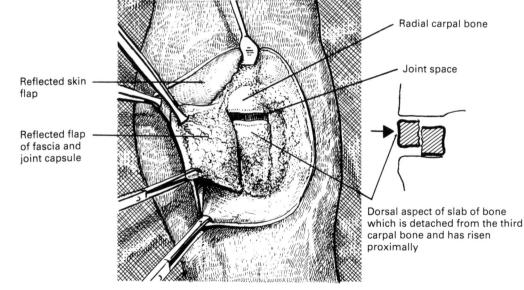

Reflected skin flap

Reflected flap of fascia and joint capsule

Radial carpal bone

Joint space

Dorsal aspect of slab of bone which is detached from the third carpal bone and has risen proximally

Fig. 10.16. Repair of a slab fracture of the third carpal bone. A skin flap is formed as in Fig. 10.13 and the underlying fascia and joint capsule are incised to expose the fracture.

The incision is closed by replacing the reflected fascia and co-apting it and the joint capsule with a series of interrupted synthetic absorbable sutures which are laid individually before tying them. The skin flap is replaced and sutured with mattress sutures using monofilament nylon.

Carpal arthroscopy

Two portals of entry are required for the arthroscopic removal of chip fractures from the radiocarpal or the intercarpal joint. In either case the instrument portal is placed nearest the fragment and the arthroscope portal is situated on the opposite side of the joint. The lateral portal is situated between the tendons of the extensor carpii radialis and the common digital extensor muscles, while the medial portal is medial to the extensor carpii radialis tendon. Care should be taken not to damage the tendon sheaths when making the stab incisions through the skin.

The fragment is identified with a probe, before grasping it with a pair of forceps and freeing it with a twisting action. Intracapsular fragments and non-articular osteophytes are normally left *in situ*. The skin incisions are closed with simple interrupted sutures of monofilament nylon.

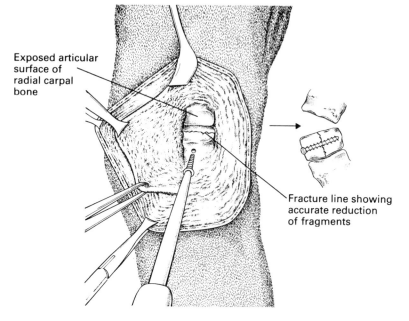

Fig. 10.17. With the carpus flexed the gap between the slab of bone and the third carpal bone is cleared of all blood clot and detritus. By flexing the carpus the fragment moves distally and can be accurately repositioned. The fragment is then immobilized and firmly compressed in position with a 3.5-mm cortical lag screw.

Metacarpus

FRACTURE OF A SPLINT BONE

Although a splint bone may be fractured at any point throughout its length the most common site is the distal extremity of the medial splint bone of a thoracic limb. If there is marked displacement with non-union or healing is accompanied by excessive new bone formation which impinges on the suspensory ligament or flexor tendons then the splint bone should be removed. Since the splint bone is an integral and weight bearing bone of the carpus it should not be totally removed but as much as possible of its proximal extremity preserved.

Removal of a medial splint bone

The horse is restrained in lateral recumbency with the affected leg ventral (Figs 10.18–10.22).

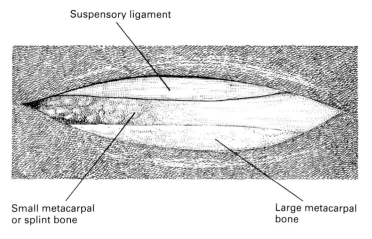

Fig. 10.18. The skin is incised tne length of, and parallel with, the caudal border of the splint bone. It is then reflected to reveal the caudal and medial aspect of the large metacarpal bone, the splint bone and the suspensory ligament.

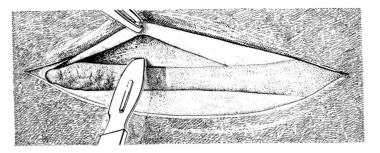

Fig. 10.19. The fascia along the caudal aspect of the splint bone is incised and the suspensory ligament dissected free and retracted to expose the whole length of the splint bone.

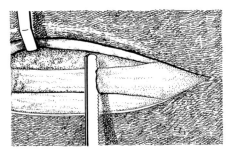

Fig. 10.20. With a hack-saw blade the splint bone, proximal to the fracture, is sawn through at an oblique angle. This results in the development of new bone between the cut surface and the metacarpal bone instead of the formation of an exostosis.

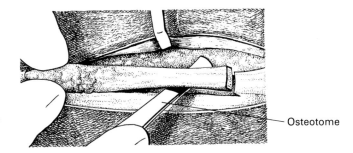

Osteotome

Fig. 10.21. The splint bone is separated from the metacarpal bone by breaking down the interosseous attachments with an osteotome and gently lifting it free. The splint bone should not be severed or freed with a chisel and hammer. The blows can result in a fissure fracture of the metacarpal bone which becomes a complete or even open fracture as the horse takes weight on the leg when getting up.

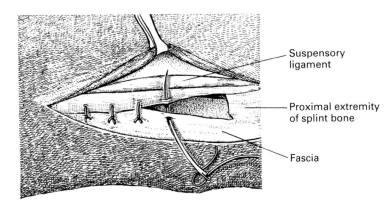

Suspensory ligament

Proximal extremity of splint bone

Fascia

Fig. 10.22. The incision is closed by co-apting the fascia to the edge of the suspensory ligament with a series of interrupted sutures using synthetic absorbable suture material and the skin with interrupted sutures of monofilament nylon.

Removal of a 'splint'

When a medial splint is very large and continually being struck by the opposite foot, the only remedy is its removal. The horse is restrained in lateral recumbency with the affected leg ventral (Figs 10.23–10.26).

An exostosis involving either of the two small metacarpal or splint bones (metacarpal bones II and IV) is colloquially referred to as a 'splint'.

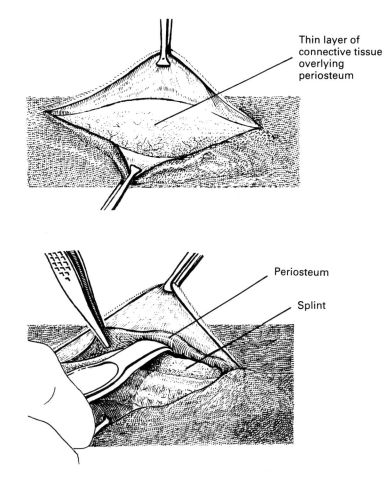

Fig. 10.23. The skin is incised longitudinally over the splint and reflected to expose a thin layer of connective tissue and periosteum.

Fig. 10.24. The connective tissue and periosteum are incised longitudinally the length of the splint and reflected from the bone using a periosteal elevator.

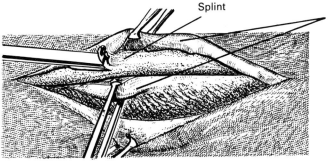

Fig. 10.25. Using a bone chisel and mallet the splint is excised and fashioned level with the small and large metacarpal bones.

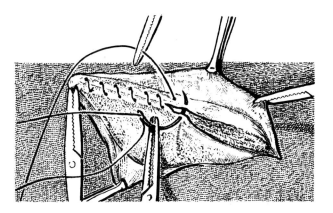

Fig. 10.26. The periosteum and connective tissue are co-apted using a continuous suture of 3 metric synthetic absorbable material and the skin with interrupted sutures of monofilament nylon.

Fetlock joint

FRACTURE OF A PROXIMAL SESAMOID BONE

Fracture of a proximal sesamoid bone is most frequently seen in racehorses. Following conservative methods of treatment many horses become sound but this improvement is short lived as the horse invariably goes lame during training or when raced. The most common fracture is of the apex of the bone and this is treated by the removal of the bone fragment. In such cases, up to a third of the proximal end of the bone can be removed with good results (Figs 10.27–10.32).

Transverse fractures of the middle and lower third of a proximal sesamoid bone may be treated by an open reduction and immobilization with a lag screw, or the fracture plane may be packed with cancellous bone (Figs 10.33–10.34).

The incision is closed by co-apting the collateral ligament with mattress sutures using fine synthetic absorbable suture material and the subcutaneous tissues and skin in the customary manner.

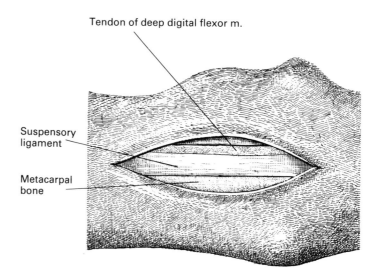

Fig. 10.27. A skin incision is made some 7.5 cm long from just below the button of the splint bone parallel with the palmar border of the metacarpal bone to the base of the fractured sesamoid bone. The skin is reflected to expose the palmar border of the metacarpal bone, suspensory ligament and edge of the tendon of the deep digital flexor. The figure shows the lateral aspect of the left fetlock joint.

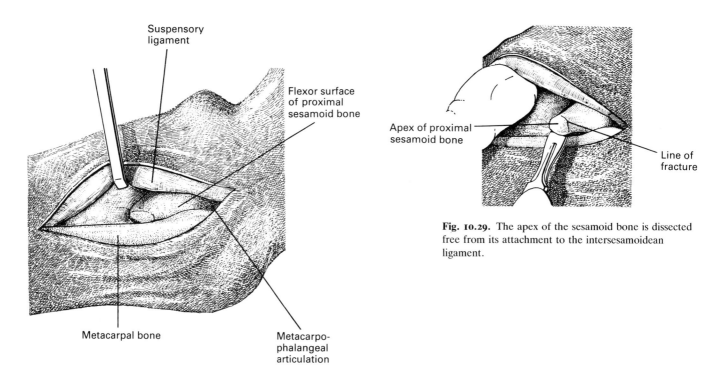

Fig. 10.28. The fascia between the metacarpal bone and suspensory ligament is incised and the incision extended distally to meet the collateral ligament of the fetlock joint. This exposes the joint capsule which is incised in like manner. The fetlock joint is now flexed and the suspensory ligament retracted to bring into view the apex and flexor surface of the sesamoid bone.

Fig. 10.29. The apex of the sesamoid bone is dissected free from its attachment to the intersesamoidean ligament.

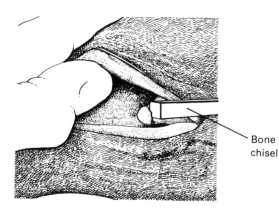

Fig. 10.30. The apex is separated along the fracture line with a bone chisel or osteotome.

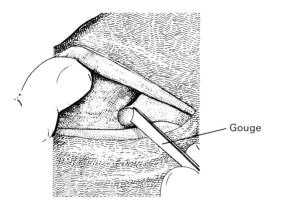

Fig. 10.31. The apex is finally separated from all its attachments with a gouge and removed.

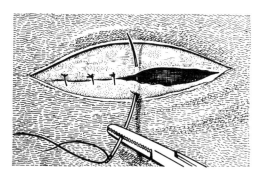

Fig. 10.32. The wound is closed by co-apting the joint capsule and fascia with interrupted sutures using synthetic absorbable suture material and the skin with interrupted sutures using monofilament nylon.

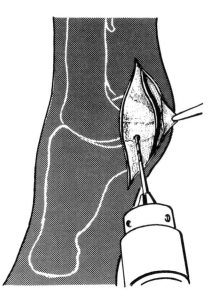

Fig. 10.33. With the horse recumbent and lying so that the fractured sesamoid bone is uppermost, the fracture is exposed by a longitudinal skin incision just dorsal to the plantar artery. The skin edges are reflected to expose the plantar artery, vein and nerve which are retracted in a plantar direction. The base of the sesamoid bone is then exposed by dividing the collateral ligament transversely and freeing the attachments of the deep sesamoidean ligaments by blunt dissection. This enables the bone to be firmly held in bone-holding forceps and a hole drilled from the posterior border of its base, directed slightly obliquely towards the apex.

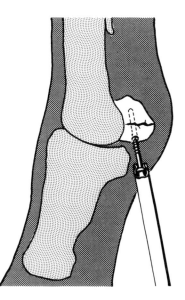

Fig. 10.34. A lag screw is then driven which pulls the two halves of the bone tightly together.

Phalanges

FRACTURE OF THE FIRST PHALANX

Fractures of the first phalanx commonly occur in the front leg and range from simple fractures with little displacement or chip fractures of the dorsal edge of the proximal articular surface to grossly comminuted fractures. Simple fractures may be complete or incomplete, sagittal or spiral and may involve both articular surfaces of the bone (Figs 10.35–10.36).

Chip fractures of the dorsal edge of the proximal surface of the first phalanx result in intermittent lameness and are treated by the removal of the detached piece of bone. This is best performed arthroscopically but may be successfully achieved via a dorsal arthrotomy (Figs 10.37–10.40).

Fractures of the second phalanx are rare. Fractures of the third phalanx are not uncommon and non-articular fractures have a good prognosis when treated conservatively by rest and fitting a bar shoe with heel clips to prevent expansion of the foot when weight is taken. Intra-articular fractures in horses under 3 years of age can be satisfactorily treated on the same lines but in older horses the fracture requires to be immobilized with an ASIF cortical lag screw. Careful preparation is necessary to reduce contamination during surgery and it is advisable to soak the foot in strong iodine solution for 48 hours before wrapping it in a sterile adhesive plastic drape.

An area of horn is removed with a 13.5-mm drill bit and the fracture immobilized with a 4.5-mm cortical lag screw. The screw should not impinge

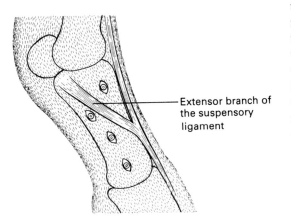

Fig. 10.35. Immobilization of a split pastern. Non-displaced fractures can be immobilized with two, three or possibly four, lag screws inserted through stab incisions, using the extensor branch of the suspensory ligament as a landmark. The screws are placed at right angles to the fracture line and parallel with the articular surfaces. The proximal fragment is overdrilled when using cortical screws to achieve compression at the fracture site.

Extensor branch of the suspensory ligament

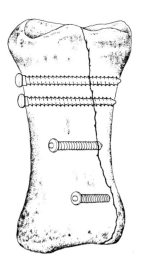

Fig. 10.36. Immobilization of a spiral fracture of the first phalanx. The lag screws must be placed at right angles to the fracture plane to ensure adequate compression. This requires careful planning and a thorough pre-operative radiographic examination.

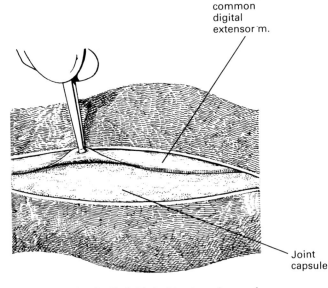

Tendon of common digital extensor m.

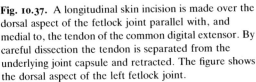

Joint capsule

Fig. 10.37. A longitudinal skin incision is made over the dorsal aspect of the fetlock joint parallel with, and medial to, the tendon of the common digital extensor. By careful dissection the tendon is separated from the underlying joint capsule and retracted. The figure shows the dorsal aspect of the left fetlock joint.

on the sensitive laminae on the opposite side of the hoof and should be removed as soon as healing is complete.

Complete transverse fractures which do not extend beyond 1 cm from the tip of the extensor process respond well to the removal of the detached piece of bone (Figs 10.41 – 10.42).

The incision is closed by co-apting the tendon and joint capsule together with interrupted sutures using synthetic absorbable suture material and the skin in the customary manner.

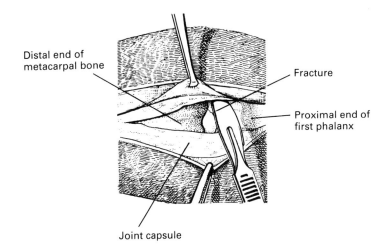

Fig. 10.38. The joint capsule is incised and its attachments to the dorsal and proximal surface of the first phalanx dissected free.

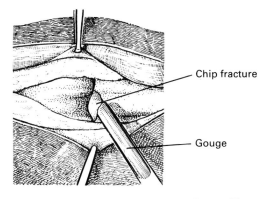

Fig. 10.39. Slight flexion of the fetlock joint provides adequate exposure for the examination of the joint and removal of the fragment of bone using either a gouge or bone-nibbling forceps.

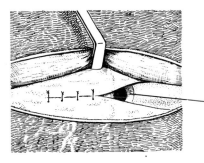

Fig. 10.40. The joint capsule is closed with interrupted sutures using synthetic absorbable suture material. The extensor tendon is repositioned and the skin incision closed with interrupted sutures using monofilament nylon.

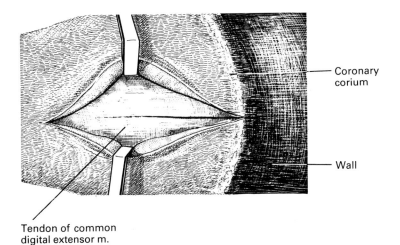

Fig. 10.41. A longitudinal and midline incision is made from the pastern joint and extended distally through the coronary corium to the wall of the hoof. The skin edges are retracted to expose the expanded portion of the tendon of the common digital extensor which is incised together with the joint capsule.

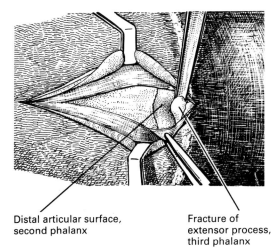

Fig. 10.42. The edges of the incised tendon are forcibly retracted and its attachments to the extensor process dissected free. This enables the fragment of bone to be detached with a gouge and removed.

The foot

OPERATION FOR SANDCRACK

A sandcrack is a fissure in the wall of the hoof and treatment is directed to removing the pressure at the free extremity and to immobilizing the edges of the crack (Fig. 10.43).

The grooves must be cut to the depth of the white zone if they are to relieve pressure on and immobilize the edges of the sandcrack effectively, and it is a matter of choice whether a hoof saw, hot iron or drawing knife is used to fashion them. The bearing surface of the wall immediately under a complete crack must be pared away to prevent any pressure at this point from the shoe.

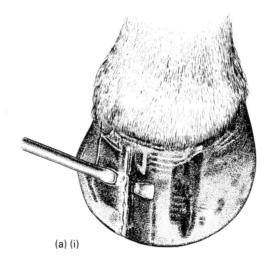

(a) (i)

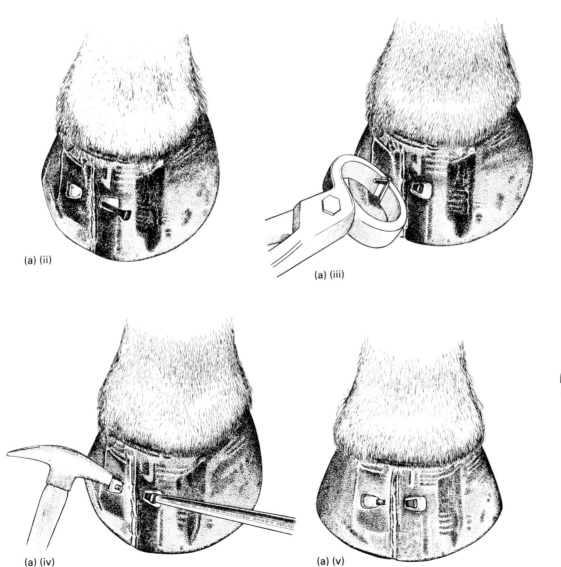

(a) (ii)

(a) (iii)

(a) (iv)

(a) (v)

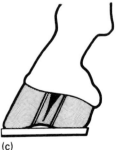

(b)

(c)

THORACIC LIMB — HORSE/THE FOOT 185

GROOVING THE WALL

A number of techniques are employed to obtain expansion at the heels and to relieve pressure within the foot. The method of grooving the wall shown in Fig. 10.44 is both simple and effective.

OPERATION FOR QUITTOR

Necrosis of a lateral cartilage is termed 'a quittor' and is characterized by one or more sinuses discharging at the coronet.

Treatment is directed towards removal of all necrotic and diseased tissue, the provision of drainage and the control of infection so that the wound can heal by granulation. The time-honoured method of attaining these ideals necessitated removal of a section of the horn and reflecting a flap of the coronary corium and skin. This established free drainage but the development of a false quarter. The great advance in controlling infection has led to less drastic methods to effect a cure.

The operation (Fig. 10.45) should be performed under general anaesthesia and with a tourniquet to control haemorrhage. Post operation the wound is packed with vaseline gauze and dressed every 2—3 days. Healing is by granulation which may become exuberant and have to be controlled by cauterization to enable the skin edges to unite.

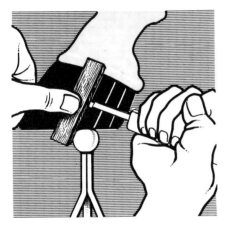

Fig. 10.44. With the foot resting on a tripod three or four parallel grooves are cut at 2-cm intervals from the coronet to the bearing surface. These grooves are placed on both the medial and lateral aspects of the heels, extend down to the white line and each is 0.5 cm wide. They are easily fashioned using a drawing knife and if the wall is very hard it can be softened by cold water footbaths for 1 hour twice daily for 2—3 days.

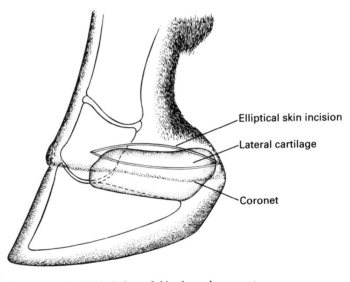

Elliptical skin incision

Lateral cartilage

Coronet

Fig. 10.45. An elliptical piece of skin above the coronet, which includes the discharging sinus or sinuses. is removed to expose the cartilage. The edges of the wound are retracted, all necrotic cartilage dissected free and a thorough debridement of the surrounding tissues carried out.

Fig. 10.43. (*Opposite*). (a) *Immobilizing the edges of a deep sandcrack using a standard horseshoe nail*: (i) After paring the edges of the sandcrack a special tool, heated to a dull red heat, is used to fashion a bed for the nail on either side of the sandcrack. If only one nail is required then the beds are sited just above the centre of the sandcrack with the inner edge of the bed about 6 mm from the edge of the sandcrack. If two nails are used then the proximal one is inserted 12 mm below the coronet and the other 18 mm below it. (ii) A horseshoe nail, slightly bent on flat, is driven across the sandcrack and driven home using the point of a buffer as a punch. (iii) The point of the nail is turned over and cut off with pincers. (iv) The turned over end of the nail is tapped into position while the head of the nail is kept in position with the end of a handle of the pincers. (v) Procedure completed, the edges of a deep sandcrack are immobilized with a horseshoe nail.

Due to the comparative thinness and flat surface of the horn at the quarters, deep sandcracks cannot be satisfactorily immobilized using either clips or horseshoe nails. These methods are only suitable for toe sandcracks.

(b) *Superficial and incomplete*: Two grooves are cut from the coronet in the form of a V to meet at the lower limit of the crack.

(c) *Superficial and complete*: Two parallel grooves are cut, one on each side of the crack, from the coronet to the bearing surface.

Thoracic limb — dog

DRAPING A LEG FOR SURGERY

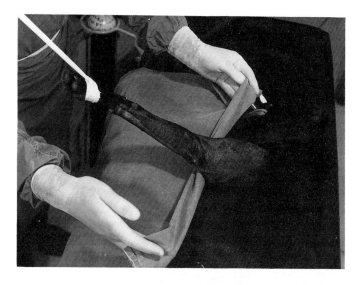

Fig. 10.46. After the leg has been clipped it is held by a tape, disinfected and a sterile towel is placed beneath it.

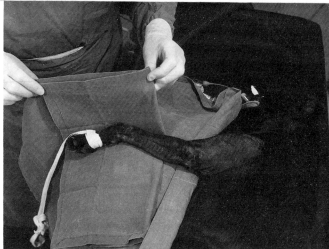

Fig. 10.47. A second towel is placed on top of the first towel with its upper edge resting just distal to the proposed incision and the leg lowered onto the towel.

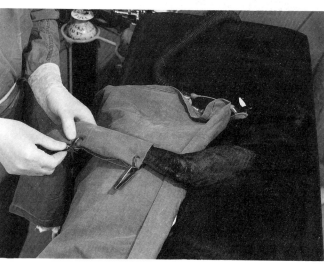

Fig. 10.48. The extremity of the leg is wrapped in the second towel which is retained in position with towel clips. This permits the leg to be manipulated during surgery without any risk of contamination.

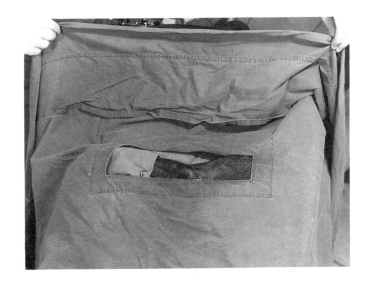

Fig. 10.49. A laparotomy sheet, with a rectangular hole in the centre, is placed over the leg and unfolded.

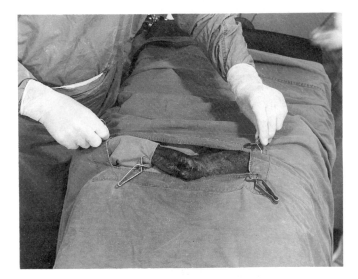

Fig. 10.50. The hole is positioned with its upper edge resting just proximal to the operation site and retained with a towel clip at each extremity.

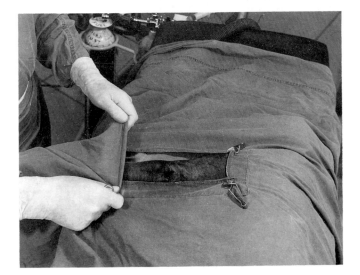

Fig. 10.51. The lower edge of the hole is folded over to complete the isolation of the operation site and retained with two towel clips.

Shoulder joint

CAUDO-LATERAL APPROACH

The caudo-lateral approach (Figs 10.52–10.55) to the shoulder is frequently used to remove osteochondritis dissecans lesions from the caudal aspect of the humeral head. The joint is irrigated with saline and the joint capsule co-apted with horizontal mattress sutures of 3 metric absorbable suture material. The muscles are repositioned and sutured to their tendon insertions using horizontal mattress sutures of similar material. The subcutaneous tissue and skin are closed in the usual manner.

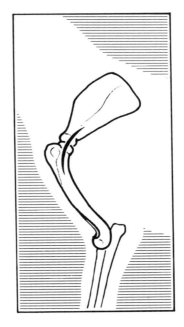

Fig. 10.52. To perform an arthrotomy of the left shoulder joint, the dog is placed in lateral recumbency with the affected leg uppermost. A slightly curved skin incision is made which extends from a point just proximal and caudal to the acromion process of the scapula down to the upper third of the humerus.

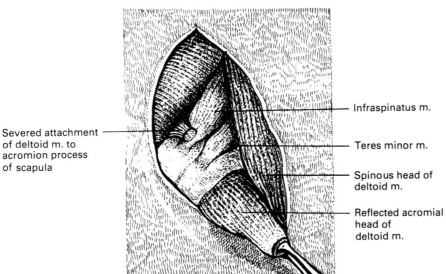

Severed attachment of deltoid m. to acromion process of scapula

Infraspinatus m.

Teres minor m.

Spinous head of deltoid m.

Reflected acromial head of deltoid m.

Fig. 10.53. The acromial head of the deltoid muscle is separated by blunt dissection, severed about 1 cm from its attachment to the acromion process and reflected ventrally. This exposes the tendons of the infraspinatus and teres minor muscles crossing the lateral aspect of the shoulder joint. Alternatively, the spinous and acromial heads of the deltoid muscle may be retracted with Gelpi retractors without severing the acromial head.

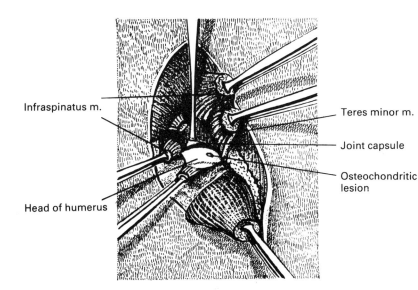

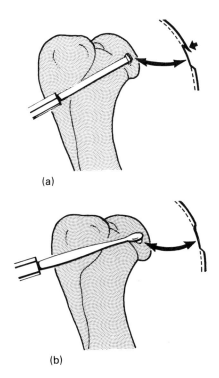

Fig. 10.54. The tendons of insertion of the infraspinatus and teres minor muscles are severed about 1 cm from their attachments to the greater tuberosity and reflected to expose the joint capsule. The more experienced surgeon will reflect these muscles by placing a pair of Gelpi retractors between them, rather than transecting them. The thickened joint capsule is incised transversely midway between its points of attachment to ensure that adequate tissue is left on either side for repair. At the caudal extremity of the incision, care must be taken not to damage the branches of the circumflex artery and vein or axillary nerve.

Fig. 10.55. The caudal articular surface of the humeral head can now be inspected but to obtain satisfactory exposure of the lesion it is generally necessary to extend the joint and rotate the head of the humerus laterally. The loosely attached flap of cartilage is lifted off with dressing forceps (a), any attached areas being broken down with an osteotome. The exposed subchondral bone is then curetted and any cartilage not firmly attached at the periphery of the lesion is removed likewise (b).

DISLOCATION OF THE SHOULDER JOINT

Dislocation of the shoulder joint is most frequently lateral and although easily reduced by a closed reduction it remains unstable. If redislocation occurs then an open reduction and stabilization of the joint is necessary (Figs 10.56–10.61).

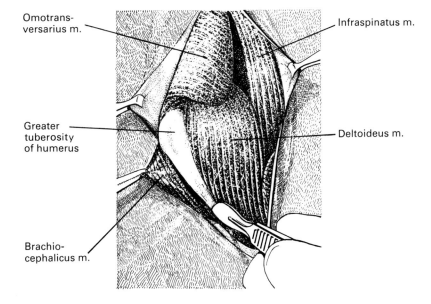

Fig. 10.56. The shoulder joint is approached from the lateral aspect by a curved skin incision which extends from the upper third of the spine of the scapula down over the greater tuberosity of the humerus and terminates towards the middle of the humerus. The skin edges are reflected and the brachiocephalicus and deltoideus muscles separated to expose the lateral aspect of the proximal extremity of the humerus.

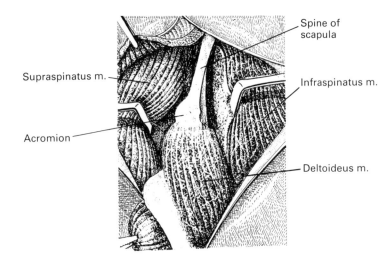

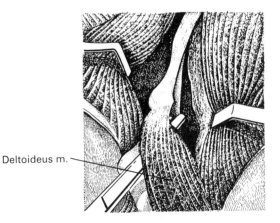

Fig. 10.57. The attachments of the omotransversarius, supraspinatus and infraspinatus muscles to the spine of the scapula are separated and the muscles retracted to expose the acromion.

Fig. 10.58. The ventral surface of the deltoideus muscle is freed carefully by blunt dissection to conserve its attachment to both the acromion and humerus.

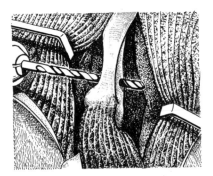

Fig. 10.59. A tunnel is drilled, using a 3-mm twist drill, transversely through the spine and close to the blade of the scapula approximately 1.5−2.0 cm from the acromion.

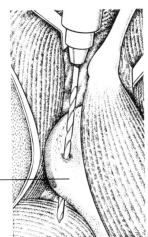

Fig. 10.60. A tunnel is drilled obliquely through the proximal extremity of the humerus from a point about 1.5 cm below the crest of the greater tuberosity to emerge through the lateral ridge.

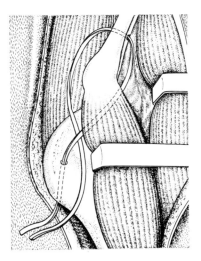

Fig. 10.61. (*Left*). A length of 0.6-cm nylon tape is passed up the humeral tunnel, under the attachment of the deltoideus muscle, through the hole in the scapular spine and brought down under itself. Finally the ends of the tape are pulled sufficiently tight to stabilize the joint and tied. The muscles are repositioned and the subcutaneous fascia closed with a continuous suture of synthetic absorbable suture material. The skin is co-apted with interrupted sutures of monofilament nylon.

Humerus

FRACTURE OF THE HUMERAL SHAFT

Overriding fractures of the shaft of the humerus are virtually impossible to reduce by closed methods or to immobilize by external fixation. Following an open reduction the fracture may either be repaired with an intramedullary pin or a bone plate and screws.

Repair with an intermedullary pin

The intramedullary pin selected is of a diameter equal to the medullary cavity at its narrowest point and of a length which extends from the cranio-lateral extremity of the greater tuberosity to just above the supratrochlear foramen. When the fracture involves the distal third of the shaft, a smaller diameter pin should be selected and driven into the medial condyle of the distal humerus.

Figures 10.62–10.65 show the procedure for repairing a fracture with an intermedullary pin. The pin is finally aligned and pushed into the cancellous bone of the distal fragment (Fig. 10.65).

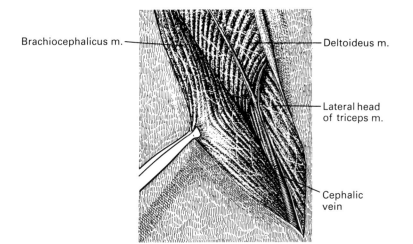

Fig. 10.62. The skin is incised on the cranio-lateral aspect of the limb along a line joining the greater tuberosity and epicondyle. The skin is reflected to expose the brachiocephalicus, deltoideus and lateral head of the triceps muscle and the cephalic vein. The figure shows the left thoracic limb.

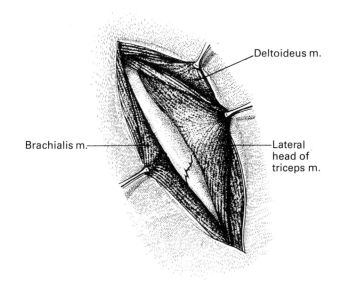

Fig. 10.63. The lateral head of the triceps and the brachialis muscle are separated along their line of cleavage and retracted to expose the lateral aspect of the shaft of the humerus. In fractures of the distal extremity, care must be taken to identify the radial nerve.

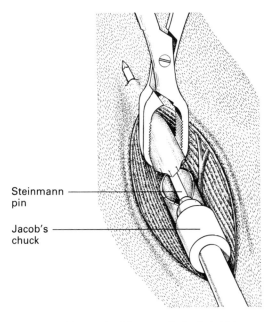

Fig. 10.64. The proximal fragment is firmly held by bone-holding forceps and the intramedullary pin, fitted in a Jacob's chuck, is passed up the medullary cavity and rotated through the cancellous bone until the point emerges on the cranio-lateral surface of the greater tuberosity and lies subcutaneously. The overlying skin is incised and the pin extruded a further 5.0–7.5 cm.

The fracture site is held securely in bone-holding forceps to prevent its disruption while the pin is broken off. The point at which the pin is to be broken off is determined from pre-operation radiographs and the site is prepared by sawing completely around and through about two-thirds its thickness.

The muscles and skin are co-apted in the usual manner.

Repair with a bone plate and screws

The shortness and curvature of the humeral shaft makes contouring a bone plate to its lateral aspect difficult and time consuming. Thus the fracture is best treated by performing an open reduction and fixation with a bone plate and screws on the medial aspect of the limb (Figs 10.66–10.67).

The muscles and skin are co-apted in the usual manner.

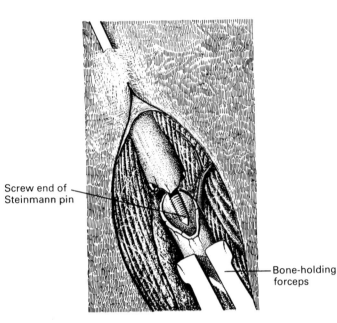

Screw end of Steinmann pin

Bone-holding forceps

Fig. 10.65. The chuck is removed and attached to the protruding proximal end of the intramedullary pin. The pin is then carefully drawn up the proximal fragment using a rotary movement, until the point is protruding just beyond the fracture line. With the distal fragment held in bone-holding forceps and the intramedullary pin used to manipulate the proximal fragment, the fracture is reduced and the protruding point of the intramedullary pin manoeuvred into the medullary cavity of the distal fragment. Final alignment is made and the pin pushed into the cancellous bone of the distal fragment until the point comes to rest just above the supratrochlear foramen. The use of a screw-ended pin was previously thought to improve pin stability, but this is doubtful and the pin may fracture if it is subjected to bending forces at its threaded/non-threaded junction.

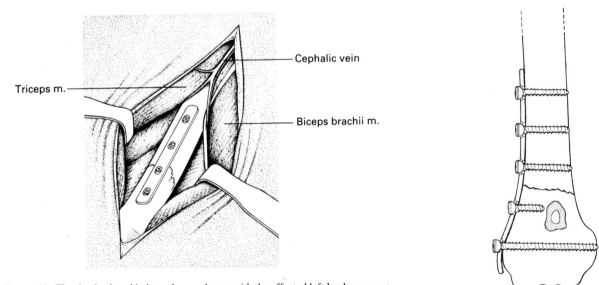

Triceps m.

Cephalic vein

Biceps brachii m.

Fig. 10.66. The dog is placed in lateral recumbency with the affected left leg lowermost. To obtain adequate exposure of the distal and medial aspects of the shaft of the humerus the dog's thorax requires to be slightly rotated upwards and the limb pulled at right angles to the vertebral column and retained under traction. A longitudinal skin incision is made from the distal third of the humerus to the elbow joint. The biceps brachii and medial head of the triceps muscle are divided along their line of cleavage, between the branches of the cephalic vein, to expose the fracture. The fracture is reduced by manipulation and immobilized with a bone plate with at least two screws on either side of the fracture line.

Fig. 10.67. Cranio-caudal view of a distal fracture of the shaft of the humerus. Note the position of the distal screws. Care must be taken when selecting the site for driving them that they do not enter the supratrochlear foramen, thereby obstructing the anconeal process of the olecranon and preventing normal extension of the elbow joint.

Elbow joint

UNUNITED ANCONEAL PROCESS

Failure of the anconeal process to unite with the olecranon results in intermittent lameness which becomes permanent as an osteoarthritis develops. This condition is treated by removing the detached or displaced piece of bone (Figs 10.68–10.72).

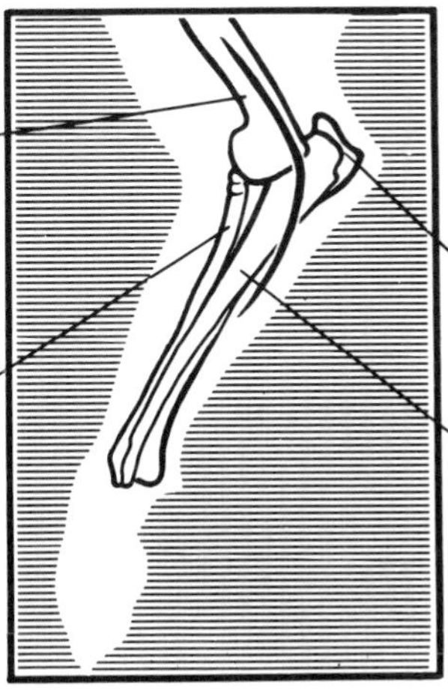

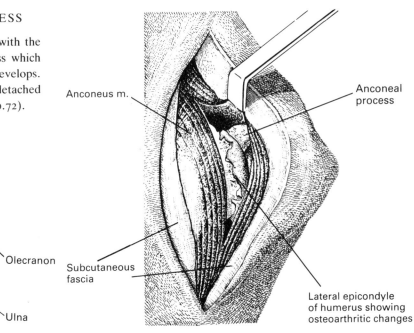

Fig. 10.70. The fascia, anconeus muscle and joint capsule are incised, and, with the joint flexed, are retracted to expose the lateral epicondyle of the humerus and the ununited anconeal process.

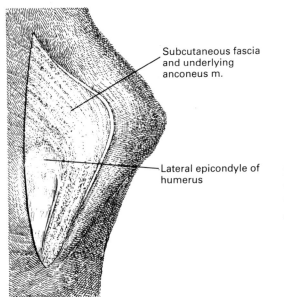

Fig. 10.68. The dog is positioned in lateral recumbency with the affected leg uppermost and supported on a sandbag. The joint is exposed via a curved skin incision extending from the distal and posterior extremity of the humerus to the upper third of the ulna.

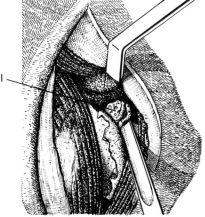

Fig. 10.71. The anconeal process is removed by separating it along its line of fusion using a gouge or osteotome and severing any caudal attachments to the joint capsule with scissors.

Fig. 10.69. The edges of the skin are reflected. The lateral epicondyle of the humerus and the anconeus muscle lie under the subcutaneous fascia.

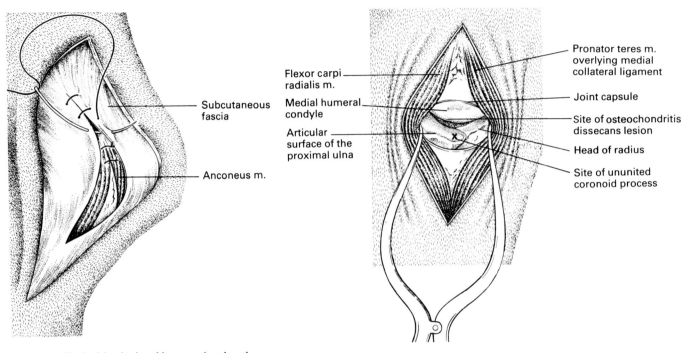

Fig. 10.72. The incision is closed by co-apting the edges of the anconeus muscle with interrupted sutures of absorbable synthetic material. The subcutaneous fascia is closed with a continuous suture of similar material and the skin closed in the usual manner.

Fig. 10.73. Exposure of the medial aspect of a left elbow. A skin incision is made from the lower third of the humerus, extending over the medial epicondyle of the humerus to terminate at the upper third of the radius. The incision is continued through the fascia overlying the superficial digital flexor, flexor carpi radialis and pronator teres muscles. The latter two muscles are separated by blunt dissection and retracted with Gelpi retractors. The joint capsule is incised and the Gelpi retractors repositioned. The joint is then flexed and the coronoid process or articular flap on the medial humeral condyle removed with a gouge.

The incision is closed by co-apting the joint capsule with simple interrupted sutures of synthetic absorbable suture material. The overlying fascia and subcutaneous tissues are closed with continuous sutures of similar material and the skin in the customary manner. Post operation it is advisable to support the elbow joint in a bandage for 7–10 days.

UNUNITED CORONOID PROCESS AND OSTEOCHONDRITIS DISSECANS OF THE MEDIAL HUMERAL CONDYLE

An ununited or fragmented coronoid process and osteochondritis dissecans of the medial humeral condyle are common causes of elbow lameness in young, rapidly growing large dogs. If surgery is required, the treatment in both cases is to expose the medial aspect of the elbow joint and remove the osteochondral fragments (Fig. 10.73). The dog is restrained in lateral recumbency, lying on the affected leg, with a sandbag placed under the elbow. To obtain satisfactory exposure the elbow must be flexed and the carpus inwardly rotated, using the sandbag as a fulcrum.

In most cases a muscle splitting approach can be used but if additional exposure is required the medial collateral ligament can be transected, with or without transection of the pronator teres muscle. Any transected structures must be carefully sutured when the arthrotomy is repaired.

FRACTURE OF THE LATERAL HUMERAL CONDYLE

The lateral condyle has a comparatively frail neck of bone which curves laterally away from the main shaft and is weakened on its medial aspect by the supratrochlear foramen. Any stress which causes a fracture of the lateral condyle deprives the trochlea of its lateral support, and it fractures through the supratrochlear foramen. The condyle is displaced and normal function of the joint can only be restored by open reduction and fixation.

Repair with a transfixion screw

Open reduction and fixation using a transfixion screw is shown in Figs 10.74–10.80. Closure of the wound is effected by replacing the muscles and co-apting them with interrupted sutures of synthetic absorbable material and the skin in the usual manner.

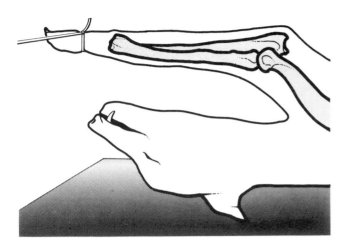

Fig. 10.74. The dog is positioned in dorsal recumbency with the leg drawn forwards. The joint is approached by a longitudinal skin incision over the point of the elbow.

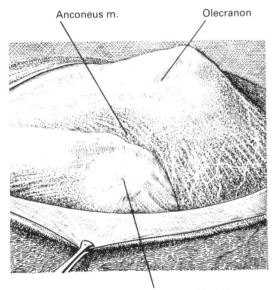

Anconeus m.   Olecranon

Lateral epicondyle of humerus

Fig. 10.75. The skin is reflected medially and laterally to expose disrupted subcuticular tissue and antebrachial fascia. Beneath can be identified the olecranon, anconeus muscle and loose lateral epicondyle.

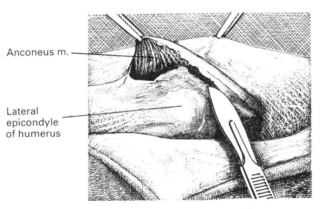

Anconeus m.

Lateral epicondyle of humerus

Fig. 10.76. The detached epicondyle is isolated by severing the attachments of the anconeus muscle.

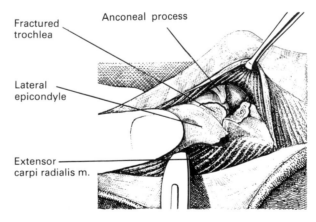

Fractured trochlea   Anconeal process

Lateral epicondyle

Extensor carpi radialis m.

Fig. 10.77. The attachments of the extensor carpi radialis muscle are severed. This permits the detached epicondyle to be freely manipulated while remaining attached to the radius by the lateral digital extensor and extensor carpi ulnaris muscles.

Fractures of the lateral condyle which are under 24 hours old may be repaired by closed reduction, immobilizing them with a lag screw placed through a stab incision.

It is helpful in these cases to hold the reconstructed trochlea in position with a retaining clamp (Figs 10.81–10.82). The clamp acts as a drill guide which ensures that the drill hole passes centrally through the trochlea and allows the screw to be driven without disturbing the reconstructed trochlea.

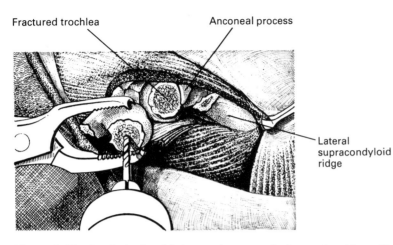

Fig. 10.78. The detached epicondyle is rotated to expose the fractured trochlea and held in Frosch bone-holding forceps while a hole is drilled through the centre of the trochlea using a standard 4.0-mm twist drill.

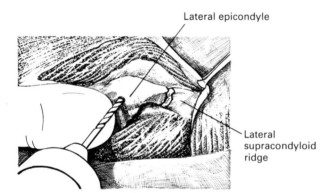

Fig. 10.79. The detached epicondyle is accurately reduced and using the drill hole as a guide, a hole is drilled through the medial trochlea.

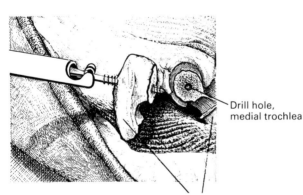

Fig. 10.80. A 4.4-mm transfixion screw is driven through the displaced epicondyle until its point just emerges. The epicondyle is now accurately reduced by inserting the point of the screw into the drill hole of the medial trochlea. Final alignment is made and the screw driven through the medial trochlea to obtain good immobilization. During the final tightening of the screw, care must be taken to ensure that the alignment of the supracondyloid ridge is not disrupted. Provided the non-threaded portion of the screw crosses the fracture plane, compression is produced at the fracture site as the screw is tightened.

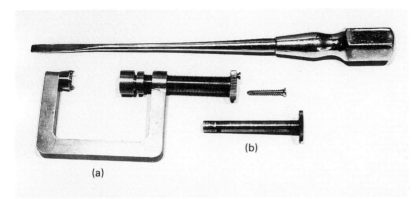

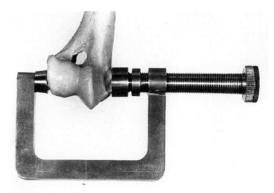

Fig. 10.81. Components of the retaining clamp. (a) Retaining clamp with adjusting screw which is hollow to take the screwdriver and screw. (b) Sleeve which fits into the adjusting screw of the retaining clamp and acts as the drill guide.

Fig. 10.82. Clamp in position to retain a detached medial epicondyle. Note that the clamp requires to be slightly angulated to drill the trochlea along its true medio-lateral axis.

Repair with ASIF screws using the lag screw principle

The fracture is reduced and immobilized with condylar clamps (Fig. 10.83a). Interfragmentary compression is achieved either with a fully threaded cortical screw or a partially threaded cancellous screw (Fig. 10.83b,c). To counteract rotational forces it may be necessary to drive an additional Kirschner wire up the lateral condyle.

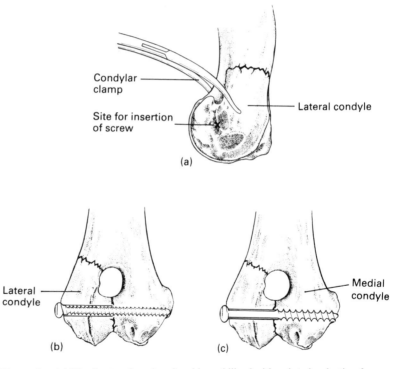

Fig. 10.83. (a) The fracture is reduced and immobilized with pointed reduction forceps or condylar clamps. (b) Repair with a fully threaded cortical screw. The lateral condyle is overdrilled so the screw is free to slide through this part of the bone before it grips the medial condyle. (c) Repair with a partially threaded cancellous screw. The shank of the screw is of a smaller diameter than the threaded portion, thus creating compression as the screw is tightened.

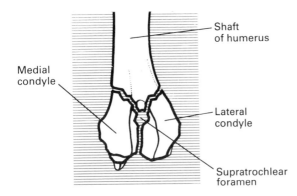

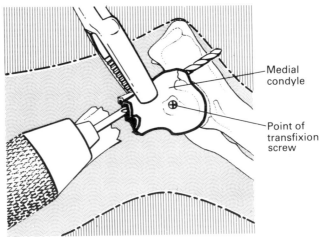

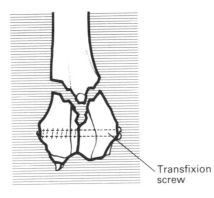

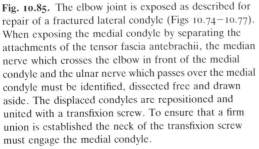

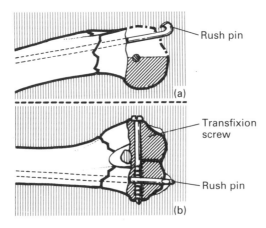

Fig. 10.84. A typical intercondylar fracture of the distal extremity of the humerus. The condyles are separated and detached from the shaft of the humerus. Repair is carried out in two stages: (i) repairing the fractured trochlea by joining the two condyles, and (ii) anchoring the strong medial condyle to the shaft.

Fig. 10.86. The medial condyle is held in Frosch bone-holding forceps and a hole drilled down its long axis to emerge at the origin of the flexors of the carpus and digits.

Fig. 10.85. The elbow joint is exposed as described for repair of a fractured lateral condyle (Figs 10.74–10.77). When exposing the medial condyle by separating the attachments of the tensor fascia antebrachii, the median nerve which crosses the elbow in front of the medial condyle and the ulnar nerve which passes over the medial condyle must be identified, dissected free and drawn aside. The displaced condyles are repositioned and united with a transfixion screw. To ensure that a firm union is established the neck of the transfixion screw must engage the medial condyle.

Fig. 10.87. The supracondylar fracture is reduced and immobilized with a Rush pin. The pin is inserted through the medial condyle to enter the medullary cavity of the humerus and driven home until the hooked end engages the distal end of the medial condyle. This is satisfactory for small dogs but larger dogs require plate fixation. (a) Medial view, and (b) cranial view.

INTERCONDYLAR FRACTURE OF THE HUMERUS

A similar but greater stress than that which causes a fracture of the lateral condyle results in both the medial and lateral condyles being sheared from their attachment to the diaphysis. This gives rise to an intercondylar fracture which is commonly referred to as a T or Y fracture.

Repair using a lag screw and Rush pin

See Figs 10.84–10.87.

Repair using a bone plate

The fracture is most easily exposed by a caudal approach and osteotomy of the olecranon (Fig. 10.88). The triceps muscle is reflected proximally and the intercondylar fracture repaired with a lag screw. The supracondylar fracture is reduced and immobilized with a plate applied to the caudal aspect of the medial condyle (Fig. 10.89). In giant breed dogs, a second plate can be applied to the caudal aspect of the lateral condyle. The osteotomized olecranon is repaired using a tension band technique (see Fig. 10.92).

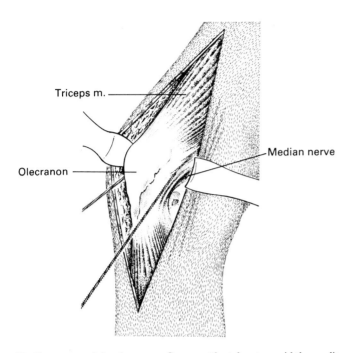

Triceps m.

Olecranon

Median nerve

Fig. 10.88. Osteotomy of the olecranon. Care must be taken to avoid the median nerve which is cranial to the osteotomy.

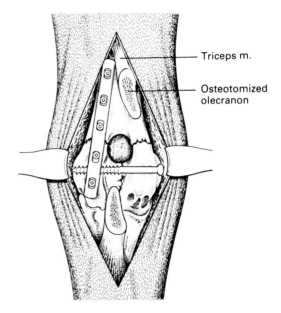

Triceps m.

Osteotomized olecranon

Fig. 10.89. The intercondylar fracture is repaired with a lag screw and the medial condyle immobilized with a bone plate applied to its caudal aspect.

Radius and ulna

FRACTURE OF THE OLECRANON

The most common site of fracture is at the lower end of the semilunar notch. Due to the pull of the triceps muscle, reduction of the fracture cannot be maintained except by internal fixation using the tension band principle. Either two intramedullary pins and a figure-of-eight wire, or a bone plate and screws can be used (Figs 10.90–10.93).

FRACTURE OF THE RADIUS AND ULNA

Complete and overriding fractures of the radius and ulna are extremely difficult to reduce and align accurately by closed methods. Unless accurate reduction and alignment are attained together with rigid immobilization, mal-union and non-unions can result. For these reasons, and because it is essential that a dog's radius should be in perfect alignment, these fractures are most satisfactorily treated by an open reduction and internal fixation with a bone plate and screws.

To ensure that an accurate alignment of the leg is obtained it is necessary to be able to see and manipulate the forepaw. Disinfection of the digits is essential to prevent contamination of the surgical

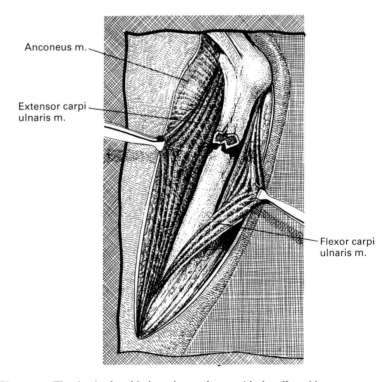

Anconeus m.

Extensor carpi ulnaris m.

Flexor carpi ulnaris m.

Fig. 10.90. The dog is placed in lateral recumbency with the affected leg uppermost. The fracture is exposed by a caudo-lateral skin incision extending from above the point of the elbow to some 5 cm distal to the fracture. The extensor carpi ulnaris and flexor carpi ulnaris muscles are separated and retracted to expose the fracture site and the lateral surface of the olecranon and ulna.

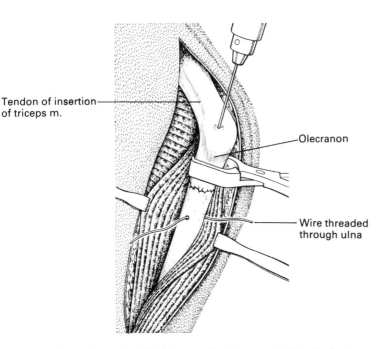

Tendon of insertion of triceps m.

Olecranon

Wire threaded through ulna

Fig. 10.91. A small tunnel is drilled through the olecranon distal to the fracture and a length of wire threaded through it. The fracture is reduced and a small intramedullary pin or Kirschner wire is drilled from the point of the olecranon distally.

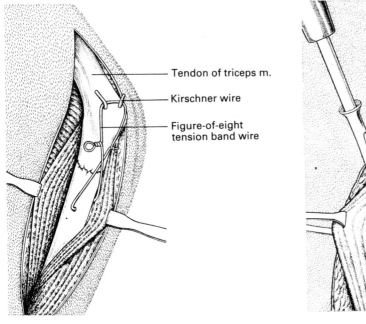

Tendon of triceps m.

Kirschner wire

Figure-of-eight tension band wire

Fig. 10.92. A second pin is driven parallel to the first. The stainless steel wire is taken around the pins and tightened as shown. The loop enables both sides of the wire to be tightened independently. The ends of the pins are bent over, cut short and rotated so that they finish flush with the tendon of the triceps.

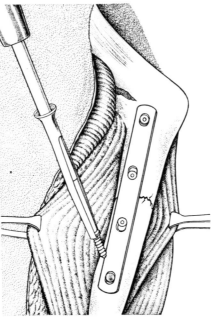

Fig. 10.93. An alternative technique, particularly applicable when fractures are comminuted, is to immobilize the fracture with a laterally applied bone plate.

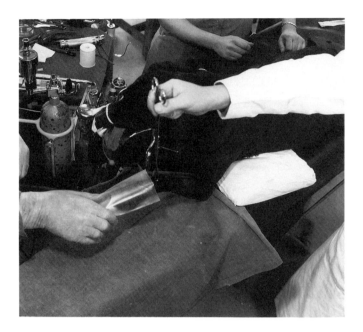

Fig. 10.94. The leg is held in tissue forceps, disinfected in the usual way, a drape placed beneath it and a nylon bag put over the digits.

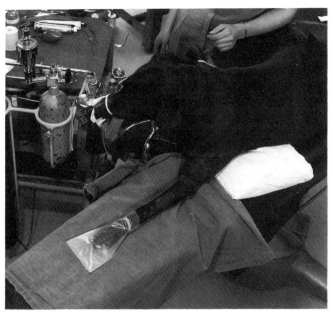

Fig. 10.95. The nylon bag is tied in position with a tape and the leg draped by passing it through a hole in a laparotomy sheet.

field. This presents difficulties and whatever method is employed it is not without its disadvantages, but the problem can be overcome by putting the disinfected foot into a sterile nylon autoclave bag (Figs 10.94–10.95).

The radius is approached from the cranial aspect by a midline skin incision and its shaft exposed (Fig. 10.96). The fractured ends are isolated and freed by blunt dissection and realigned (Fig. 10.97).

FRACTURE OF DISTAL EXTREMITY OF THE RADIUS

Fractures of the distal extremity of the radius are difficult to immobilize with a standard bone plate if the distal fragment is small. In the smaller breeds non-union is a frequent complication and the fractures are best repaired with ASIF miniplates or special T plates. If these are unavailable they can be treated with an intramedullary pin inserted via the antebrachio-carpal joint (Figs 10.98–10.101). In either instance, packing the fracture site with cancellous bone is advised.

The incision is closed with the joint extended. The joint capsule and fascia are co-apted with a continuous suture using synthetic absorbable suture material, the tendons are repositioned and the

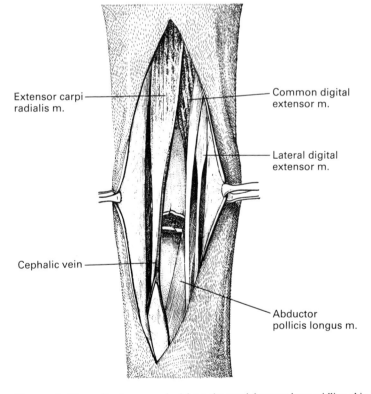

Extensor carpi radialis m.

Common digital extensor m.

Lateral digital extensor m.

Cephalic vein

Abductor pollicis longus m.

Fig. 10.96. The radius is approached from the cranial aspect by a midline skin incision extending from just below the elbow to a little above the carpus. The skin is reflected and the cephalic vein isolated and retracted medially. The shaft of the radius is exposed by separating the extensor carpi radialis and common digital extensor muscles along their line of cleavage. Isolation and freeing the fractured ends by blunt dissection presents little difficulty.

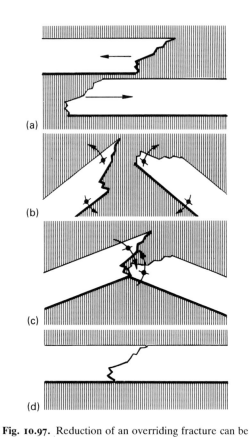

Fig. 10.97. Reduction of an overriding fracture can be difficult especially if it is of several days standing and accompanied by muscle contracture. This is easily overcome by elevating the two ends (b), fitting them together (c) and pressing them back into normal alignment (d).

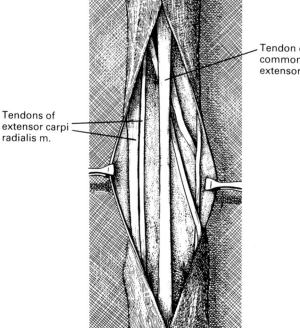

Fig. 10.98. The distal extremity of the radius is exposed by a longitudinal skin incision over the cranial aspect of the carpus extending from the lower third of the radius to the proximal extremity of the metacarpus.

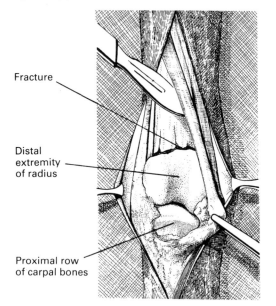

Fig. 10.99. The tendons of the extensor carpi radialis and common digital extensor are separated along their line of cleavage and retracted. The fractured ends are freed by blunt dissection, reduced and aligned. The fascia and joint capsule are incised and the antebrachiocarpal joint flexed to expose the articular surfaces.

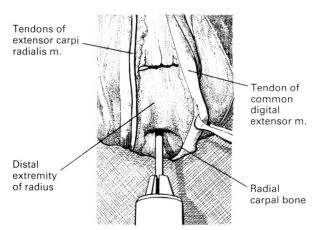

Fig. 10.100. An intramedullary pin is inserted via the distal articular surface of the radius. In some cases it is helpful first to drill a hole before inserting the pin.

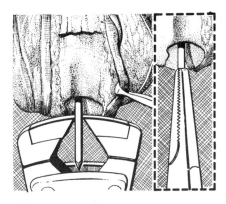

Fig. 10.101. The pin is driven half to two-thirds up the medullary cavity of the radius. It is then withdrawn, 0.5 cm cut off and driven home flush with or below the surface of the articular cartilage.

skin closed in the usual manner. Post operation the joint is supported in a cast until healing is established.

THORACIC LIMB DEFORMITIES

For a dog to develop normally the radius and ulna must grow in unison. In the larger breeds of dogs, deformities of their legs often develop during their period of rapid growth.

Premature closure of the distal ulnar growth plate, while the radius continues to grow at its normal rate, has a 'bow-string' effect, and is followed by a cranial bowing of the radius with lateral deviation of the foot. This deformity can be corrected by removing 1.5−2 cm of the middle of the shaft of the ulna (Figs 10.102−10.103).

In severe cases, it is necessary to prevent further growth of the medial aspect of the radial distal growth plate by stapling (Fig. 10.104).

Segmental ulnar ostectomy and transepiphyseal stapling is best performed before the dog is 6 months old, so as to capitalize on its remaining growth potential. Significant straightening of the limb is unlikely after this age.

Cuneiform osteotomy

A mal-union fracture of the radius and ulna with gross distortion or an uncorrected growth deformity can be realigned by a cuneiform osteotomy (Figs 10.105−10.106).

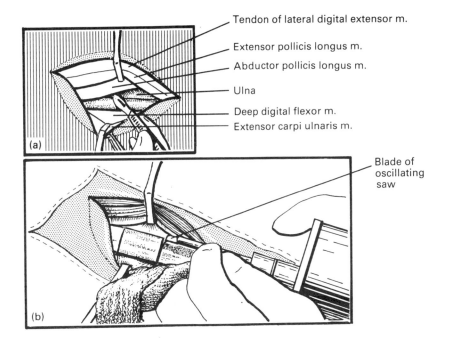

Tendon of lateral digital extensor m.

Extensor pollicis longus m.

Abductor pollicis longus m.

Ulna

Deep digital flexor m.

Extensor carpi ulnaris m.

Blade of oscillating saw

Fig. 10.102. (a) A longitudinal skin incision is made along the palpable lateral border of the shaft of the ulna. The lateral digital extensor and extensor carpi ulnaris muscles are separated by blunt dissection to expose the shaft of the ulna which is isolated by freeing the attachments of the abductor pollicis muscle. (b) Using an oscillating saw a 1.5−2-cm section of the ulna is removed. Care must be taken that no periosteum remains as this stimulates healing and leads to rapid bridging of the gap which is not the purpose of the resection.

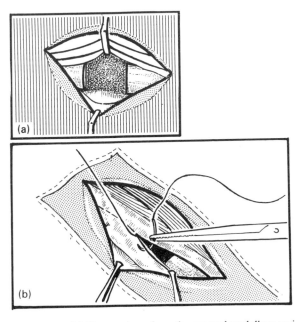

Fig. 10.103. (a) Haemorrhage from the exposed medullary cavity of the gap in the ulna is considerable and can be controlled by plugging it with absorbable gelatin sponge. (b) The resection is protected by co-apting over it the lateral digital extensor and extensor carpi ulnaris muscles with a continuous suture and the skin is then sutured in the usual manner.

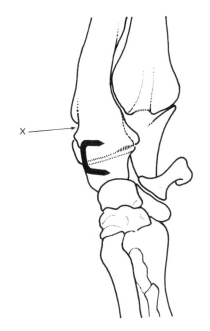

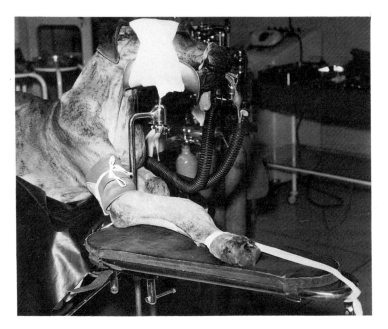

Fig. 10.104. As a rule one staple bridging the growth plate on the medial aspect is adequate but if considered necessary a second staple can be placed cranio-medially. Care must be taken in locating the exact position of the growth plate with a needle, as the notch X can easily be mistaken for it. It is always advisable to check radiologically that the staples are correctly positioned. (For details of the technique of inserting staples see Fig. 10.10.)

Fig. 10.105. The dog is supported in ventral recumbency, an Esmarch's bandage and tourniquet applied and the leg supported on an extension board. The leg is prepared in the usual manner, a nylon bag tied over the foot and the limb draped by passing it through the hole in a laparotomy sheet. This enables the leg to be freely manipulated during the operation.

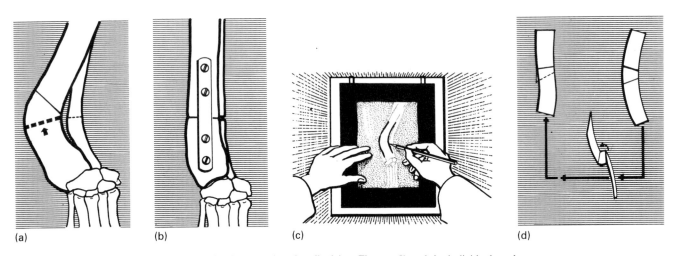

(a)   (b)   (c)   (d)

Fig. 10.106. (a) The cranial shaft of the radius is exposed as described (see Fig. 10.98) and the individual tendons dissected free. A wedge of bone is removed from the radius at the point of maximum curvature using an osteotome, and the ulna is severed with bone-cutting forceps. If available, an oscillating saw will make these osteotomies quicker and less traumatic.

During these procedures care must be taken to conserve the blood supply to the foot. Also it should be noted that the radius cannot be aligned until the ulna is divided. When cutting the wedge it is an advantage to make the distal saw-cut parallel to the antebrachio-carpal joint and to angulate the proximal saw-cut to fashion the size of the wedge to be removed.

(b) The radius is aligned and immobilized with a bone plate and screws. This operation results in some shortening of the leg which is directly related to the size of wedge removed.

(c–d) The size of the osteotomy to be performed can be accurately predetermined by making a tracing of the outline of the deformed bone from radiographs taken pre-operatively, cutting it out, and then folding it over at the point of maximum curvature to produce a straight bone.

Carpus

FRACTURE OF THE ACCESSORY CARPAL BONE

A small chip fracture of the ventral border of the accessory carpal bone is a relatively common injury in Greyhounds. If the chip is small it should be excised carefully (Figs 10.107–10.109). Larger slab fractures should be immobilized with a 1.5-mm screw.

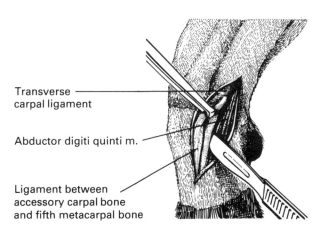

Transverse carpal ligament

Abductor digiti quinti m.

Ligament between accessory carpal bone and fifth metacarpal bone

Fig. 10.108. The ligament and digiti quinti muscle are separated along their line of cleavage and the incision extended to sever the carpal transverse ligament.

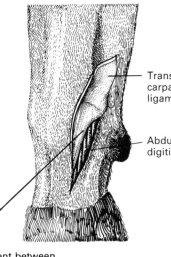

Transverse carpal ligament

Abductor digiti quinti m.

Ligament between accessory carpal bone and fifth metacarpal bone

Fig. 10.107. A skin incision approximately 4 cm long is made obliquely across the lateral aspect of the accessory carpal bone and the skin edges reflected to expose the carpal transverse ligament, the ligament between the accessory carpal bone and the fifth metacarpal bone and the abductor digiti quinti muscle.

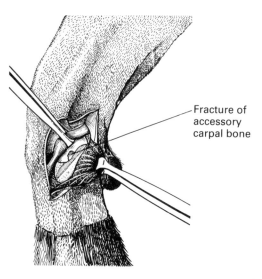

Fracture of accessory carpal bone

Fig. 10.109. The ligament and muscle are retracted and their attachments to the accessory carpal bone dissected free to expose the ventral border of the bone. The detached piece of bone is dissected free and any bony projections are removed with bone-nibbling forceps and the incision closed in the usual manner.

Phalanges

SUBLUXATION OF THE PROXIMAL INTERPHALANGEAL JOINT

This injury is especially common in Greyhounds. It may vary from a Type I sprain associated with stretching or tearing of one collateral ligament to a Type III sprain with rupture of both collateral ligaments, with or without avulsion chip fractures.

Type I sprains should be supported in a padded bandage for 3–4 weeks and the nail trimmed to reduce leverage on the affected joint. In Type II luxations, one of the collateral ligaments is completely severed and must be repaired with horizontal mattress sutures of non-absorbable material or polydioxanone. The joint should be supported for 6 weeks post-operatively. Type II luxations which remain as persistently painful joints and Type III sprains may be treated by amputation of the digit or arthrodesis of the affected joint (Figs 10.110–10.113).

The articular surfaces are debrided and the joint immobilized in a normal standing position with a horizontal mattress suture of stainless steel wire. Additional stability can be attained by using a small bone plate applied to the dorsal aspect of the phalanges or with a Kirschner wire inserted across the joint.

Arthrodesis of the proximal interphalangeal joint

See Figs 10.110–10.112.

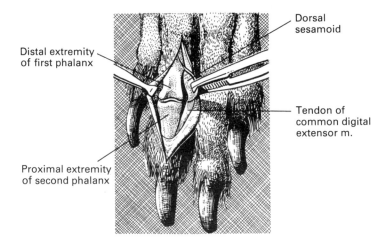

Fig. 10.110. The joint is exposed by a longitudinal skin incision over its dorsal aspect. The tendon of the digital extensor muscle together with the sesamoid bone is freed and held to one side.

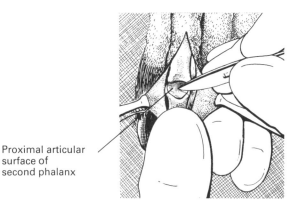

Fig. 10.111. The joint is flexed and the articular cartilage curetted off the ends of the bones.

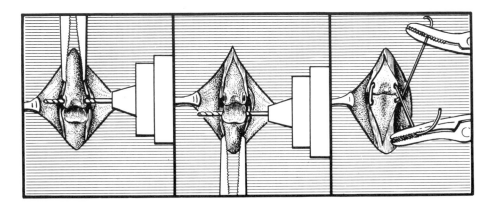

Fig. 10.112. Using a 1.5-mm drill the distal extremity of the first phalanx and the proximal extremity of the second phalanx are drilled transversely so that the drill enters and emerges at the points of origin and insertion of the collateral ligaments respectively. A monofilament stainless steel wire is threaded through the holes and then, with the joint in the normal standing position, twisted tightly. The twisted end is cut off short and pressed flat against the lateral aspect of the second phalanx. The extensor tendon and sesamoid bone are repositioned and the skin closed in the usual manner.

Arthrodesis using a Kirschner wire

Both the methods described for arthrodesing this joint have their advocates. In practice, the wire suture tends to break before arthrodesis is established but the Kirschner wire although it is technically more difficult to insert, provides better immobilization of the joint (Fig. 10.113). Further strength can be provided by employing a figure-of-eight tension band wire over the dorsal aspect of the joint.

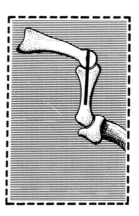

Fig. 10.113. Kirschner wire used to immobilize the proximal interphalangeal joint.

Pelvic limb — horse

Stifle joint

UPWARD FIXATION OF THE PATELLA

Intermittent upward fixation of the patella occurs in all types of horses of all ages but more especially in ponies and young stock. When the stifle joint is extended the patella rides upwards on the trochlea and slips over its rim (Fig. 10.114). This results in a temporary fixation which is followed almost immediately by release of the patella.

The operation most frequently performed to alleviate this condition is desmotomy of the medial patellar ligament. It is designed to release the tension on the accessory cartilage and to prevent it hooking over the trochlea. Relief is obtained by either severing or resecting 1.5—2.5 cm of the medial patellar ligament.

It is customary to perform the operation with the horse standing under local analgesia. The ligament is located by palpation and a stab incision is made through the skin and underlying fascia just medial to its midpoint. Through this incision a tenotome is passed on flat, under the medial ligament and then turned on edge to sever it. The authors prefer, however, to expose the ligament with the horse under general anaesthesia, and remove a 1.5—2.5-cm section of its length (Fig. 10.115).

OSTEOCHONDRITIS DISSECANS

In the horse, osteochondritis dissecans most

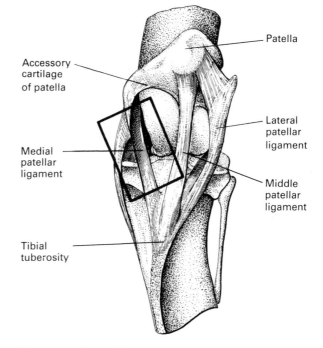

Fig. 10.114. The medial patellar ligament is an extension of the accessory cartilage of the patella. The cartilage becomes hooked over the medial trochlea of the femur during upward fixation. The figure shows a cranial view of the left stifle joint.

frequently affects the lateral trochlear ridge of the distal femur. The results of conservative treatment are generally poor and entail a rest of at least 6 months before the result can be assessed. Surgical

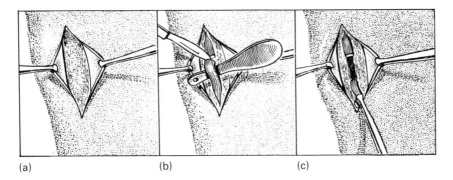

(a)   (b)   (c)

Fig. 10.115. The horse is placed in dorsal recumbency and the hind leg extended. Using the tibial tuberosity as a landmark the medial patellar ligament is located by palpation. (a) A skin incision 4–5 cm long is made parallel with the medial edge of the ligament and midway between the tibial tuberosity and the accessory cartilage of the patella. This exposes the underlying fascia. (b) The fascia is incised and the medial patellar ligament is picked up with a tenaculum and brought out through the incision. (c) The ligament is divided and 1.5–2.5 cm removed. If this does not result in the normal free movement of the patella when the stifle joint is flexed and extended, then it is necessary to incise the aponeurosis of the gracilis and sartorius muscles which blend with the medial patellar ligament, at the midpoint of the incision to the depth of 1.5 cm. The incision is closed by co-apting the fascia and skin with three or four interrupted sutures of synthetic absorbable suture material and monofilament nylon respectively.

treatment is the method of choice; the majority of cases return to normal work.

With the horse in lateral recumbency, and the affected leg uppermost and extended, an arthrotomy of the femoropatellar joint is performed, between the lateral and middle patellar ligaments, to expose the lateral trochlear ridge.

A skin incision, 10–12 cm in length is made extending from the base of the patella between the lateral and middle patellar ligaments to the tibial crest. The superficial and deep fascia is next incised to expose the cranial fat pad. This is either incised likewise or an eliptical portion removed to expose the joint capsule which is then incised to expose the lateral trochlear ridge.

Any detached pieces or fragments of cartilage are removed and the lesion curetted leaving it with a smooth cartilaginous edge. If the crater is not haemorrhagic then four to six holes (2 mm diameter) should be drilled into the underlying cancellous bone to promote vascularization.

Prior to closure, the joint is flushed with isotonic saline solution. The arthrotomy is closed by co-apting the joint capsule and the edge of the fat pad with a continuous suture and the superficial and deep fascia together with interrupted sutures using a 4 metric synthetic absorbable suture material, and the skin with mattress sutures using monofilament nylon. The incision is protected by over-sewing a gauze pad.

Post-operatively, the horse should be rested for 3 months before being returned gradually to work.

CYST OF THE MEDIAL FEMORAL CONDYLE

Horses treated conservatively with 6 months rest result in recovery in approximately 50 per cent of cases. Surgical treatment is indicated in those cases

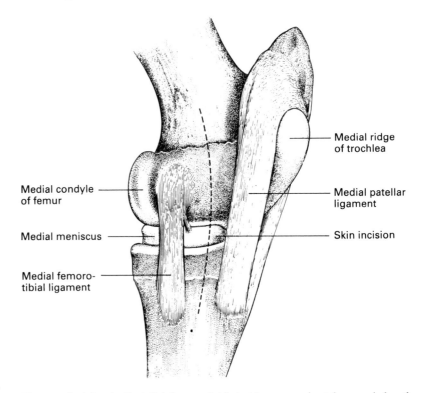

Medial ridge of trochlea

Medial patellar ligament

Skin incision

Medial condyle of femur

Medial meniscus

Medial femoro-tibial ligament

Fig. 10.116. A longitudinal slightly curved skin incision, approximately 15 cm in length, is made between the medial femorotibial ligament and the medial straight patellar ligament. The incision is continued through the connective tissue and fascia to expose the joint capsule, which is then incised longitudinally.

which are severely lame when first examined and those which remain lame after conservative treatment.

Treatment comprises a medial arthrotomy of the femorotibial joint, removing the inverted cartilage from around the opening of the cyst, and curetting the cyst to remove its lining and any detritus (Figs 10.116–10.117). This is followed by packing the cavity firmly with an autogenous cancellous bone graft obtained from the contralateral tuber coxae. In approximately 60 per cent of cases the cavity is subsequently filled with either normal bone or a mixed fibrocancellous bone, the cyst opening is obliterated by fibrocartilage and a normal functioning joint is re-established.

The operation is performed under general anaesthesia with the horse lying on its side with the affected leg ventral and the uppermost leg extended forwards.

Packing the cyst

Pieces of cancellous bone are firmly packed into the cavity, using a punch, until it is completely filled without encroaching on the edges of the surrounding articular cartilage.

The incision is closed by co-apting the joint capsule with a continuous suture and the fascia with interrupted sutures using 3 metric synthetic absorbable material, and the skin with mattress sutures of monofilament nylon.

Obtaining the autogenous cancellous bone graft

The cancellous bone graft is obtained from the

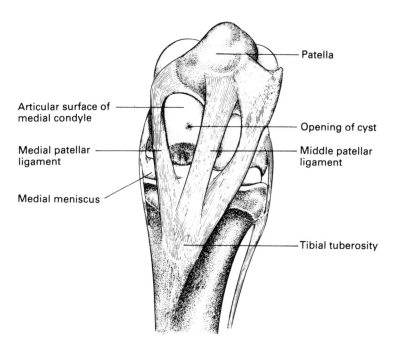

Fig. 10.117. The medial femorotibial and medial patellar ligaments are retracted and the joint slowly flexed to bring the opening of the cyst into view and positioned for curettage and packing.

contralateral tuber coxae (Figs 10.118–10.119). A 10–12-cm incision is made along the middle of the quadrangular mass forming the tuber coxae. The subcutaneous tissues are incised and the fat either reflected or removed to expose the periosteum. The incision is closed by co-apting the periosteum and subcutaneous tissues with a continuous suture using 3 metric synthetic absorbable material and the skin with mattress sutures of monofilament nylon.

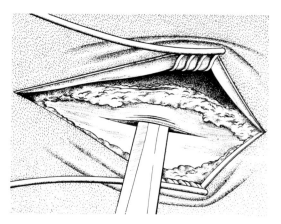

Fig. 10.118. The periosteum is incised longitudinally and reflected with a periosteal elevator.

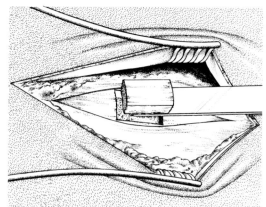

Fig. 10.119. A rectangular piece of cortical bone, measuring 1.5 × 3.0 cm is removed with an osteotome to expose the underlying cancellous bone, pieces of which are removed with a gouge and immediately wrapped in a blood-soaked swab.

Hock joint

BONE SPAVIN DISEASE

Bone spavin is a degenerative joint disease of the 'low motion' joints of the hock, usually involving the distal intertarsal and tarso-metatarsal joints. Occasionally the proximal intertarsal joints are involved.

Non-surgical treatment in the form of exercise with or without the use of non-steroidal anti-inflammatory drugs can result in spontaneous bony ankylosis of the joints and remission of the lameness. This is unpredictable, however, and may take a long time.

Arthrodesis of the distal intertarsal and tarso-metatarsal joints is an alternative method of treatment which is indicated in cases in which the degenerative joint disease changes are characterized by osteolysis with no, or only minimal, periosteal reaction. The principle of the procedure is the surgical destruction of approximately 60 per cent of the opposing articular surfaces thereby inducing a rigid ankylosis.

The operation is performed under general anaesthesia with the horse in lateral recumbency and the affected leg undermost. The joint or joints to be drilled are located on the cranio-medial aspect of the hock just caudal to the saphenous vein using 23 gauge hypodermic needles; correct positioning being checked radiographically. A 5-cm vertical skin incision is made exposing the cunean tendon from which a 2-cm section is removed. Drilling of the distal intertarsal joint is commenced through a stab incision in the ligaments and joint capsule, using a 3.5-mm bit, preferably in a hand drill. The direction of this first track is checked radiographically soon after it is begun to ensure it is along the plane of the joint. If found to be correct, it is used as a guide for all subsequent drill tracks. Depending on the size of the horse, three to four tracks, radiating from the original drill hole (Fig. 10.120) are sufficient to destroy the required amount of articular cartilage. Care should be taken to avoid excessive drilling which can lead to joint instability and much greater post-operative discomfort. The procedure is repeated on the tarsometatarsal joint if this is involved also. After removing any bone debris by flushing with sterile saline, the wound is closed in two layers. Parenteral antibiotics and oral phenylbutazone are administered for 5 days post-operatively. The horse is confined to a box for 1 month, with walking exercise in hand during the second 2 weeks. Thereafter exercise is progressively increased provided it does

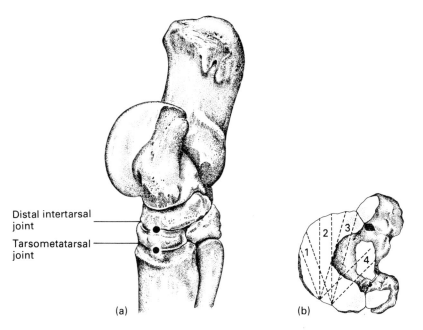

Distal intertarsal joint

Tarsometatarsal joint

(a)   (b)

Fig. 10.120. (a) Medial aspect of the hock, and (b) 1–4: drill tracks.

not cause the animal undue discomfort. Approximately 75 per cent of horses return to soundness 5–10 months after surgery.

STRINGHALT

Stringhalt is an involuntary flexion of one or both hind legs during progression. The aetiology is unknown but in many cases the condition can be relieved by removing 15–18 cm of the tendon of the lateral digital extensor (Fig. 10.121).

The operation is performed with the horse in lateral recumbency and the affected leg uppermost. A longitudinal skin incision on line with the point of the hock and 7.5–10 cm in length is made along the muscle belly of the lateral digital extensor. The underlying layer of thick fascia is incised to expose the muscle which is isolated by blunt dissection. The identity of the muscle is confirmed by pulling on it and noting movement at its distal attachment to the tendon of the long digital extensor. Next the tendon of the lateral digital extensor is exposed by a 2.5-cm skin incision just proximal to its junction with the tendon of the long digital extensor. It is isolated by blunt dissection and severed. Finally, traction is applied to the proximal portion and the severed tendon pulled up through the incision. The tendon is then severed proximally together with 7.5–10 cm of muscle belly.

In some cases extraction of the tendon is difficult due to adhesions where it crosses the hock and they have to be broken down.

After removal of the tendon the fascia at the proximal incision is co-apted with a continuous suture using 3 metric synthetic absorbable material and then both skin incisions with interrupted sutures using monofilament nylon. It is important that the horse is given walking exercise, which is gradually increased, from the day following operation to prevent the formation of adhesions during wound healing.

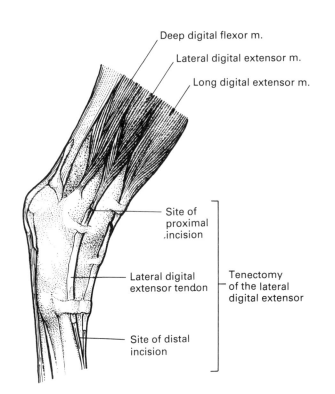

Deep digital flexor m.

Lateral digital extensor m.

Long digital extensor m.

Site of proximal incision

Lateral digital extensor tendon

Tenectomy of the lateral digital extensor

Site of distal incision

Fig. 10.121. Lateral aspect of the right hock. Note the proximal and distal sites for performing tenectomy of the lateral digital extensor.

Pelvic limb — dog

Pelvis

Fracture of the pelvis is a relatively common sequel to road accidents. In the absence of serious nerve injury which may cause either hind leg paralysis or bladder dysfunction, the majority of dogs with pelvic injuries make remarkably good recoveries in spite of very extensive bone damage.

In certain cases where there is gross bone displacement, particularly when the fractures are bilateral or the acetabulum is involved, open reduction and internal fixation is necessary (Fig. 10.122). The surgical exposure of the ilium is along the long axis of its ventral border, incising the aponeurosis of the tensor fascia lata ventrally and the sartorius muscle cranially. The exposure is continued by subperiosteal elevation and dorsal reflection of the middle and deep gluteal muscles. Exposure of the acetabulum is best performed by osteotomy of the great trochanter. The osteo-

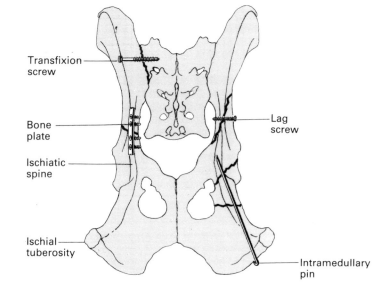

Transfixion screw

Bone plate

Ischiatic spine

Ischial tuberosity

Lag screw

Intramedullary pin

Fig. 10.122. Some common fractures of the pelvis in the dog which, when accompanied by gross bone displacement, are most satisfactorily treated by open reduction and fixation by the methods indicated.

tomized portion is subsequently repaired with a lag screw or tension band wire.

Fixation may be achieved by the use of transfixion and lag screws, or by the application of small bone plates. Ischial fractures may be immobilized by means of an intramedullary pin inserted at the ischial tuberosity and lodged in the ischiatic spine. Acetabular fractures are best repaired with a care-fully contoured bone plate. An ASIF reconstruction plate is ideal since it can be contoured in three planes.

Most pelvic fractures cause a reduction in the size of the pelvic inlet, and this must be borne in mind when dealing with the condition in the breeding bitch.

Hip joint

AMPUTATION OF THE FEMORAL HEAD

Excision arthroplasty is frequently employed in the treatment of fractures of the femoral neck, osteoarthritis and ischaemic necrosis of the femoral head. A false joint is established which, especially in small dogs, functions most efficiently.

A number of methods are practised to expose the hip joint but in the authors' experience the cranio-lateral approach has much to commend it (Figs 10.123–10.129). This method provides a good exposure, enabling the joint capsule to be accurately co-apted to ensure the formation of a satisfactory false joint.

The joint capsule is co-apted with horizontal mattress sutures using absorbable synthetic suture material. The tenotomized portion of the deep gluteal muscle is similarly repaired, followed by co-aptation of the biceps femoris and the tensor fascia lata by a continuous suture. The skin incision is closed in the usual manner.

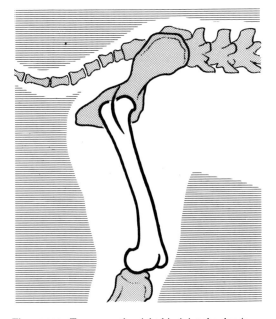

Fig. 10.123. To expose the right hip joint the dog is restrained in lateral recumbency with the affected hip joint uppermost. The joint is exposed by a curved skin incision commencing from a point 2.5–5.0 cm above the greater trochanter and extending distally along the line of the femur to terminate at its upper third.

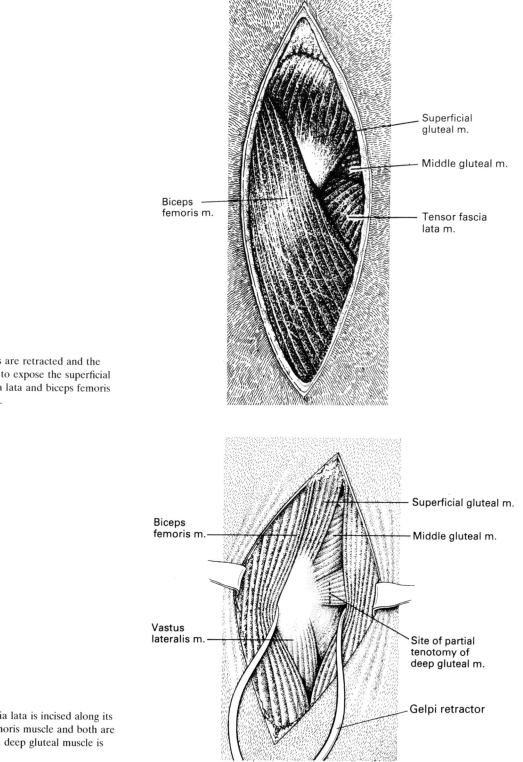

Superficial
gluteal m.

Middle gluteal m.

Tensor fascia
lata m.

Biceps
femoris m.

Fig. 10.124. The skin edges are retracted and the subcutaneous fat separated to expose the superficial gluteal muscle, tensor fascia lata and biceps femoris muscle in the right hind leg.

Biceps
femoris m.

Vastus
lateralis m.

Superficial gluteal m.

Middle gluteal m.

Site of partial
tenotomy of
deep gluteal m.

Gelpi retractor

Fig. 10.125. The tensor fascia lata is incised along its attachment to the biceps femoris muscle and both are retracted. The tendon of the deep gluteal muscle is partially tenotomized.

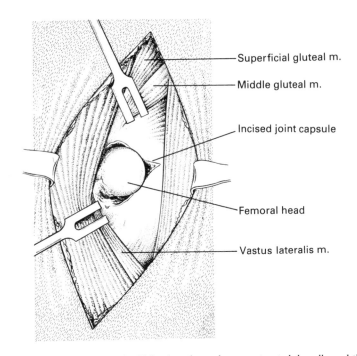

Superficial gluteal m.

Middle gluteal m.

Incised joint capsule

Femoral head

Vastus lateralis m.

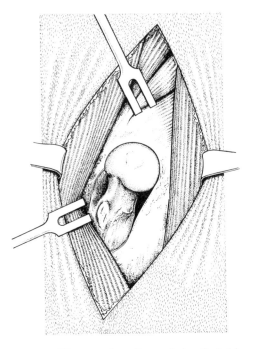

Fig. 10.126. The superficial and middle gluteal muscles are retracted dorsally and the vastus lateralis is retracted caudally. The joint capsule is incised about two-thirds of the way around the circumference of the acetabulum and some 0.3 cm from its attachment to the rim. The stifle is externally rotated through 90° so that the femoral head is disarticulated. It may be necessary to divide the teres ligament with curved scissors in order to achieve this.

Fig. 10.127. The vastus lateralis muscle is reflected from its origin on the lateral aspect of the proximal femur with a periosteal elevator to expose the femoral neck.

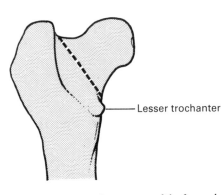

Lesser trochanter

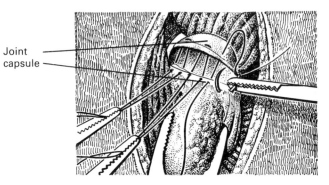

Joint capsule

Fig. 10.128. Direction of osteotomy of the femoral neck. The osteotome or saw is directed distally to the lesser trochanter.

Fig. 10.129. The joint capsule is closed with two or three mattress sutures using synthetic absorbable suture material. All the sutures are laid before tying them.

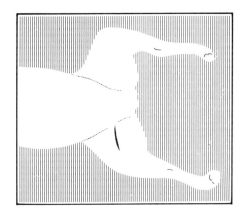

Fig. 10.130. Site of skin incision for exposing the pectineus muscle of the right leg. The dog is placed in dorsal recumbency with the affected leg abducted to expose the medial aspect of the thigh.

PECTINECTOMY

Resection of the pectineus muscle (Figs 10.130–10.32) is employed for the treatment of hip dysplasia. It reduces the tension and improves abduction and extension of the joint but does not allay the progressive development of osteoarthritic changes.

The subcutaneous tissues are co-apted with a continuous suture using 3 metric synthetic absorbable suture material and the skin with interrupted sutures using monofilament nylon.

TRIPLE PELVIC OSTEOTOMY

Triple pelvic osteotomy is used to improve joint congruency in skeletally immature dogs with subluxation of their femoral heads due to hip dysplasia. The acetabular portion of the pelvis is isolated by osteotomy of the pubis, ischium and ilium and rotated to improve the dorsal cover of the femoral head (Fig. 10.133).

The pubis is exposed by performing a pectinectomy (Figs 10.130–132) and sectioned with an osteotome. A portion of the pubic bone may be removed, but if the osteotomy is made close to the medial face of the acetabulum this is generally unnecessary.

The dog is then placed in lateral recumbency and the ischium exposed by subperiosteally elevating the internal obturator and the semimembranosus and quadratus femoris muscles from its dorsal and ventral surfaces respectively. An embryotomy wire is carefully passed through the obturator foramen to section the ischium.

A lateral approach is made to the wing of the

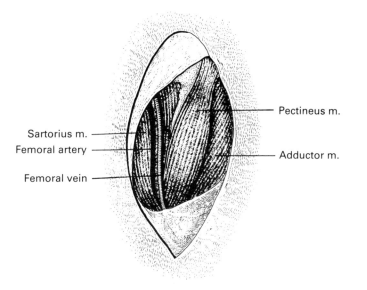

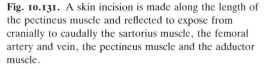

Sartorius m.
Femoral artery
Femoral vein
Pectineus m.
Adductor m.

Fig. 10.131. A skin incision is made along the length of the pectineus muscle and reflected to expose from cranially to caudally the sartorius muscle, the femoral artery and vein, the pectineus muscle and the adductor muscle.

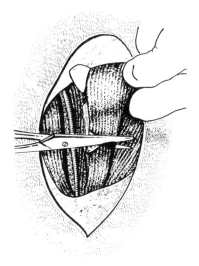

Fig. 10.132. Using blunt dissection and with due care not to injure the femoral artery or vein the pectineus muscle is separated from its neighbours. Experience has shown that satisfactory results are obtained by simply resecting 4–5 cm of its central portion.

ilium, elevating the middle gluteal muscle from its ventral attachment to the tensor fascia lata. The ileum is osteotomized at right angles to the long axis of the pelvis with an oscillating saw or osteotome, freeing the acetabular portion of the pelvis. (Fig 10.133b). This is rotated to increase the dorsal cover of the femoral head and immobilized with a pre-contoured bone plate (Fig. 10.133c). This plate is twisted around its long axis to match the angle required to rotate the acetabulum sufficiently to eliminate dorsal subluxation of the femoral head.

Post-operatively, the dog is restricted to lead exercise until the osteotomies have healed.

SUBTROCHANTERIC FEMORAL OSTEOTOMY

An alternative technique for improving joint congruency in dysplastic dogs is a subtrochanteric femoral osteotomy. This is indicated where the angles of inclination and anteversion of the femoral neck are increased producing coxa valgus. The inclination angle is the angle that the femoral neck makes with the diaphysis when the femur is viewed in a standard ventrodorsal radiographic projection of the pelvis with the femora extended and parallel and the stifles vertical. The normal angle is approximately 145°. The angle of anteversion is the angle that the femoral neck makes with the diaphysis in the horizontal plane. This can be established trigonometrically from measurements taken from ventrodorsal and lateral radiographs of the pelvis and femur.

A subtrochanteric femoral osteotomy involves removal of a wedge of bone from the medial aspect of the femur (Fig. 10.134a) so as to create varisation of the femoral neck. The osteotomy is immobilized with an ASIF double hook plate (Fig. 10.134c) which provides a very secure three point anchorage in the greater trochanter. Careful pre-planning is required to determine the size of the wedge and the osteotomy angle. The optimum post-surgical inclination angle is about 135°.

DISLOCATION OF THE HIP JOINT

Dislocation of the hip joint is very common in the dog. In the majority of cases, provided the acetabulum and femoral head are not dysplastic, a closed reduction by direct traction is satisfactory but if this fails, or if dislocation persistently recurs after repeated reductions then it is necessary to perform an open reduction with fixation (Figs 10.135–10.138).

To retain the head of the femur in the acetabulum the ruptured ligamentum teres is replaced by a prosthesis of braided nylon which is anchored

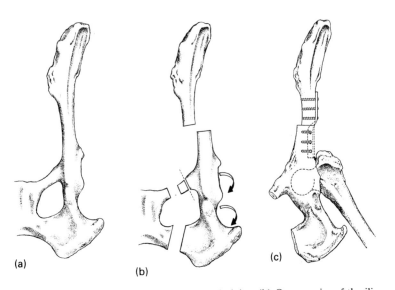

(a) (b) (c)

Fig. 10.133. (a) Hemipelvis with dysplastic hip joint. (b) Osteotomies of the ilium, pubis and ischium permit rotation of the acetabular segment. (c) The ilial osteotomy is immobilized with a pre-contoured bone plate.

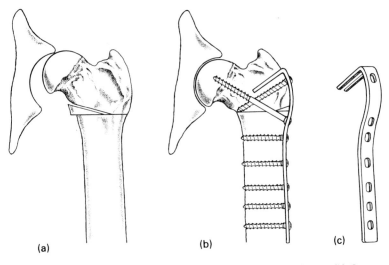

(a) (b) (c)

Fig. 10.134. (a) Wedge removed from the medial aspect of the femur. (b) Osteotomy repaired with double hook plate (c).

behind the acetabular fossa by means of a 'toggle pin'.

The hip joint is exposed by the method described (see Figs 10.124–10.126). The acetabulum is carefully inspected and any blood clot, granulation tissue and remnants of the joint capsule or ligamentum teres removed.

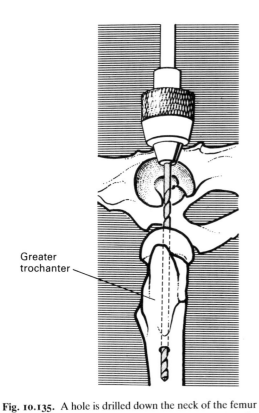

Greater
trochanter

Fig. 10.135. A hole is drilled down the neck of the femur from the point of origin of the ligamentum teres, i.e. the fovea capitis, to emerge at the base of the greater trochanter.

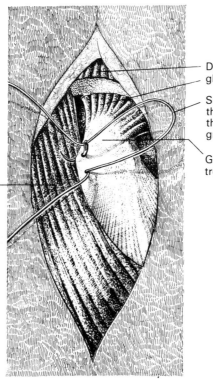

(a)

(b)

(c)

Acetabular
fossa

Head of
femur

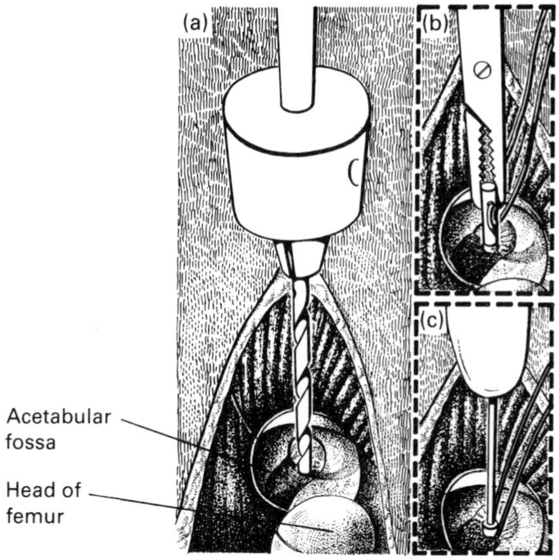

Fig. 10.136. (a) Using a larger drill bit, a hole is drilled through the centre of the acetabular fossa and care taken that the point only just penetrates into the pelvic cavity and does not injure the underlying organs. (b) A 'toggle pin' of slightly smaller diameter than the hole drilled and threaded with braided nylon is inserted into the hole. (Braided nylon: dogs under 15 kg, size 3.5 metric; over 15 kg, size 5 metric.) (c) With a fine probe the toggle pin is pushed through the drill hole until it lies free in the pelvic cavity. The braided nylon is then tensed to bring the toggle pin flush against the medial surface of the acetabulum.

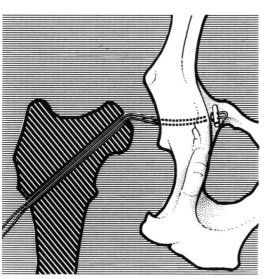

Fig. 10.137. The ends of the braided nylon are threaded through the drill hole in the femoral neck. The head of the femur is repositioned in the acetabulum and the braided nylon pulled taut.

Deep
gluteal m.

Suture being passed
through small hole drilled
through base of
greater trochanter

Greater
trochanter

Biceps
femoris m.

Fig. 10.138. The ends of the braided nylon are tensed to ensure that the head of the femur fits into the acetabulum before passing each end in opposite directions through a hole drilled across the base of the greater trochanter, and securely tying it to its fellow.

Femur

FRACTURE OF THE FEMORAL SHAFT

Fractures of the shaft of the femur are the most common of all fractures encountered in the dog. Owing to the large and powerful muscle groups surrounding the shaft it is impossible to perform effectively a closed reduction or attain external immobilization. The majority of cases are treated by intramedullary fixation, but if the medullary cavity is excessively wide, the shaft has a marked curvature, or the fracture is grossly comminuted then internal fixation with a bone plate is the method of choice.

Exposure of the fracture is shown in Figs 10.139–10.141.

Figures 10.142–10.146 depict a Venables bone plate since these are still widely used. They are neither as strong or versatile as ASIF dynamic compression plates, nor do they permit axial compression as depicted in Fig. 10.8. Nevertheless, provided a plate of adequate size is applied correctly it will provide a rigid form of internal fixation.

Finally, the incision is closed with interrupted sutures (Figs 10.147–10.148).

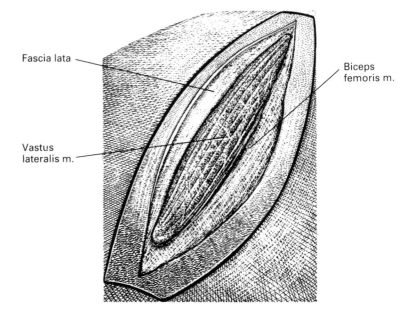

Fig. 10.140. The skin edges are reflected to expose the fascia lata, which is incised along the line of its attachment to the biceps femoris to reveal the vastus lateralis muscle.

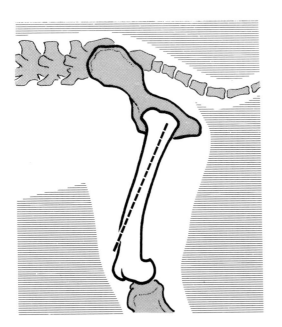

Fig. 10.139. To expose the lateral aspect of the shaft of the femur the dog is placed in lateral recumbency with the affected leg uppermost. The skin is incised practically the whole length of the femur, along the line joining the greater trochanter and the cranial aspect of the stifle joint.

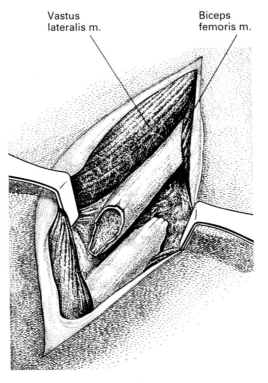

Fig. 10.141. The vastus lateralis and biceps femoris muscles are separated by blunt dissection and retracted to expose the fracture. Blood clots and any detached fragments of bone are removed from the site of fracture.

218

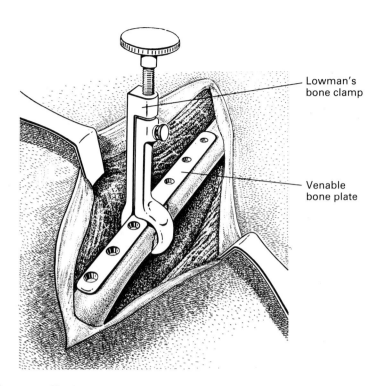

Lowman's
bone clamp

Venable
bone plate

Fig. 10.142. The fractured ends of the bone are freed of muscle attachments and the fracture reduced and aligned. Following reduction, the bone plate is carefully positioned on the lateral surface of the shaft and retained in position with a bone clamp. A Lowman's self-retaining bone clamp is depicted here.

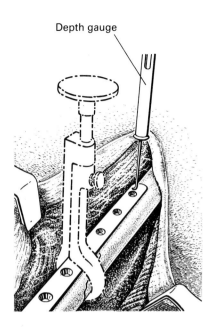

Depth gauge

Fig. 10.144. A screw depth gauge is used to determine accurately the length of screw required. The hooked end is passed down through both drill holes to engage on the outside of the distal cortex, and the adjustable sleeve is fixed against the proximal cortex. The gauge is removed, and the length of screw required read off from the scale or the screw can be measured against the protruding end. The diameter of the shaft of a long bone varies considerably throughout its length, so all screws have to be individually selected after measuring each drill hole.

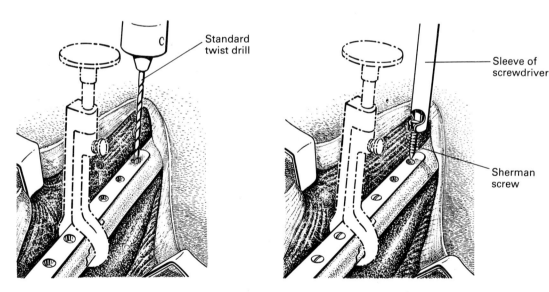

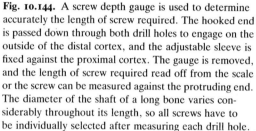

Standard
twist drill

Sleeve of
screwdriver

Sherman
screw

Fig. 10.143. A hole is drilled at right angles to the shaft of the bone and through both cortices with a 2.8-mm twist drill using a hole in the plate as a guide. Care must be taken that the drill does not come in contact with the plate as this results in the transfer of metallic particles which leads to corrosion and tissue reaction.

Fig. 10.145. A standard 3.5-mm Sherman type orthopaedic screw is driven. The second screw to be driven on either side of the fracture fixes the plate in position.

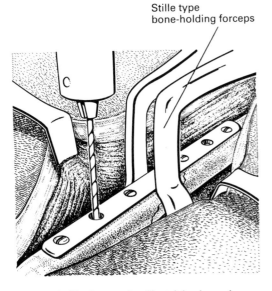

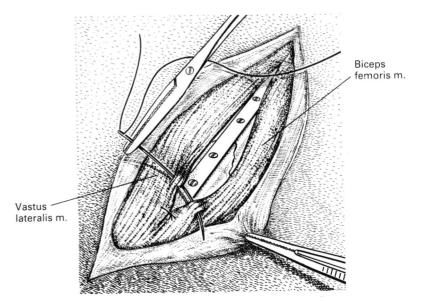

Fig. 10.146. If a Lowman's self-retaining bone clamp cannot be satisfactorily employed then the bone plate can generally be held in position with Stille type bone-holding forceps.

Fig. 10.147. At the distal extremity of the incision the vastus lateralis muscle is retained in position under the biceps femoris muscle with one or two interrupted sutures.

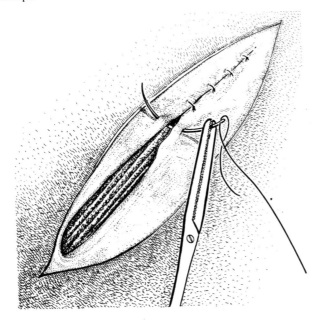

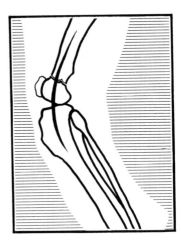

Fig. 10.149. The dog is positioned in lateral recumbency with the affected leg uppermost. The site is exposed via a parapatellar skin incision which extends from the distal third of the femur to the proximal third of the tibia.

Fig. 10.148. The fascia lata and fascia of the biceps femoris muscle are co-apted with interrupted sutures.

FRACTURES OF THE DISTAL FEMUR

In young dogs a fracture of the distal epiphysis of the femur, and in adult dogs a supracondylar fracture, are not uncommon. In both cases the condyles rotate caudally and the distal extremity of the shaft is displaced cranially.

In these cases an open reduction and fixation are essential. Numerous methods have been recommended to immobilize these fractures but the authors find that a small bone plate attached to the lateral surface maintains perfect alignment and immobilization of the supracondylar fracture (Figs 10.149–10.153).

Distal femoral physeal fractures should not be bridged with a bone plate and most of these fractures can be repaired very successfully with crossed Kirschner wires or small intramedullary pins. All implants should be removed as soon as healing is complete so as not to create a growth deformity.

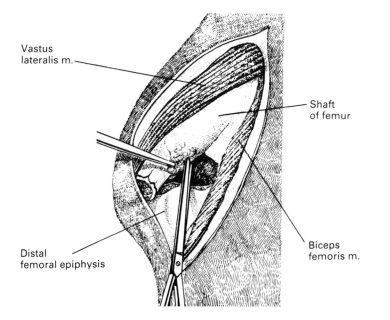

Vastus
lateralis m.

Shaft
of femur

Distal
femoral epiphysis

Biceps
femoris m.

Fig. 10.150. The vastus lateralis and biceps femoris muscles are separated along their line of cleavage and the incision is extended distally through the fascia of the femoropatellar joint and joint capsule. The distal extremity of the shaft of the femur and the detached epiphysis are isolated by blunt dissection.

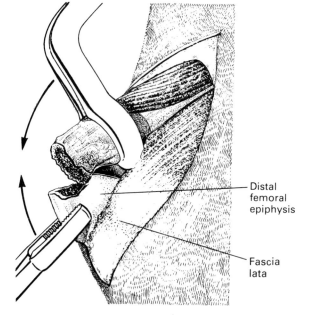

Distal
femoral
epiphysis

Fascia
lata

Fig. 10.151. With the shaft of the femur held in Stille type bone-holding forceps and the detached epiphysis in Frosch bone-holding forceps the bones are aligned, brought into contact and the fracture reduced by extending the joint.

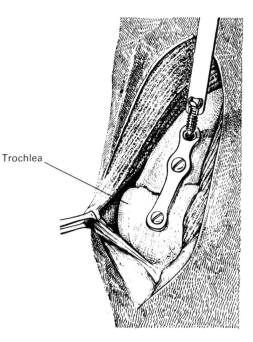

Trochlea

Fig. 10.152. A three-holed bone plate is fixed on the lateral aspect by driving two screws into the distal end of the shaft and one through the condyles. If the fracture involves the physis, it should be repaired with small intramedullary pins or crossed Kirschner wires and the implants removed in 4–6 weeks so that they do not interfere with normal growth.

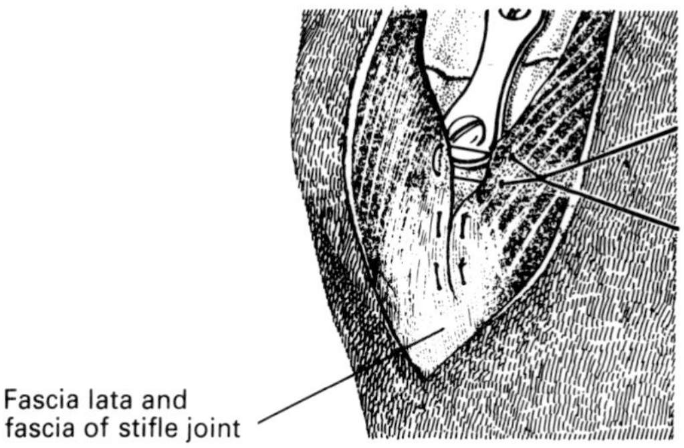

Fascia lata and
fascia of stifle joint

Fig. 10.153. It is important when closing the incision to ensure the patella has been accurately repositioned in the trochlea groove and securely retained in position by co-apting the fascia and joint capsule opposite the patella with mattress sutures using synthetic absorbable suture material.

Stifle joint

RUPTURE OF THE CRANIAL CRUCIATE LIGAMENT

Rupture of the cranial cruciate ligament results in a mechanical instability of the joint, which is followed by degenerative osteoarthritis. The object of treatment is to stabilize the joint. This is attained by replacing the ruptured ligament with a prosthesis.

Patsaama's technique

Many modifications of Patsaama's original method have been suggested but in all cases the prosthesis is inserted through femoral and tibial bone tunnels and anchored at either end. Figures 10.154–10.164 depict skin being used as the prosthesis.

To ensure that the skin prosthesis crosses the intercondyloid fossa in the position originally occupied by the intact cranial cruciate ligament it is necessary to drill two holes. They are referred to as the femoral and tibial tunnels, respectively, and it is essential they emerge in the intercondyloid fossa at the exact points of attachment of the ligament.

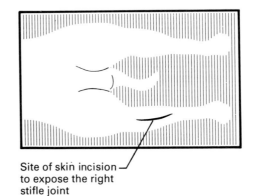

Site of skin incision to expose the right stifle joint

Fig. 10.154. The dog is positioned in dorsal recumbency with the affected leg extended and resting on a sandbag.

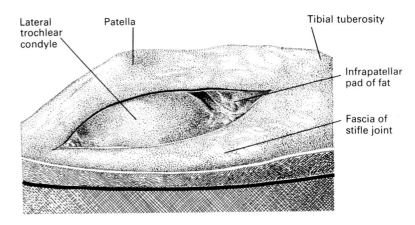

Lateral trochlear condyle — Patella — Tibial tuberosity — Infrapatellar pad of fat — Fascia of stifle joint

Fig. 10.155. The stifle joint is approached from the lateral aspect by a parapatellar skin incision extending from the lower third of the femur to the upper third of the tibia. This exposes the underlying fascia which is incised together with the joint capsule to open the joint.

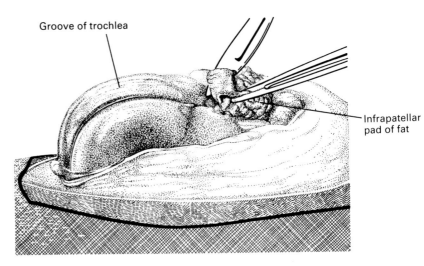

Groove of trochlea — Infrapatellar pad of fat

Fig. 10.156. The patella is dislocated medially to expose the trochlea and infrapatellar pad of fat.

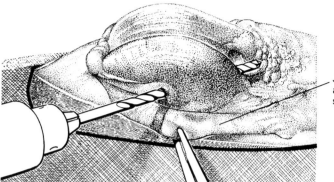

Joint capsule and fascia of stile joint

Fig. 10.157. The femoral tunnel is drilled from just above the origin of the lateral collateral ligament. It emerges on the medial surface of the lateral condyle at the point of attachment of the cranial cruciate ligament.

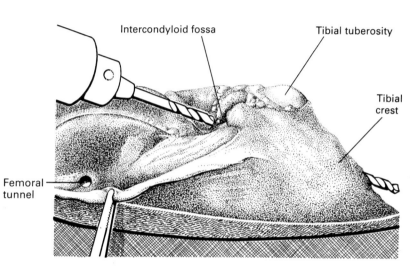

Intercondyloid fossa

Tibial tuberosity

Tibial crest

Femoral tunnel

Fig. 10.158. With the stifle joint in maximum flexion the tibial tunnel is drilled from the intercondyloid fossa to emerge towards the distal extremity of the tibial crest.

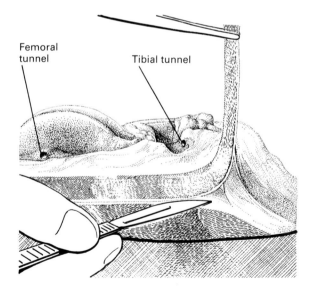

Femoral tunnel

Tibial tunnel

Fig. 10.159. The skin transplant is cut the length of and parallel with the edge of the incision. Its width varies from 3 mm for small dogs to 5 mm for large dogs.

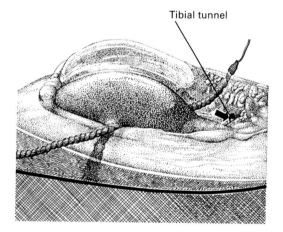

Tibial tunnel

Fig. 10.160. The skin is passed through the femoral and tibial tunnels by twisting it up and attaching a length of monofilament wire to one end. The wire is first passed through the femoral tunnel and the skin pulled through. The wire is then continued down the tibial tunnel followed by the skin.

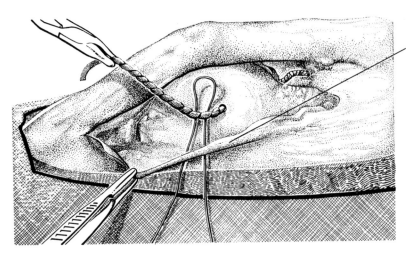

Joint capsule
and fascia
of stifle joint

Fig. 10.161. The patella is repositioned in the trochlea. The skin transplant at the femoral tunnel is anchored by suturing it to the joint capsule and fascia with two mattress sutures using monofilament nylon. Any excess of skin is cut off.

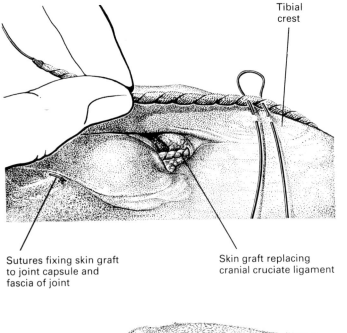

Tibial
crest

Sutures fixing skin graft
to joint capsule and
fascia of joint

Skin graft replacing
cranial cruciate ligament

Fig. 10.162. The stifle is extended. The skin transplant is pulled tight and its end reflected back over the tibial crest and attached to the fascia with two mattress sutures using monofilament nylon.

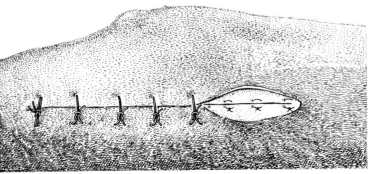

Fig. 10.163. The joint capsule and fascia are co-apted with mattress sutures and the skin incision is closed with interrupted sutures using monofilament nylon.

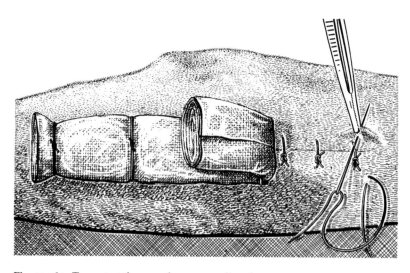

Fig. 10.164. To protect the wound a gauze pad can be oversewn.

'Over the top' technique

An alternative technique, the so-called 'over the top' technique, was described by Arnoczky. This involves fashioning the prosthesis from the medial fascia of the stifle and the medial third of the straight patellar ligament (including a quadrant of the patella). The distal end of the prosthesis remains attached to the tibia and the free end is passed through the joint to emerge over the lateral femoral condyle proximal to the lateral fabella. It is pulled taut and anchored to the dense femoro-fabellar ligament and adjacent periosteum of the femur. The advantages of this technique over Patsaama's method are the lack of bone tunnels on which the prosthesis may fray, the graft retains a vascular supply from its distal attachment and it is sounder biomechanically.

Numerous variations of Arnoczky's original technique are employed. In the authors' experience the procedure shown in Figs 10.165–10.169 provides satisfactory results.

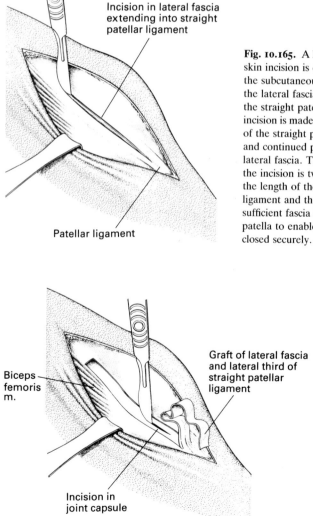

Incision in lateral fascia extending into straight patellar ligament

Patellar ligament

Fig. 10.165. A lateral parapatellar skin incision is continued through the subcutaneous fascia to expose the lateral fascia of the stifle and the straight patellar ligament. An incision is made in the lateral third of the straight patellar ligament and continued proximally into the lateral fascia. The total length of the incision is two to three times the length of the straight patellar ligament and there should be sufficient fascia left lateral to the patella to enable the joint to be closed securely.

Biceps femoris m.

Graft of lateral fascia and lateral third of straight patellar ligament

Incision in joint capsule

Fig. 10.166. A second incision is made parallel to the first so that a graft 1.0–1.5 cm in width is created. It is left attached distally. The joint capsule is then incised along a similar line.

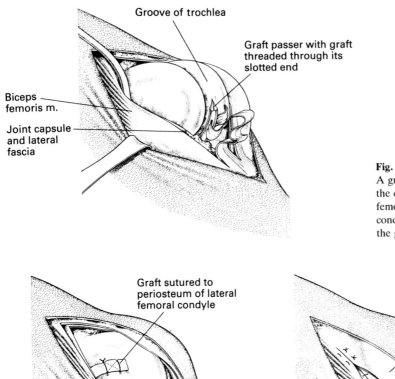

Groove of trochlea

Graft passer with graft threaded through its slotted end

Biceps femoris m.

Joint capsule and lateral fascia

Fig. 10.167. The patella is luxated medially and the joint flexed. A graft passer is inserted within the joint and pushed through the caudo-lateral aspect of the joint capsule, through the dense femorofabellar ligament, so that it emerges between the femoral condyles lateral to the caudal cruciate ligament. The free end of the graft is threaded through the graft passer.

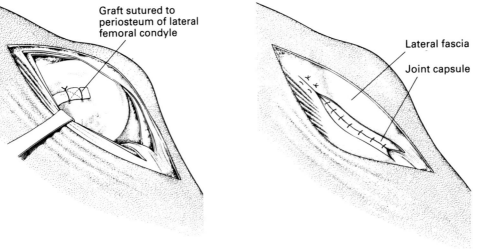

Graft sutured to periosteum of lateral femoral condyle

Lateral fascia

Joint capsule

Fig. 10.168. The graft is pulled taut and anchored with doubled 3.5-mm monofilament nylon to the adjacent dense fascia and the periosteum of the lateral femoral condyle.

Fig. 10.169. The joint capsule is closed with cruciate mattress sutures of synthetic absorbable material. The lateral fascia is repaired with horizontal mattress sutures of similar material and subcutaneous tissues and skin are routinely closed.

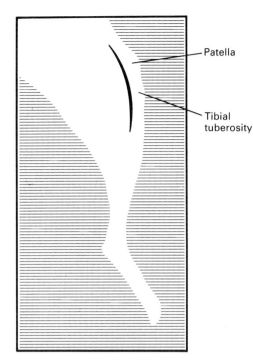

Fig. 10.170. To replace a ruptured medial collateral ligament the dog is placed in lateral recumbency with the affected leg ventral. The ligament is exposed via a lightly curved parapatellar skin incision which extends from the lower third of the femur to the upper third of the tibia.

RUPTURE OF A COLLATERAL LIGAMENT OF THE FEMOROTIBIAL JOINT

The collateral ligaments may be either torn from their insertions or ruptured. These injuries interfere with the normal stability of the joint, and cannot be treated either by external immobilization or by repair of the torn ligament. Replacement of the collateral ligament with wire is a practical method of treatment (Figs 10.170–10.172).

In most cases the wire breaks, but by the time this occurs considerable peri-articular fibrous tissue has been laid down which adequately stabilizes the joint, and unless the ends of the broken wire cause irritation or pain, it need not be removed.

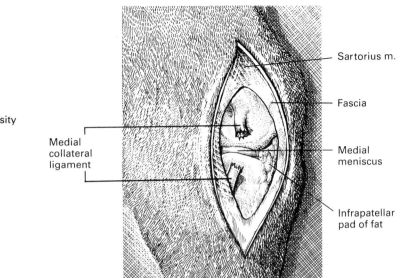

Fig. 10.171. The underlying sartorius muscle and fascia are incised the length of the incision and retracted. The remnants of the collateral ligament are isolated by dissection and their origins exposed.

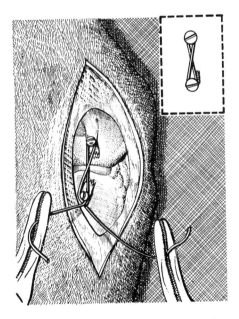

Fig. 10.172. A 12-mm standard Sherman screw is inserted into the condyle of the femur at the point of origin of the ligament and a second screw just below the medial condyle of the tibia. These two screws are then joined by a strand of monofilament wire (0.8–1.0 mm) placed around them in the manner of a figure-of-eight. To stabilize the joint effectively the wire has to be drawn just tight enough to permit only 80 per cent of the normal range of flexion and extension.

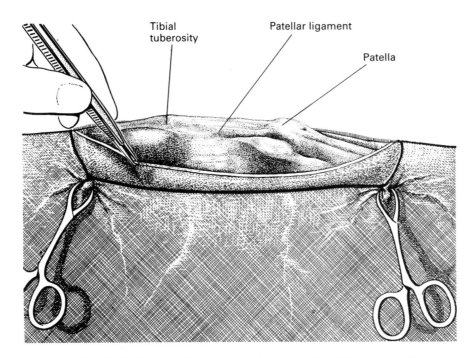

Tibial tuberosity

Patellar ligament

Patella

Fig. 10.173. A longitudinal skin incision is made over the cranial aspect of the stifle joint extending from the distal extremity of the femur to the upper third of the tibia. The skin is reflected to both sides and the underlying connective tissue is incised to expose the patella, patellar ligament and tibial tuberosity.

DISLOCATION OF THE PATELLA

The commonest cause of medial dislocation of the patella, either permanent or intermittent, is a congenital defect. It may be due to a curvature of the distal extremity of the femur, medial displacement of the tibial tuberosity or abnormalities of the trochlea. The object of treatment is to retain the patella in the trochlea and this is attained by either transplanting the tibial tuberosity to re-align the pull of the quadriceps, patella and patellar ligament, by fashioning a new trochlea or by performing a capsulectomy. Mild cases may be corrected by a capsulectomy but the majority require the tibial tuberosity to be transplanted laterally and reinforced with a capsulectomy. In severe cases these measures may have to be combined with fashioning a new trochlea. In these cases the patella is invariably flat and must be trimmed to shape to fit into the depth of the reconstructed trochlea.

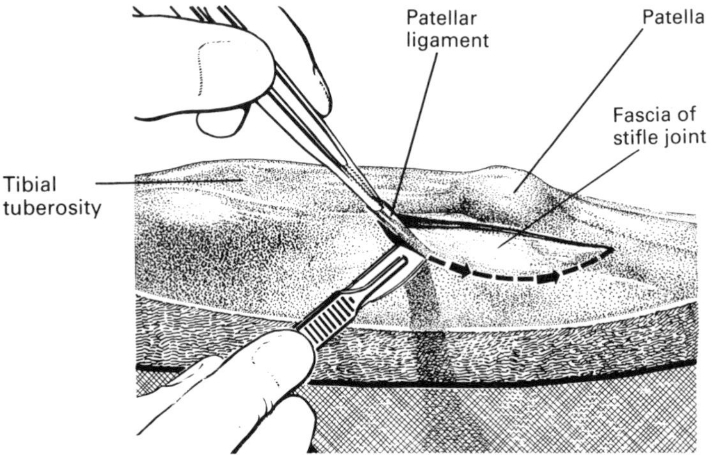

Capsulectomy

The dog is restrained in dorsal recumbency with the affected leg extended and resting on a sandbag. First, a skin incision is made (Fig. 10.173) and the skin reflected so a second incision can be made through the fascia and joint capsule (Fig. 10.174).

Patellar ligament

Patella

Fascia of stifle joint

Tibial tuberosity

Fig. 10.174. An incision 2.5–5 cm in length is made through the fascia and joint capsule just lateral to the patella. This forms the base line for the removal of an elliptical segment. This incision is closed with mattress sutures using synthetic absorbable suture material. The first suture is placed opposite the middle of the patella and pulled tight. An attempt is then made to push the patella medially. If this succeeds the elliptical incision is enlarged until manual dislocation is not possible. Then closure is completed.

This incision is closed as described then the original incision is closed by first co-apting the subcutaneous tissues with interrupted sutures using synthetic absorbable material and then the skin in the usual manner.

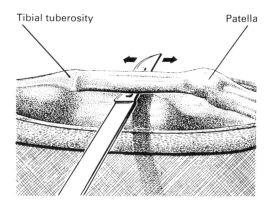

Fig. 10.175. The patellar ligament is isolated by passing the blade of a scalpel beneath it and severing the fascial attachments between the patella and the tibial tuberosity.

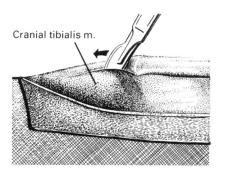

Fig. 10.176. The attachment of the cranial tibialis muscle to the tibial crest is incised.

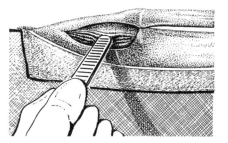

Fig. 10.177. The cranial tibialis muscle is separated from the tibial crest by blunt dissection.

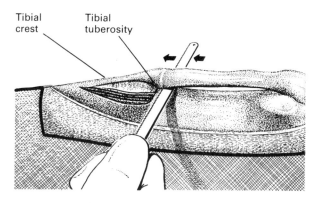

Fig. 10.178. The tibial tuberosity together with the patellar ligament is sawn off with a hack-saw blade.

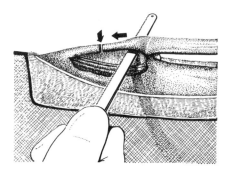

Fig. 10.179. Two saw-cuts are made to remove the tibial tuberosity: one parallel with the tuberosity and the other placed distal and at right angles to the tuberosity.

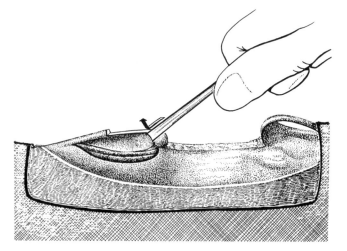

Fig. 10.180. A niche is gouged out of the proximo-lateral aspect of the tibia to form a bed for the transplant.

Lateral transposition of the tibial tuberosity

The patella, patellar ligament and tibial tuberosity are exposed as described (see Fig. 10.173). The procedure is shown in Figs 10.175–10.182.

After completing the transplant the stability of the patella is tested. If it can still be dislocated medially then in addition a capsulectomy is performed.

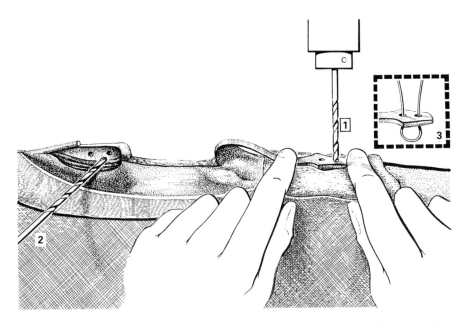

Fig. 10.181. (1) The tibial tuberosity is reflected, held securely on a swab, and two holes drilled through it, 0.3–0.5 cm apart, with a 1.5-mm twist drill. (2) With the same size drill two holes are drilled transversely through the proximal aspect of the tibial crest in a latero-medial direction. (3) A strand of monofilament stainless steel wire (size 0.8–1.0 mm) is threaded through the holes in the tibial tuberosity.

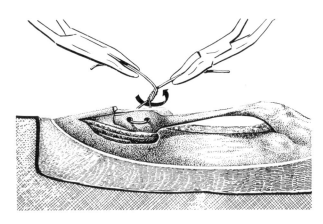

Fig. 10.182. The tibial tuberosity is transplanted by rotating it through 90° and passing the wires through the holes in the tibia. It is then fitted into the prepared bed by pulling the wires tight and twisting up the ends. The twisted end is cut off to leave about 0.3–0.5 cm which is pressed flat against the bone.

Tibia

EPIPHYSEAL SEPARATION OF THE TIBIAL TUBEROSITY

Efficient joint function is not re-established unless the detached tibial tuberosity is reduced. An open reduction and fixation with two Kirschner wires and a figure-of-eight tension band wire is recommended (Figs 10.183–10.185).

The implants should be removed as soon as healing is established. It is particularly important to remove the figure-of-eight wire so as not to interfere with normal growth.

FRACTURE OF THE TIBIAL SHAFT

Fractures of the shaft of the tibia are invariably overriding and often open. A closed reduction is difficult and, owing to the shape of the leg, casts provide inadequate support. These cases may be treated by open reduction and internal fixation with a bone plate applied to the caudo-medial aspect of the shaft.

Although there are disadvantages inherent in the use of an intramedullary pin, many cases are

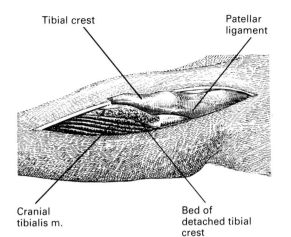

Fig. 10.183. The detached tibial tuberosity is exposed via a longitudinal skin incision extending from the patella to the upper third of the tibia.

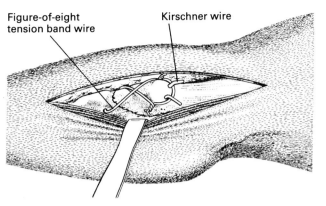

Fig. 10.185. The detached tuberosity is carefully repositioned and immobilized with two Kirschner wires and a figure-of-eight tension band wire.

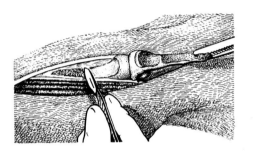

Fig. 10.184. After displacement, the epiphyseal breach rapidly fills with granulation tissue. To reduce the tibial tuberosity accurately it is necessary to remove this tissue carefully.

satisfactorily treated by this method. The pin should be driven in in a normograde fashion, i.e. started on the cranial aspect of the tibial tuberosity, driven distally through the proximal fragment, the fracture site and into the distal fragment. This ensures the proximal end of the pin does not enter the stifle joint. Additional rotational stability can often be provided with cerclage wires, especially when the fracture is oblique or spiral (Figs 10.186–10.187).

The subcutaneous tissue is co-apted with interrupted sutures of synthetic absorbable material and the skin sutured in the usual manner.

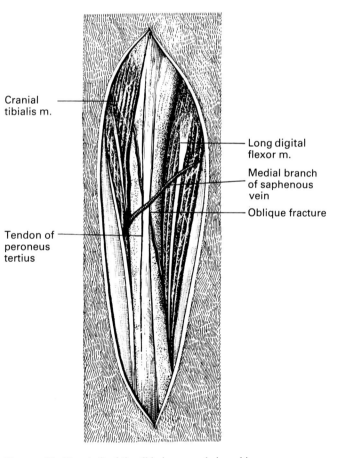

Fig. 10.186. The shaft of the tibia is exposed via a skin incision along its medial aspect. The subcutaneous tissues have to be incised and dissected off the shaft to expose the fracture effectively.

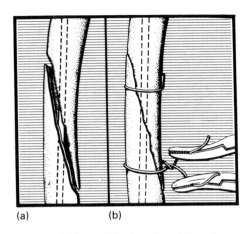

Fig. 10.187. (a) Immobilization of an oblique fracture with an intramedullary pin tends to push the edges of the fracture apart. (b) The edges of the fracture are brought together and a satisfactory reduction maintained by placing one or two cerclage wire loops around the bone.

SEPARATION OF THE DISTAL EPIPHYSIS OF THE TIBIA

In these cases the shaft of the tibia is displaced cranially, and is treated by an open reduction and fixation with two Kirschner wires (Fig. 10.188).

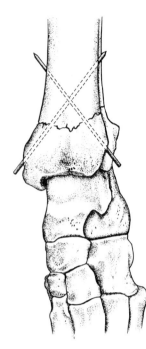

Fig. 10.188. The displaced epiphysis is reduced and the fracture immobilized with two Kirschner wires.

Hock joint

DISLOCATION OF THE TALOCRURAL JOINT

Dislocations of the talocrural joint occur in both the dog and cat. If it remains stable following a closed reduction it is immobilized in a cast but if it redislocates then it is necessary to perform an internal fixation and replace the torn collateral ligaments (Figs 10.189–10.190).

The incision is closed in the usual manner and the joint supported in a cast. The wire sutures are left *in situ* indefinitely. In some cases they break, but by the time this occurs considerable peri-articular fibrous tissue has been laid down which adequately stabilizes the joint, and unless the ends of a broken wire cause irritation or pain it need not be removed.

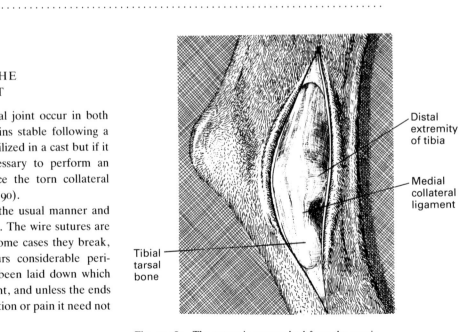

Distal extremity of tibia

Medial collateral ligament

Tibial tarsal bone

Fig. 10.189. The tarsus is approached from the cranio-medial aspect by a slightly curved skin incision extending from the lower third of the tibia to the upper end of the metatarsal bones. The medial collateral ligament has a short and long component and generally both must be replaced.

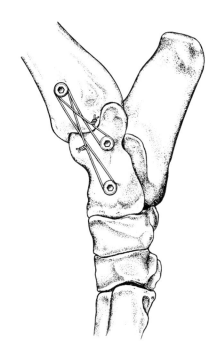

Fig. 10.190. Position of the screws and figure-of-eight wires to replace the short and long medial collateral ligaments of the talocrural joint.

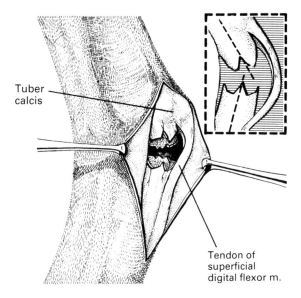

Fig. 10.191. The fracture is exposed via a skin incision on the plantaro-lateral aspect of the hock joint which extends from just above the tuber calcis to the mid-tarsus.

Tuber calcis

Tendon of superficial digital flexor m.

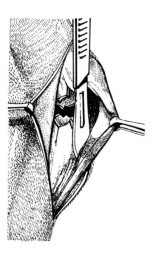

Fig. 10.192. The tendon of the superficial digital flexor muscle is dissected from the bone and retracted.

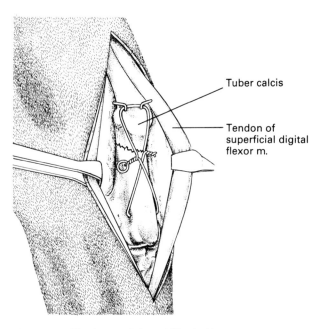

Tuber calcis

Tendon of superficial digital flexor m.

Fig. 10.193. The fracture is immobilized with two Kirschner wires and a figure-of-eight wire.

FRACTURE OF THE TUBER CALCIS OF THE CALCANEUS

It is impossible to maintain an accurate reduction of the calcaneus without internal fixation due to the pull of the Achilles tendon. The distractive force of the Achilles tendon must be counteracted with a figure-of-eight tension band wire on the plantar aspect of the tuber calcis to avoid the development of a non-union (Figs 10.191–10.193).

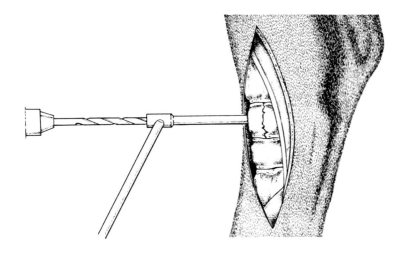

Fig. 10.194. The dorsal slab is drilled with a 2.7-mm drill through a drill sleeve. Drilling ceases when the drill bit reaches the fracture plane.

FRACTURE OF THE CENTRAL TARSAL BONE

Fractures of the central tarsal bone are common in the Greyhound and may vary from a fissure with no displacement or dorsal extrusion of a fragment, to a comminuted fracture with collapse of the joint. A displaced dorsal fragment is treated by replacing the fragment and retaining it in position with a lag screw (Figs 10.194–10.197) followed by support in a cast.

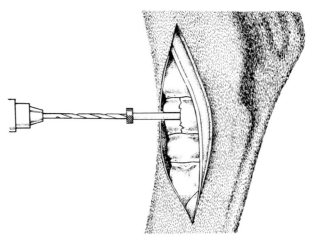

Fig. 10.195. The body of the central tarsal bone is drilled with a 2.0-mm drill through a drill insert and the depth of the hole measured.

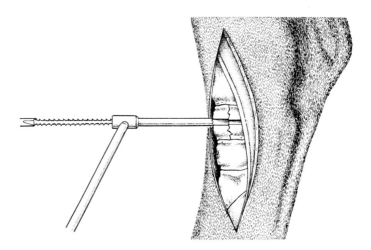

Fig. 10.196. Threads are cut into the body of the bone with 2.7-mm bone tap.

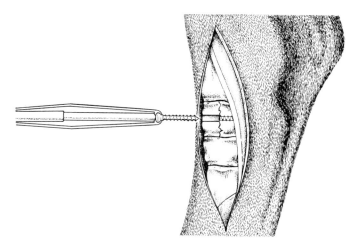

Fig. 10.197. A 2.7-mm screw of appropriate length is inserted. The fracture is compressed as the screw is tightened.

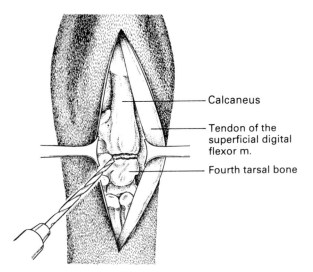

Calcaneus

Tendon of the superficial digital flexor m.

Fourth tarsal bone

Fig. 10.198. The articular surfaces of the calcaneo-quartal joint are drilled and curetted so as to destroy them.

SUBLUXATION OF THE PROXIMAL INTERTARSAL JOINT

Rupture of the plantar ligament causes collapse of the tarsus with resulting hyperflexion of the hock when weight is taken. Closed reduction followed by external fixation provides immediate stabilization but when the cast is removed and weight taken a degree of hyperflexion inevitably ensues which prevents normal joint function. Arthrodesis of the calcaneo-quartal joint is the only way to return the dog to satisfactory locomotor efficiency (Figs 10.198–10.199).

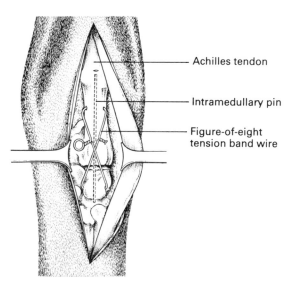

Achilles tendon

Intramedullary pin

Figure-of-eight tension band wire

Fig. 10.199. A transverse hole is drilled with a 1.5-mm drill bit through the plantar process of the fourth tarsal bone and a length of stainless steel wire threaded through it. A second tunnel is drilled through the calcaneus approximately one-third of its length from its proximal end and a second piece of stainless steel wire inserted. The proximal intertarsal subluxation is reduced and a drill hole is started on the proximal surface of the tuber calcis. The fibres of the Achilles tendon are divided longitudinally in order that the drill bit is unimpeded. The drill is directed down the medullary canal of the calcaneus and across the calcaneo-quartal joint. The drill is removed and a small Steinmann pin is driven down its track and countersunk below the surface of the tuber calcis. The two pieces of wire are twisted in a figure-of-eight so as to form a tension band on the plantar aspect of the joint.

Orthopaedic instruments

In bone surgery, plates, screws, pins and wire are used. Few metals can be left in the body without causing a severe tissue reaction but three have been found satisfactory for surgical implants. First, stainless steel of the SMO or EAN58J variety which is an austinitic stainless steel containing about 18 per cent chromium, 8 per cent nickel, and 2−4 per cent molybdenum. Secondly, vitallium or vinertia, a non-ferrous alloy containing 65 per cent cobalt, 30 per cent chromium, and 3 per cent molybdenum and thirdly, titanium, an element which is very light.

The choice of metal for bone plates, screws, etc. is very much a matter of personal preference. The authors have found the stainless steel implants to be entirely satisfactory, being inert in tissues, corrosion resistant and having the necessary mechanical strength.

Different metals should not be used in contact with one another. A stainless steel bone plate should not be held in place with vitallium screws as electrolytic and chemical reactions will cause corrosion of the implants. This results in local tissue reaction which may be followed by wound breakdown or the non-union of a fracture.

BONE PLATES

Bone plates are designed to provide maximum strength with minimal dimensions and are contoured slightly to accommodate the curvature of the bone. Three variations are in common use: (i) compression plates, of which there are many sizes and variations (Figs 10.200−10.201), (ii) the Venable bone plate, and (iii) the Sherman plate.

Compression plates

ASIF dynamic compression plates range from the broad 18-hole 4.5 mm to the three-hole 2-mm miniplate. The holes are elliptical so that when eccentrically placed screws are tightened the bone moves relative to the plate and the fracture line is compressed.

A wide variety of special plates is available in the ASIF system making these plates very versatile.

Non-compression plates

See Figs 10.202−10.205.

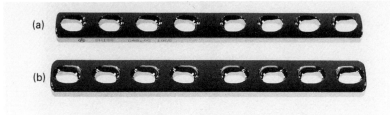

Fig. 10.200. Regular (a) and broad (b) 3.5-mm dynamic compression plates.

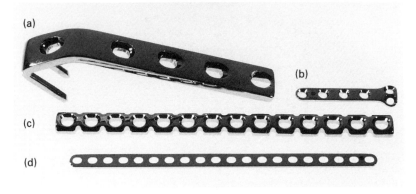

Fig. 10.201. Some special ASIF plates: (a) a double hook plate; (b) a T plate; (c) a reconstruction plate; and (d) a veterinary cuttable plate.

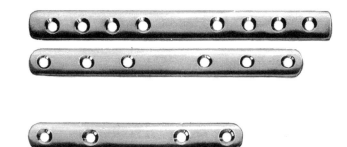

Fig. 10.202. *Venable bone plate.* This plate has no constrictions between the screw holes and is relatively strong. For this reason it is the most satisfactory bone plate for general veterinary orthopaedics when ASIF plates are unavailable. They are obtainable in eight lengths from 38 mm to 127 mm.

Length (mm)	Holes
38*	4
45*	4
64	4
76	4
90	4
102	6
114	6
127	8

Note. These bone plates are drilled and countersunk to accept 4-mm bone screws with the exception of the plates marked (*) which take a 3.6-mm screw.

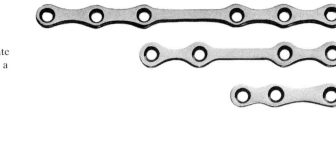

Fig. 10.203. *Sherman bone plate.* The shape of this plate is not conducive to strength, and it has therefore only a limited application in veterinary orthopaedics. It is obtainable in lengths from 25.4 mm to 140 mm and is drilled and countersunk to accept 4-mm screws.

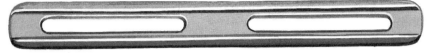

Fig. 10.204. *Eggers contact splint.* Basically a bone plate but with slots in place of the normal screw holes. It is designed to assist the longitudinal muscle pull and pressure of weight bearing to maintain the fractured ends in close contact. It is obtainable in lengths from 38 mm to 127 mm. The slot accepts a 4-mm screw.

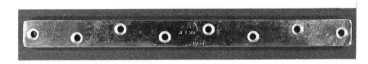

Fig. 10.205. *Heavy duty bone plate.* This plate is 4.8 mm thick and obtainable with either screw holes or slots to the following lengths: 150 mm, 180 mm and 205 mm. It is drilled and countersunk to accept 4-mm bone screws. This plate is useful for the fixation of fractures in large dogs.

BONE SCREWS

Sherman screws

Sherman screws have either fine or coarse threads and the screw slot may be either the plain slot, the Phillip's recessed head or the cross slot. The threads extend the full length of the screw to enable purchase to be obtained on both cortices of the bone. The maximum holding power of the screw is obtained when the size of the drill hole is approximately 85 per cent of the outside diameter of the screw. If the drill hole is too large it reduces the holding power of the screw and if too small the bone tends to split.

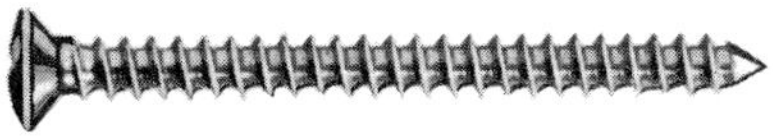

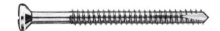

Fig. 10.207. *Transfixion screw.* This is a partially threaded self-tapping screw and is used for drawing together two bone fragments. The length of the smooth shaft near the head enables the loose fragment to be drawn up against the fixed or larger fragment. It is obtainable in the following sizes:

Diameter (mm)	Lengths (mm)
4.4	44.5, 51.0, 57.0, 63.5, 70.0, 76.0

Recommended sizes of twist drills to be used for various screws:

	Screw, outside diameter (mm)	Drills, outside diameter (mm)
Transfixion screw	4.4	4.0
Sherman screw	2.8	2.3
	3.6	2.8
	4.0	3.2

Fig. 10.206. *Sherman bone screw* (coarse thread 20 threads per inch (t.p.i.) with plain slot). This is a standard orthopaedic screw, and is self-tapping, with a truncated end. It is obtainable in the following sizes:

Diameter (mm)	Lengths (mm)
2.8	9.5, 12.7, 15.9, 19.0, 22.2, 25.4, 28.5, 31.5, 35.0, 38.0
3.6 and 4.0 (20 t.p.i.)	9.5, 12.7, 15.9, 19.0, 22.2, 25.4, 28.5, 31.5, 35.0, 38.0, 41.5, 44.5, 47.5, 51.0, 57.0, 63.5, 70.0, 76.0

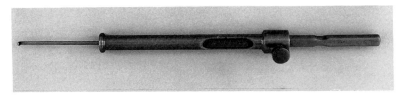

Fig. 10.208. *Screw depth gauge.* Used to determine the length of screw needed to penetrate a bone. The hooked end of the gauge is inserted into the drilled hole and hooked over the distal bone surface. The sleeve is then pushed against the bone or bone plate, fixed in position by tightening the screw and the gauge withdrawn. The calibrations on the stem indicate the length of screw required.

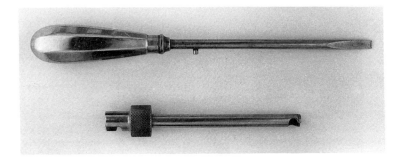

Fig. 10.209. *Screwdriver with holding sleeve.* This combination facilitates the driving of screws which are firmly locked to the end of the sleeve. This dispenses with supporting the screw in screw-holding forceps or with the fingers. When the screw is three-quarters driven the sleeve is removed and the screw driven home in the usual manner.

ASIF bone screws

This screw (Fig. 10.210) is used in cortical bone. It has a round end and therefore requires a precut thread to be cut in the bone with a bone tap.

Diameter (mm)	Lengths (mm)	Drill bit size (mm)	Tap size (mm)
1.5	6–20	1.1	1.5
2.0	6–24	1.5	2.0
2.7	6–40	2.0	2.7
3.5	10–110	2.5	3.5
4.5	14–110	3.2	4.5
5.5	24–100	4.0	5.5

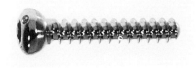

Fig. 10.210. ASIF cortical bone screw.

Cancellous bone screw

This screw (Fig. 10.211) is used in cancellous bone and has deeper threads.

Diameter (mm)	Lengths (mm)	Drill bit size (mm)	Tap size (mm)
3.5	10–60	2.0	3.5
4.0	10–50	2.5	—
6.5	30–110	3.2	6.5

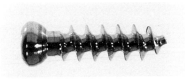

Fig. 10.211. ASIF cancellous bone screw.

DRILLS

ASIF bone drills

ASIF bone drills have a quickfit locking system which enables a rapid change of drill bit.

Bone taps (Fig. 10.212) are used to cut a thread in the bone when using screws that are not self-tapping. This enables the thread of the screw to match the thread in the bone and improves its pull-out strength.

A countersink (Fig. 10.213) increases the area of contact between the screwhead and bone, thus spreading the force over a greater area.

Tap guides (Fig. 10.214) protect the soft tissues from the sharp threads of the bone taps. They also discourage lateral movement of the tap as it cuts through the bone.

Drill sleeves (Fig. 10.215) fit within the larger gliding hole and ensure the smaller thread or pilot hole is drilled in exactly the same direction. A 4.5-mm drill sleeve has a 4.5-mm outer diameter and 3.2-mm inner diameter.

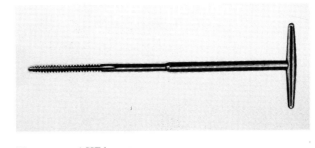

Fig. 10.212. ASIF bone tap.

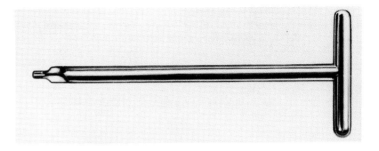

Fig. 10.213. ASIF countersink.

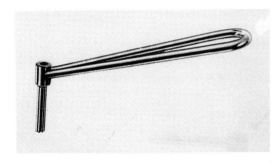

Fig. 10.214. Tap guide.

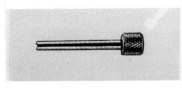

Fig. 10.215. Drill sleeve.

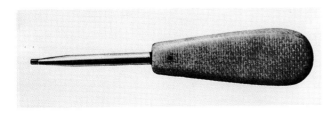

Fig. 10.216. Screwdriver for hexagonal socket heads. Most ASIF screws have hexagonal heads but different sizes require a different sized screwdriver.

Other drills

See Figs 10.217–10.219.

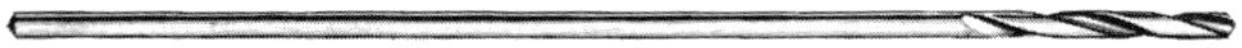

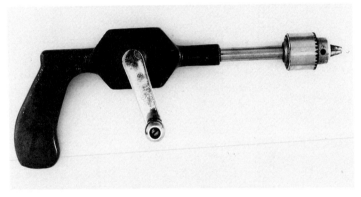

Fig. 10.217. *Drills.* Bone drills are made from either stainless steel or vitallium. Stainless steel twist drills are obtained in the following sizes:

Length (mm)	Diameters (mm)
76 and 127	1.6, 2.0, 2.4, 2.8, 3.2, 3.6, 4.0, 4.4, 4.8, 6.3

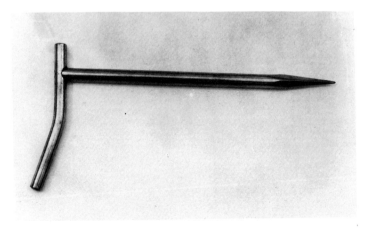

Fig. 10.218. *Pistol-grip hand drill with Jacob's chuck.* This drill has a two-to-one gear ratio and is cannulated its entire length to accommodate Steinmann pins and long-shank drills up to a 6.3-mm diameter.

Fig. 10.219. *Cortex reamer.* Used for boring holes by hand and is especially useful for starting a hole prior to drilling.

INTRAMEDULLARY PINS AND NAILS

A variety of intramedullary pins and nails (Figs 10.220–10.223) are used for the internal fixation of fractures. The most suitable metal for this type of implant is stainless steel. To secure satisfactory immobilization the pin must impact the medullary cavity.

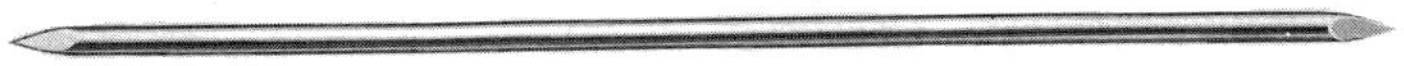

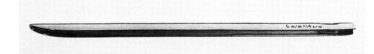

Fig. 10.220. *Steinmann pin.* This pin is the standard veterinary intramedullary pin. It is round in cross-section and pointed at both ends so that it can be inserted via the fracture site. The pins are obtainable in the following sizes:

Diameter (mm)	Lengths (mm)
1.6, 2.0, 2.4, 2.8, 3.2, 3.6, 4.0, 4.8, 6.4, 8.0	127, 150, 180, 205, 230, 255, 280, 305

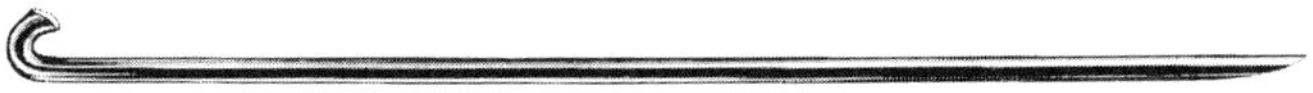

Fig. 10.221. *Rush intramedullary pin.* This pin is round in cross-section, has a 'sledge-runner' tip at one end, and a hook at the other to grip the cortex at the point of insertion. It is inserted at an oblique angle at the side of the bone and when it's 'sledge-runner' tip strikes the opposite cortex it does not penetrate it but is deflected and runs along the medullary cavity. It does not immobilize a fracture by impacting the medullary cavity but rather by the spring-like action obtained by opposing point pressures within the medullary cavity. It is obtainable in the following sizes:

Diameter (mm)	Lengths (mm)
2.4	25–102 (in 6-mm increments)
3.0	102–256 (in 13-mm increments)
4.8	203–355 (in 19-mm increments)
6.0	280–432 (in 19-mm increments)

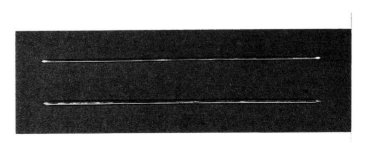

Fig. 10.222. *Kuntscher nail.* This nail is fluted and in cross-section either clover-leaf-shaped or V-shaped to enhance its grip in cancellous bone and to control rotation. The V-shaped nail is the type generally used in veterinary orthopaedics. It has a rounded point and a hole at the other end to engage the extraction hook. It is inserted by being driven into the medullary cavity via the extremity of the bone. It is obtainable in the following sizes:

Diameter (mm)	Lengths (mm)
6 and 8	140, 160, 180, 200, 240, 250, 260, 270, 280, 300, 320, 340

Fig. 10.223. (*Right*). *Kirschner wire.* This may be described as a very fine Steinmann pin. It may be obtained in stainless steel or vitallium. The former is supplied in the following sizes:

Diameter (mm)	Lengths (mm)
0.8, 1.1 and 1.5	6.25, 7.5, 8.75, 10.0, 22.5, 25.0, 30.0

ORTHOPAEDIC WIRES

See Figs 10.224–10.226.

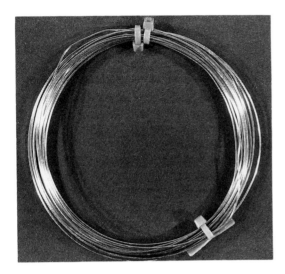

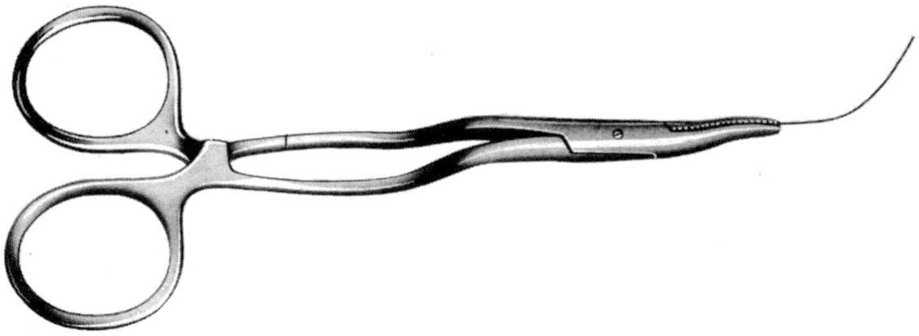

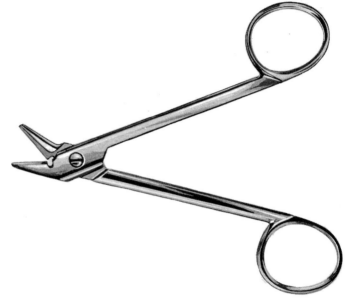

Fig. 10.225. *Wire-holding forceps*. These forceps are shaped and designed for gripping and manipulating wire.

Fig. 10.224. *Cerclage wire*. Fragments of bone can be held together with suture wire either passed through a drill hole in each fragment or by a circumferential wire loop. The ends of the wire are held in wire-holding forceps, pulled tight and secured by twisting them together, and then cutting off the twisted end with wire-cutting forceps and pressing the stump flat against the bone.

Stainless steel cerclage wire (monofilament) is obtainable in four sizes (0.8–1.5 mm diameter).

Suture wire is made from either stainless steel or tantalum and may be obtained either as a single strand (monofilament) or with several strands either twisted or braided (multifilament). Although the multifilament wire is less likely to kink and is more flexible, it is the monofilament stainless steel suture wire that is in general use in orthopaedics.

Stainless steel suture wire is available from 1.5 to 9 metric with a variety of swaged-on needles.

Fig. 10.226. *Suture-wire scissors*.

BONE-CUTTING INSTRUMENTS

See Figs 10.227–10.231.

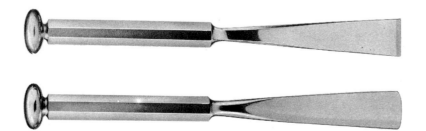

Fig. 10.227. *Chisel*. Is bevelled on one side only and used for cutting or shaping bone. It is obtainable in the following widths: 6, 8, 10, 12, 15, 20, 25 and 30 mm.

Fig. 10.228. *Gouge*. Is used for cutting out a groove or hollow in a bone. It is obtainable in the following widths: 6, 8, 10, 12, 15, 20, 25 and 30 mm.

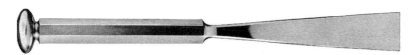

Fig. 10.229. *Osteotome*. May be described as a special type of chisel and is used for dividing bone. The edges are bevelled equally o both sides. It is obtainable in the following widths: 6, 8, 10, 12, 15, 20, 25 and 30 mm.

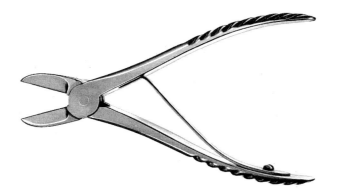

Fig. 10.230. *Liston's bone-cutting forceps*. The standard type of bone-cutting forceps, which are obtainable with either straight or curved jaws.

BONE-HOLDING INSTRUMENT

See Fig. 10.232.

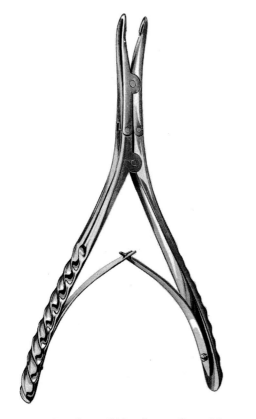

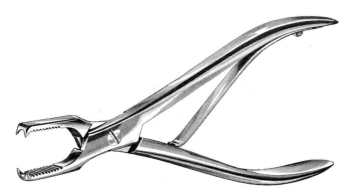

Fig. 10.232. *Frosch's bone-holding forceps*. A very useful pattern of forceps for holding and manipulating small bones.

Fig. 10.231. *Luer bone-nibbling forceps*. Powerful double-action forceps designed for removing small pieces of hard compact bone.

Section 11
Amputations

Amputation of a limb

Many small dogs and cats live normal and active lives after amputation of either a front or a hind leg, whereas farm animals and the larger breeds of dog are severely handicapped by the loss of a limb. When planning an amputation it is not necessary to fashion a stump suitable for fitting a prosthesis, and one should therefore aim to produce a short stump which will not unbalance the animal or cause it any encumbrance. The usual site to amputate a front leg is through the middle of the humerus, or for a hind leg through the middle of the femur. Forequarter amputation, removing the scapula and the humerus in their entirety, may be required in the management of some tumours. Similarly, the hindlimbs may, on occasion, be disarticulated at the hip joint.

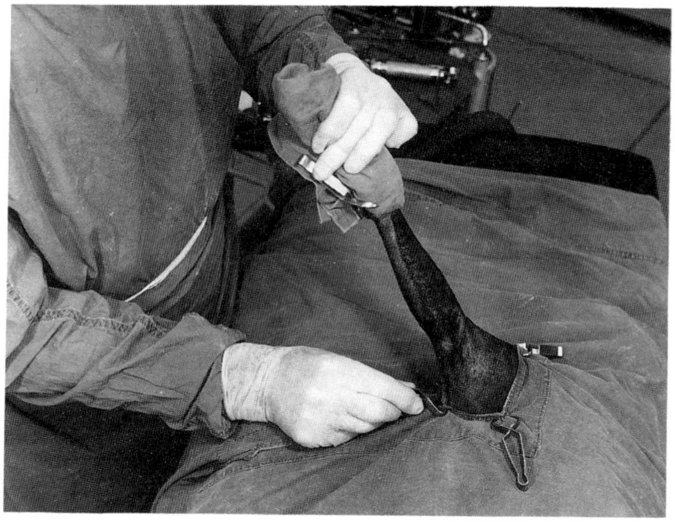

AMPUTATION OF THE THORACIC LIMB — DOG

Left thoracic limb

See Figs 11.1–11.9.

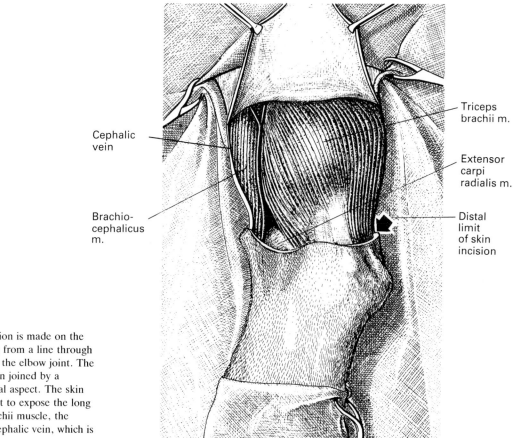

Fig. 11.1. The dog is placed in lateral recumbency with the affected leg uppermost, resting on a sandbag. The distal extremity of the leg is draped in the customary manner and passed through the opening of a laparotomy sheet to permit ease of manipulation during surgery.

Cephalic vein

Brachio-cephalicus m.

Triceps brachii m.

Extensor carpi radialis m.

Distal limit of skin incision

Fig. 11.2. A semicircular skin incision is made on the lateral aspect of the limb extending from a line through the middle of the humerus down to the elbow joint. The leg is then abducted and the incision joined by a corresponding incision on the medial aspect. The skin flap is reflected on the lateral aspect to expose the long and lateral heads of the triceps brachii muscle, the brachiocephalicus muscle and the cephalic vein, which is ligated.

247

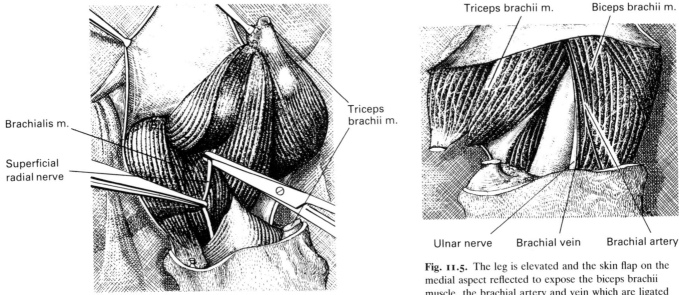

Brachialis m.

Superficial radial nerve

Triceps brachii m.

Fig. 11.3. The common tendon of insertion of the triceps brachii is severed, and the muscle mass reflected proximally to expose the brachialis muscle where it curves around the lower third of the humerus and the superficial radial nerve which is severed proximally.

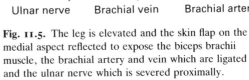

Triceps brachii m.   Biceps brachii m.

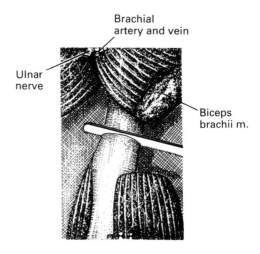

Ulnar nerve   Brachial vein   Brachial artery

Fig. 11.5. The leg is elevated and the skin flap on the medial aspect reflected to expose the biceps brachii muscle, the brachial artery and vein which are ligated and the ulnar nerve which is severed proximally.

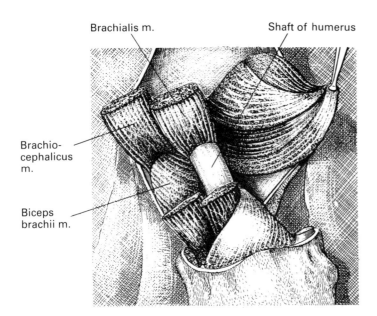

Brachialis m.   Shaft of humerus

Brachio-cephalicus m.

Biceps brachii m.

Fig. 11.4. The brachialis and brachiocephalicus muscles are severed and reflected to expose the lateral aspect of the shaft of the humerus.

Brachial artery and vein

Ulnar nerve

Biceps brachii m.

Fig. 11.6. The biceps brachii muscle is severed just proximal to where it divides to be inserted onto the radius and ulna and is reflected. The leg can now be amputated by sawing through the shaft of the humerus using a hack-saw blade.

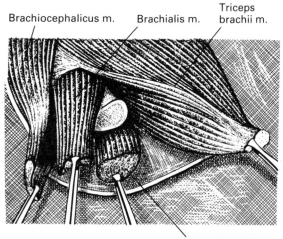

Brachiocephalicus m.   Brachialis m.   Triceps brachii m.

Biceps brachii m.

Fig. 11.7. The ends of the severed muscles are sutured together with interrupted synthetic absorbable sutures, to form a protective muscle pad over the stump of the humerus. The brachialis and biceps brachii muscles are first sutured together over the stump and then the brachiocephalicus and triceps brachii muscles.

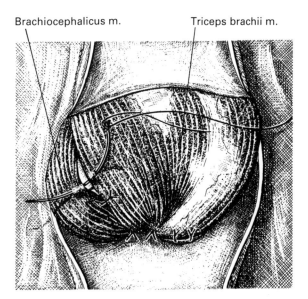

Brachiocephalicus m.   Triceps brachii m.

Fig. 11.8. After the ends of the muscles have been sutured together care must be taken to ensure that their edges are also co-apted.

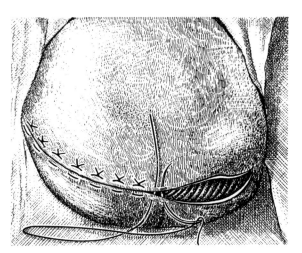

Fig. 11.9. The skin flaps are co-apted with interrupted mattress sutures using monofilament nylon.

AMPUTATION OF THE PELVIC LIMB – DOG

The leg is draped and positioned in the same manner as described for the thoracic limb.

Left pelvic limb

See Figs. 11.10–11.13.

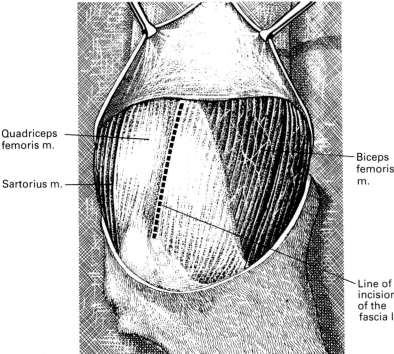

Fig. 11.10. A semicircular skin incision is made on the lateral aspect of the hind leg, extending from a line through the lower third of the thigh down to the stifle joint. The leg is then abducted and the incision joined by a corresponding incision on the medial aspect. The skin flap is reflected on the lateral aspect to expose the sartorius, quadriceps femoris, biceps femoris muscles and the fascia lata. The fascia lata is incised along the length of its attachment to the biceps femoris muscle.

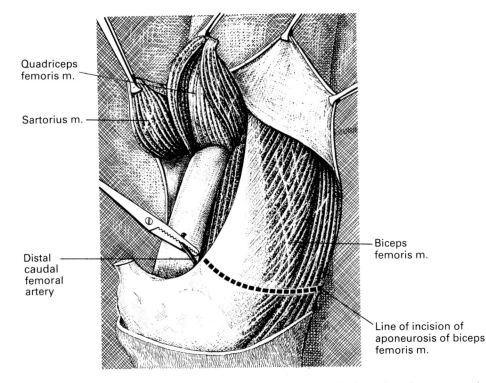

Fig. 11.11. The quadriceps femoris and biceps femoris muscles are separated by blunt dissection to expose the lateral aspect of the femur. The tendon of insertion of the quadriceps femoris muscle and the cranial belly of the sartorius muscle are severed proximal to the patella and reflected to expose the lateral aspect of the femur and the distal caudal femoral artery, which is ligated.

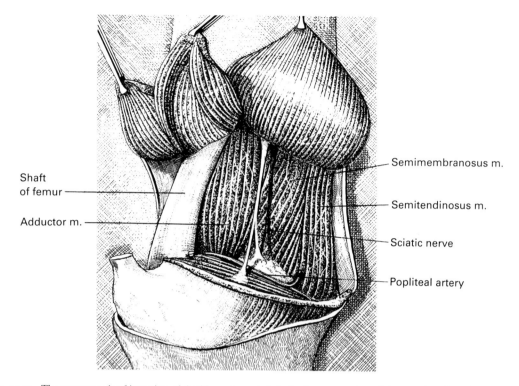

Shaft
of femur

Adductor m.

Semimembranosus m.

Semitendinosus m.

Sciatic nerve

Popliteal artery

Fig. 11.12. The aponeurosis of insertion of the biceps femoris is incised transversely and the muscle reflected to expose the popliteal artery, the sciatic nerve and the adductor, semimembranosus and semitendinosus muscles. The popliteal artery is ligated and the sciatic nerve divided proximally.

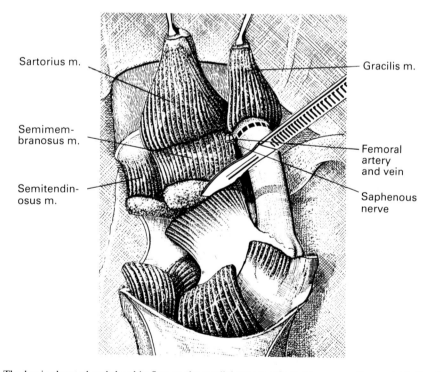

Sartorius m.

Semimem-
branosus m.

Semitendin-
osus m.

Gracilis m.

Femoral
artery
and vein

Saphenous
nerve

Fig. 11.13. The leg is elevated and the skin flap on the medial aspect reflected to expose the caudal belly of the sartorius and the gracilis muscle. These muscles are severed and reflected to expose the femoral artery and vein which are ligated and the saphenous nerve which is divided proximally. Also exposed are the semimembranosus and semitendinosus muscles which are severed together with the underlying adductor muscle to expose completely the shaft of the femur. The leg can now be amputated by sawing through the shaft of the femur using a hack-saw blade and the operation completed in the manner described for amputating the thoracic limb.

Amputation of digits

The amputation of a digit or phalanx does not seriously interfere with the locomotor efficiency of the animal. Many dogs which have had a digit amputated continue to perform satisfactorily on the race-track and in other sports, and farm animals remain as economic units within the herd or flock.

AMPUTATION OF A DIGIT – CATTLE

The most common indication for amputation of the digit is infection of the coronopedal joint which is most frequently a sequel to solar ulceration or white line abscessation at the sole–heel junction. Infection of the flexor tendon sheath and discharging sinuses above the coronary band may be further complications. Gross trauma to the digit and infection of the pastern joint are much less common indications for amputation.

The aim is to remove all necrotic and infected tissue. Provided this is achieved, the patient will be walking on the remaining digit within a few days and healing will be rapid.

The cow is cast and placed in lateral recumbency with the affected digit uppermost. Alternatively the operation may be performed with the cow standing if one of the crushes specifically designed for foot trimming is available, because these provide support for the animal and enable the limb to be adequately immobilized. Anaesthesia can be achieved simply and effectively using an intravenous regional nerve block.

Amputation (Figs 11.14–11.16) may be carried out above or below the proximal interphalangeal joint by sawing through the first or second phalanges respectively, or by disarticulation of that joint which is the method preferred by the authors.

The incision is made 0.5 cm above the coronary band and is continued through all the tissues to the underlying bone and continued in like manner to encircle the digit.

The second phalanx is exposed on its lateral aspect and the dissection is continued upwards to the proximal interphalangeal joint which is located 1.5 cm above the initial skin incision. Escape of synovial fluid indicates that the joint has been reached.

The joint is disarticulated by continuing the incision around the joint thereby transecting the extensor tendon cranially, the flexor tendon caudally and the medial collateral ligament. This is made easier by manipulating the digit.

Once the digit has been removed, the articular cartilage is removed from the distal end of the first phalanx using a scalpel or curette. Any necrotic tissue is removed by sharp dissection, and the stump of the deep flexor tendon and its synovial sheath are examined for evidence of infection.

The operation is completed by packing the wound with a non-adhesive dressing and a cotton wool pad. The foot is enclosed in cotton wool and a cotton bandage, and finally Elastoplast is applied as a pressure bandage to control haemorrhage.

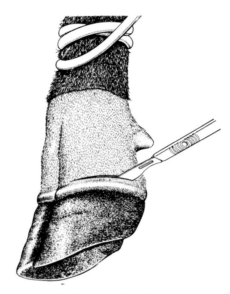

Fig. 11.14. An incision is made with a scalpel 0.5 cm above the coronary band. It is continued through all structures down to the underlying bone and continued in like manner to encircle the digit.

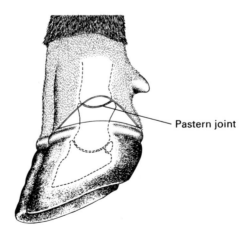

Fig. 11.15. The second phalanx is exposed by separating the surrounding reactionary fibrous tissue from it with an orthopaedic chisel.

252

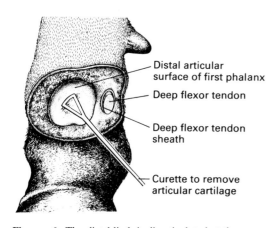

Distal articular surface of first phalanx

Deep flexor tendon

Deep flexor tendon sheath

Curette to remove articular cartilage

Fig. 11.16. The distal limb is disarticulated at the proximal interphalangeal joint and the articular cartilage of the distal surface of the first phalanx is curetted. Any necrotic tissue within the deep flexor tendon sheath must be excised before the stump is bandaged.

The stump is checked for any evidence of infection 4 days post-operatively and the dressing is renewed. Provided there are no complications, further dressings are not required.

AMPUTATION OF FIRST DIGIT OR DEW CLAW – DOG

In the thoracic limb the first digit has two phalanges and articulates with the first metacarpal bone whereas in the pelvic limb it is attached to the metatarsal bone by fibrous tissue.

It is customary to remove the first digit, when the puppy is 2–4 days old, with a pair of curved scissors. Haemorrhage is controlled by digital pressure or the application of a styptic and the wound left to heal by granulation.

If the first digit has not been removed at this early age it is advisable to leave the dog until it is over 3 months of age and perform a radical operation (Figs 11.17–11.20).

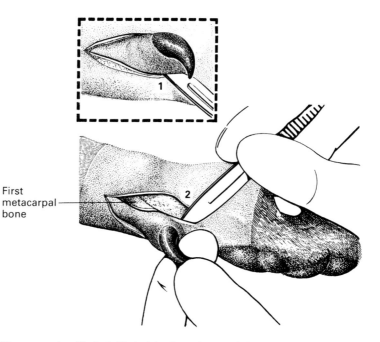

First metacarpal bone

Fig. 11.17. An elliptical skin incision is made to encircle the digit (1) and the subcutaneous tissue dissected free to expose the first metacarpal bone and proximal phalanx (2).

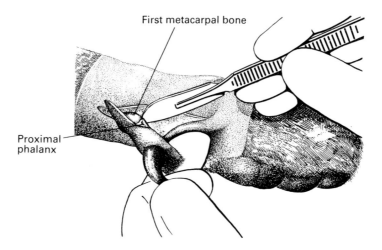

First metacarpal bone

Proximal phalanx

Fig. 11.18. The digit is retracted distally. The proximal phalanx and distal extremity of the first metacarpal bone are freed by dissection from the underlying tissues. This dissection exposes the digital artery and vein which are picked up with artery forceps and ligated.

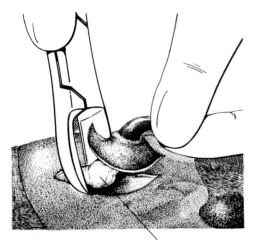

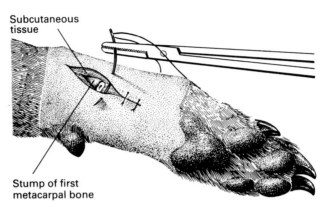

First metacarpo-phalangeal joint

Fig. II.19. The digit is amputated by severing the first metacarpal bone with bone-cutting forceps.

Subcutaneous tissue

Stump of first metacarpal bone

Fig. II.20. The incision is closed by co-apting the skin and subcutaneous tissues with a series of interrupted sutures using monofilament nylon. The wound is protected with a 'non-stick' dressing, cotton wool pad and bandages.

AMPUTATION OF DISTAL PHALANX — DOG

The success of this operation depends on the removal of the condyles of the second phalanx (Figs 11.21−11.23). If the condyles are not re-moved the dog will go lame after exercise because the pad provides insufficient protection against concussion. If they are removed the end of the bone receives no direct concussion as it is protected with a covering of fibrous tissue and does not come into direct contact with the pad.

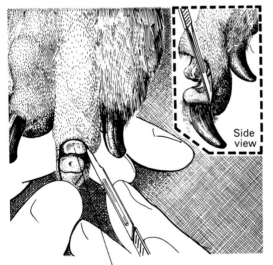

Condyle second phalanx

Fig. II.21. The nail is held in maximum flexion, a stab incision is made at right angles to the digit and as close to the base of the nail as possible, through the skin, subcutaneous tissues and into the distal interphalangeal joint. The incision is then extended to meet the pad on either side. The distal phalanx is completely disarticulated and removed by incising the skin on the ventral surface in close proximity to the pad.

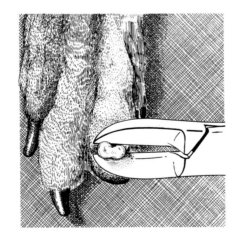

Fig. II.22. The condyles of the second phalanx are removed with bone-cutting forceps.

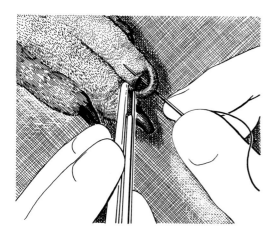

Fig. 11.23. The pad is sutured to the skin with three or four interrupted sutures using monofilament nylon. The wound is protected with a 'non-stick' dressing. A small tampon of cotton wool is placed in each interdigital space and the whole foot enclosed in a cotton wool pad and bandage.

REMOVAL OF A CLAW — DOG

When a dog turns or corners at speed it pivots on its claws. This action puts considerable stress on the interphalangeal joints. The removal of a claw is a method employed to relieve pressure on injured interphalangeal joints (Figs 11.24–11.27).

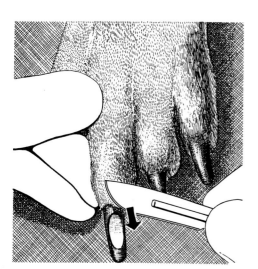

Fig. 11.24. The dorsal surface of the claw is levelled by shaving away the horn with a scalpel.

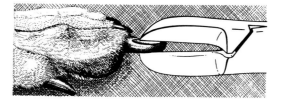

Fig. 11.25. The horn is split with bone-cutting forceps and separated from the ungual process.

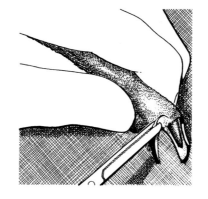

Fig. 11.26. Each section of split horn is seized with artery forceps and carefully eased away from the ungual crest of the third phalanx and the ventral surface of the corium.

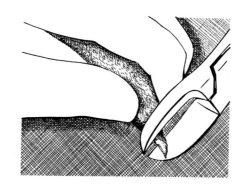

Fig. 11.27. The ungual process is removed with bone-cutting forceps, as close to the ungual crest as possible, and the surface lightly cauterized with silver nitrate.

Amputation of a tail (docking)

Docking is practised in all animals as a method of treating gross injuries and neoplasia of the tail. Docking of lambs' tails is routinely employed.

DOG

Docking of dogs' tails may be required for medical reasons. The dog is placed in ventral recumbency and its tail clipped and prepared for surgery. A tourniquet is applied at the base of the tail. The skin is incised dorsally and ventrally to create two elliptical skin flaps. The ventral and lateral coccygeal arteries are ligated or cauterized and the tail removed by disarticulation of the intercoccygeal joint proximal to the apex of the skin incision (Figs 11.28–11.32).

The end of the coccygeal vertebra is protected by suturing any available soft tissue and closing the skin with a series of interrupted mattress sutures.

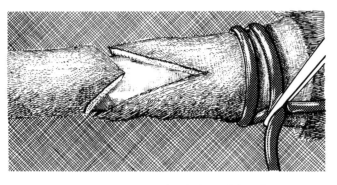

Fig. 11.28. A tourniquet is applied at the base of the tail and the skin incised so that two elliptical skin flaps are fashioned, one dorsal and one ventral.

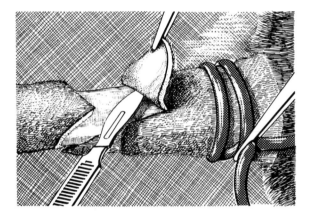

Fig. 11.29. The proximal skin flaps are reflected to expose the intercoccygeal joint proximal to the apex of the incision.

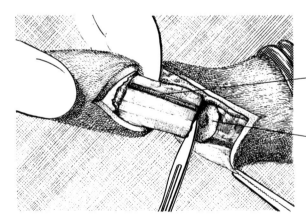

Lateral coccygeal artery

Intervertebral fibrocartilage

Fig. 11.30. The tail is removed by disarticulation and the coccygeal artery and lateral coccygeal arteries picked up and ligated.

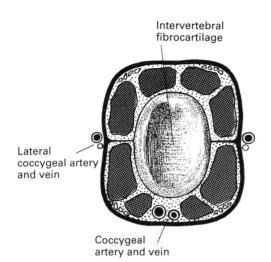

Fig. 11.31. Cross-section representation of the tail at point of disarticulation. Note the positions of the coccygeal arteries.

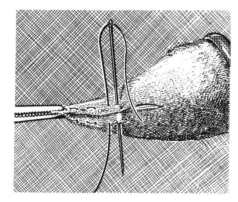

Fig. 11.32. The end of the coccygeal vertebra is protected and the wound closed by co-apting the skin flaps with interrupted mattress sutures.

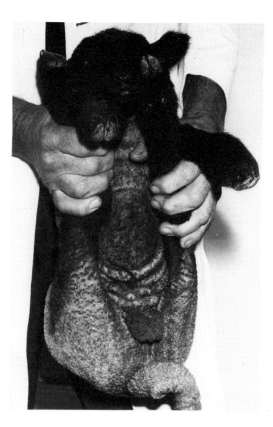

Fig. 11.33. The correct method of holding and restraining a lamb for docking.

LAMB

Lambs are generally docked when a few days old using the 'rubber ring' method (Figs 11.33–11.34). The contraction of the rubber ring produces a pressure necrosis of the underlying tissues which results in the tail separating in 10–12 days. It causes little discomfort, no haemorrhage ensues, sepsis is rare and the stump heals by granulation.

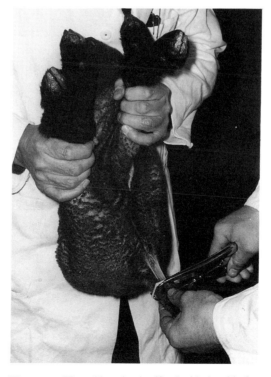

Fig. 11.34. The rubber ring is affixed with the aid of an Elastrator instrument and is adjusted to lie just distal to the caudal fold. Care should be taken not to weaken the contraction of the ring by over-stretching it.

Section 12
Miscellaneous Procedures

Repair of accidental skin wounds

Many accidental skin wounds are irregular and infected, with the skin edges either bruised or devitalized so that primary union is impossible. Bruised and infected tissue tends to slough, leaving an area which eventually heals slowly by granulation. This often leaves a large scar, devoid of hair, which gradually contracts giving rise to unsightly contraction lines.

Provided excessive amounts of skin have not been lost, these skin wounds can often be closed by direct suture, which avoids the lengthy process of healing by granulation and the subsequent unsightly scarring. Even in cases where sloughing is anticipated suturing should be attempted, as inevitably a limited amount of primary union will take place, leaving less tissue to heal by granulation.

In cases with considerable local tissue damage, it is sometimes necessary to carry out extensive wound debridement, and then to wait until healing by granulation is well established before attempting wound closure. During this process the skin edges become adherent to the underlying granulating tissue, and so lose their elasticity. Therefore, before attempting to co-apt the skin edges, it is essential to free them from the underlying tissue and to undermine the skin for some distance around the wound edges in order to produce the maximum skin mobility. It is equally important to ensure that the granulating surface is healthy, free from infection and below the level of the surrounding skin. In many wounds with irregular edges and skin retraction it is not possible to co-apt the skin edges by direct suture without first removing the exuberant granulation tissue and excising and undermining the surrounding skin (Fig. 12.1).

When dealing with extensive skin wounds which cannot be closed by direct suture, the edges of the defect may be relieved of tension by counter-incision (Fig. 12.2).

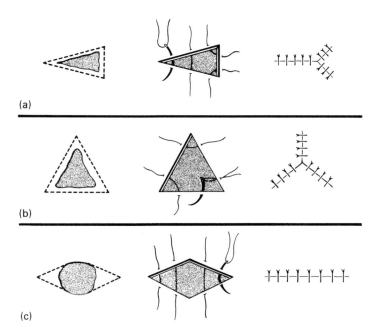

Fig. 12.1. Methods of closing irregular wounds by skin excision and direct suture.

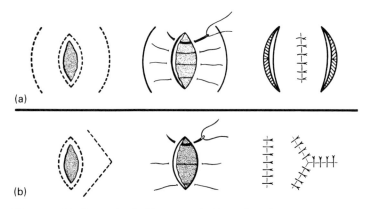

Fig. 12.2. (a) Closure by double counter-incision. The skin between the defect and the counter-incision is undermined. In many cases, after co-apting the edges of the defect it is then possible to suture together the edges of the counter-incisions, but if not they are left to heal by granulation. (b) Closure by a single counter-incision. The skin between the defect and the counter-incision is undermined, and after co-apting the defect the counter-incision is closed by Y-plasty.

Tendon injuries

Ruptures and wounds of tendons are most frequently encountered in the horse and dog. All skin wounds in the vicinity of tendons must be carefully explored as the size of the wound gives no indication of the damage to the underlying tendon. The digital flexor tendons are the tendons most frequently involved. Any wound on the caudal aspect of the limb below the carpus or hock must be viewed with the utmost concern. Little alteration will be seen in limb posture if the damage is limited to the superficial digital flexor tendon, but if the deep digital flexor is also severed, characteristic lifting of the toe is evident when weight is borne on the leg. When the suspensory or distal sesamoidean ligaments are damaged there will be marked sinking of the fetlock. The wounds are often grossly contaminated with involvement of the tendon sheath.

TENDON REPAIR

Under general anaesthesia an extensive area above and below the wound is prepared for aseptic surgery. A long skin incision is frequently necessary to expose the ends of the tendons which may have retracted a considerable distance. Before attempting to repair the tendon all frayed avascular and contaminated tissue must be removed and the ends trimmed back until normal tendon tissue is exposed. When the damage has been caused by a sharp object, such as glass, the amount of tendon which has to be removed is minimal making it feasible to join the ends by suturing using a strong non-irritating suture material such as stainless steel. However, traumatic severence of the digital flexors in the horse by over-reach wounds when the animal is moving at speed frequently results in severe fraying of the tendon ends. In these cases the considerable gap which is left between the ends of the tendon when all the irreparable tissue has been removed must be bridged by using a prosthetic material which will act as a scaffold for neontendon formation. Twisted or plaited carbon fibre and polyester fibre have been used successfully for this purpose. The fibre is embedded in T-shaped incisions in the two ends of the tendon and anchored with interrupted sutures of absorbable synthetic material (Fig. 12.3). The paratendon and subcutaneous tissues are closed separately in a simple continuous pattern and the skin with simple interrupted sutures. The wound is dressed with sterile gauze and the leg is cast in a slightly flexed position up to the level of the carpus or tarsus for 7–10 weeks. In the horse, following removal of the cast continuing support for the healing tendon is provided by a shoe with extended branches.

TENDON SUTURE

Numerous suture patterns exist for the repair of tendons but the following three will be found suitable for most occasions. Round tendons may be sutured using a locking loop pattern (Fig. 12.4) or a triple pulley suture (Fig. 12.5). Flat tendons are

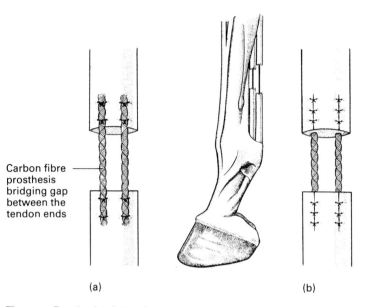

Carbon fibre prosthesis bridging gap between the tendon ends

(a)   (b)

Fig. 12.3. Repair of deficit in flexor tendons using carbon or polyester fibre prosthesis. (a) By suture with absorbable synthetic material to the surface of the tendon. (b) By implantation into ⊥-shaped incisions into the tendon and suture.

best sutured using a variation of the Ford interlocking suture (Fig. 12.6).

INFERIOR CHECK LIGAMENT DESMOTOMY

Severe contraction of the deep flexor tendon in foals which does not respond to manual stretching, paring down of the heel, and extension of the toe, can be treated successfully by desmotomy of the inferior check ligament.

With the patient in lateral recumbency under general anaesthesia, the check ligament is approached from the lateral or medial aspect in the proximal third of the metacarpus (Fig. 12.7a). Identification of the ligament is facilitated by the use of an Esmarch bandage. The skin, subcutis and deep fascia are incised along the cranial border of the deep flexor tendon (Fig. 12.7b). The groove between the check ligament and the deep flexor tendon is identified allowing the ligament to be isolated with dissecting scissors and transected (Fig. 12.7c). Fascia and skin are sutured with absorbable suture material and an elastic bandage applied from coronet to carpus. Some improvement in the position of the foot is evident immediately postoperatively but daily exercise on a hard surface is necessary to complete the stretching of the muscle – tendon unit. This process is helped by shortening the heel and applying a shoe with an extended toe.

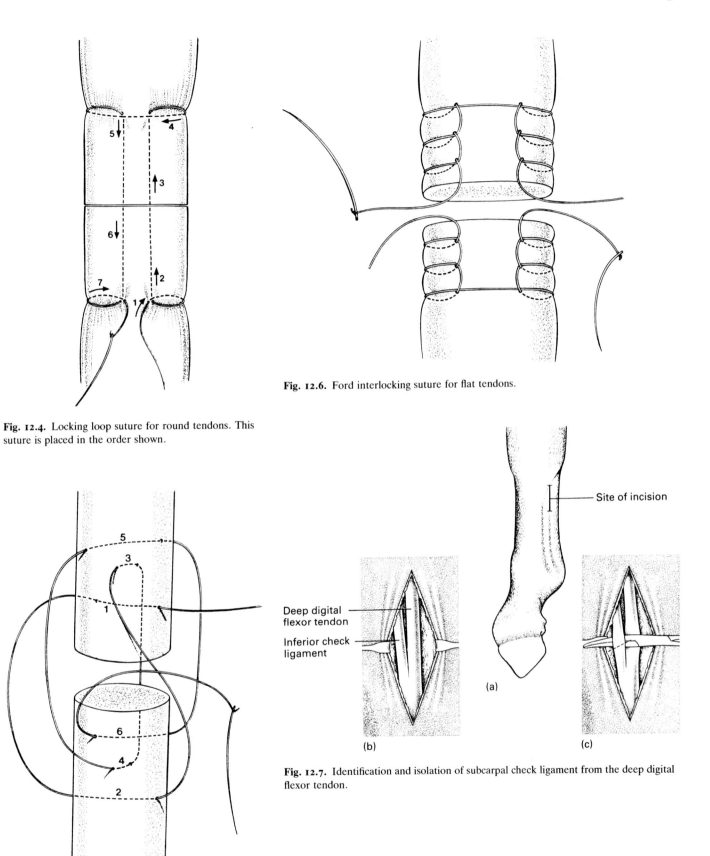

Fig. 12.4. Locking loop suture for round tendons. This suture is placed in the order shown.

Fig. 12.5. Triple pulley suture for round tendons. This is a stronger suture pattern then the locking loop.

Fig. 12.6. Ford interlocking suture for flat tendons.

Fig. 12.7. Identification and isolation of subcarpal check ligament from the deep digital flexor tendon.

Prolapse of the rectum

This condition occurs in all species, but is most common in the pig. In the majority of cases there is no obvious cause for the condition, and providing that there is no irreversible damage to the prolapsed rectum, it can easily be replaced and maintained in position by means of a purse-string suture placed around the anus.

If, however, the prolapse has been present for some time, then an intense venous congestion of the prolapsed viscus will occur. In addition, the congested and devitalized tissue may become traumatized to such a degree that amputation offers the only hope for successful treatment (Fig. 12.8). Before attempting amputation, it is necessary to pass a probe between the prolapse and the anal ring in order to ascertain that one is dealing with a rectal prolapse, and not with the terminal portion of a piece of intussuscepted small intestine.

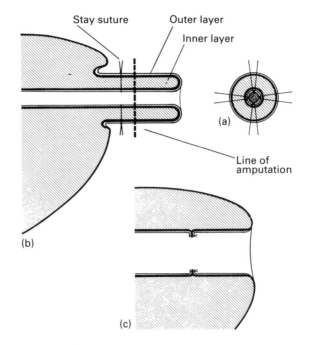

Fig. 12.8. (a) In order to prevent the inner portion of the prolapse retracting into the abdominal cavity after amputation, a stay suture should be inserted into each quadrant through all layers of the prolapse, using strong suture material of any type. (b) The rectum is amputated distal to the stay sutures, and any bleeding vessels picked up and ligated. The outer and inner layers of the amputated rectum are then sutured together, using interrupted sutures of a suitable size synthetic absorbable material. (c) The stay sutures are removed and the stump returned through the anus. A purse-string suture is inserted around the anal ring, and tied just tight enough to prevent a further prolapse, yet allowing sufficient room for defecation. It should be removed 48 hours later.

....

Excision of anal sacs — dog

The anal sacs lie on the ventrolateral aspect of the anus, deep to the external anal sphincter muscle, and their ducts open on the mucocutaneous border of the rectum. They are adequately supplied with blood from both the caudal rectal and the perineal arteries (Fig. 12.9).

In order to ensure the complete removal of the anal sac it is common practice to outline the sac with a variety of packing materials. These vary from cotton wool, wax, to plaster-of-Paris, but modern dental impression plastics are probably the most suitable for this purpose. These have a relatively short 'pot life' but long enough to enable the material to be injected into the sac through its excretory duct. After setting, the plastic remains rubber-like in texture and allows easy identification of the anal sacs. To excise the anal sacs the skin is incised over them on either side of the anal opening. By blunt dissection the sac is freed, the duct isolated, ligated with 3 metric synthetic absorbable suture material and removed. Due to the extensive blood supply, haemostasis must be of a high stan-

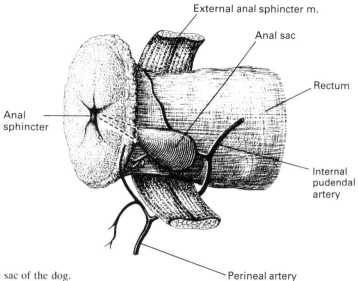

Fig. 12.9. The blood supply to the anal sac of the dog.

dard, and care must be taken to obliterate the dead space created by removal of the sac with a continuous 2 metric synthetic absorbable suture before suturing the skin.

Caslick's operation for pneumovagina — mare

In a mare of normal conformation, the caudal part of the vagina acts as a valve which prevents the aspiration of air and bacterial contaminants into the genital tract (Fig. 12.10). This valve effect may be destroyed by injury to the perineum at foaling, or impaired by defects in conformation which may be either congenital, or acquired with age. The aspiration of air and bacteria into the vagina leads to vaginitis and cervicitis, and is a serious cause of infertility in mares, particularly of Thoroughbreds.

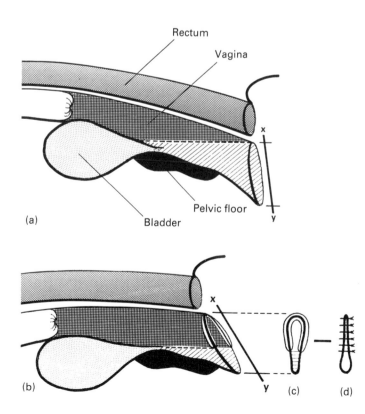

Fig. 12.10. (a) Diagrammatic representation of the normal vaginal seal. The angle of the line $x-y$ is approximately 80° and the upper commissure of the vulva is level with the floor of the pelvis, producing a valvular seal against the aspiration of air and bacteria into the anterior vagina. (b) Cranial retraction of the anus causes a forward tilting of the vulva, and draws the upper commissure of the vulva above the level of the pelvic floor, thus destroying the valvular seal. (c) A thin strip of tissue on either side of the mucocutaneous junction of the upper commissure of the vulva is dissected away to just below the level of the pelvic floor. (d) The raw surfaces are held together by sutures or metal clips until healing is complete.

In his discussion of the causes of pneumovagina in the mare, Caslick stated, 'To have a normal constriction between the vulva and vagina, the mare should have what one might term an ideal vulva. It should lie at an angle of about 80°, and the union of the upper commissure should extend below the floor of the pelvic girdle.' He went on to suggest that a simple remedy to the condition of pneumovagina would be to suture together the upper commissure of the vulva to just below the level of the pelvic floor, which would re-establish the vulval seal and thus eliminate the pneumovagina.

Within a few weeks, vaginal swabs will reveal a normal bacterial flora. The sutured upper commissure of the vulva may split during service and parturition, and in both cases will require resuturing.

Perineal reconstruction — mare

Tearing of the upper commissure of the vulva during the violent second stage of labour in the mare may rapidly progress to splitting of both the perineum and the anal sphincter, resulting in a third-degree perineal laceration with the formation of a recto-vaginal fistula (Fig. 12.11). This not only leads to faecal contamination of the vagina, but by destroying the natural seal of the posterior vagina also allows air to be aspirated into the vagina.

Early attempts to repair this very serious injury aimed at reconstructing both the roof of the vagina and the floor of the rectum at a single operation. They were frequently unsuccessful due mainly to the dry and bulky faecal bolus in the mare which overstretched and eventually tore open the suture lines. In view of this it was suggested by W.A. Aanes that the repair should be carried out in two stages (Figs 12.12–12.15):

1 To repair the vaginal roof which would function at the same time as the floor of the rectum. No attempt was to be made to close the anal sphincter.

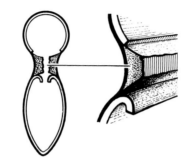

Fig. 12.12. A strip of vaginal mucous membrane is dissected free from the V-shaped shelf of connective tissue which demarcates the remains of the vaginal roof and the rectal floor. This creates a strip of raw tissue on either side of the defect.

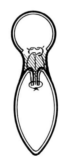

Fig. 12.13. The raw edges are drawn together by a series of interrupted sutures preferably of non-absorbable material. Insertion of these sutures is commenced at the cranial end of the defect, gradually working backwards until the roof of the vagina is closed to the level of the perineum. The free edges of vaginal mucous membrane are drawn together by a continuous synthetic absorbable suture, which is inserted simultaneously with the interrupted sutures.

This closure creates a roof to the vagina, which in turn acts as the floor of the rectum, preventing faecal contamination of the vagina. The perineum and anal sphincter are left open in order to allow the easy passage of faeces during the healing period. The mare will, however, continue to aspirate air into the vagina.

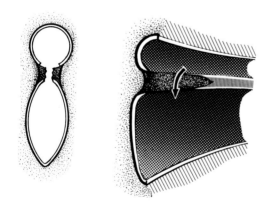

Fig. 12.11. Third-degree laceration of the perineum. Schematic section through the rectum, vagina and perineal body. The arrow indicates the passage of faeces from rectum to vagina.

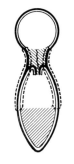

Fig. 12.14. A strip of tissue is cut from the mucocutaneous border of the upper commissure of the vulva and from the perineal scar tissue. Note that the lower margin of the strip extends below the floor of the pelvis, to ensure the reconstruction of the posterior vaginal seal.

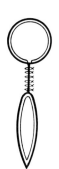

Fig. 12.15. The perineum is reconstructed by suturing together the raw edges using the same principles as that devised by Caslick (Fig. 12.10).

2 To reconstruct the vaginal seal and the perineum by using a modification of Caslick's operation (see p. 265).

In order to ensure success, the first stage of the operation is not attempted until the edges of the recto-vaginal tear are completely healed and all potentially necrotic tissue has sloughed. This means a period of 3–6 weeks following the injury. The second procedure is normally carried out within 10–14 days of the first.

....

Cryotherapy

The principle of cryotherapy is to produce tissue necrosis by freezing. The efficacy of the treatment depends partly upon the type of tissue to be frozen, but more significantly upon the type of freezing technique and the cryogen used. There are two major techniques, freezing with a cryoprobe or with a spray. Cryoprobes are suitable for small areas but where large masses or regions require freezing it is advisable to use a spray.

The cryogens in common use are gaseous nitrous oxide and liquid nitrogen. The former can only be delivered through a probe whereas liquid nitrogen can be used either as a probe or spray. Liquid nitrogen also possesses the advantage of being a much colder, and therefore more potent, cryogen. It has a boiling point of −196°C which permits rapid cooling of tissues. It is necessary to produce tissue temperatures of approximately −30°C in order to achieve adequate destruction and the best results are obtained by freezing the tissues rapidly and allowing them to thaw slowly. In practice, a double freeze–thaw cycle is employed to ensure effective destruction.

Nitrous oxide machines are designed to be attached to anaesthetic nitrous oxide bottles. These are readily available and wastage is minimal. Liquid

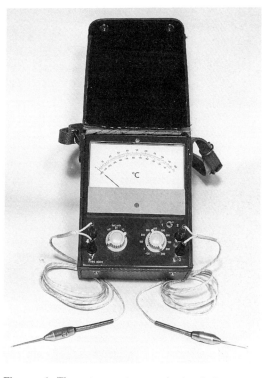

Fig. 12.16. Tissue temperature monitoring device together with tissue probes.

nitrogen is now also readily available and can be stored for extended periods in modern dewars. There is still some loss during storage due to evaporation but recent advances in the design of holding containers have largely overcome this problem.

Cryoprobes may be used in a number of ways. Contact freezing, as its name implies, entails freezing the tissue by applying the probe to its surface. Stab freezing can be performed by incising into the area to be frozen and inserting the probe into its centre. This is particularly suitable for solid masses. Large areas or big tumours may either be debulked surgically before freezing, or overlapping iceballs must be created to cover the entire region. Whatever technique is employed, it is necessary to obtain adhesion between the probe and the area before freezing is effective. This is not a problem where the surface of the area is moist but on occasions cryoadhesion must be improved by the application of a water-soluble jelly. Freezing with a spray technique is slightly less controlled but much less time-consuming and more efficient. Spray-cones are available which concentrate the cryogen to a given area and increase its effect.

Following freezing, the tissues within the iceball will either slough, or form a dry, leathery eschar which slowly detaches from the underlying tissues. Although the process of sloughing may produce an ugly and often offensive wound, the process is painless to the patient as the local nerve endings are destroyed within the iceball. Once sloughing is complete the area will heal by granulation tissue and produce relatively small amounts of scar tissue.

Cryotherapy is commonly employed for the

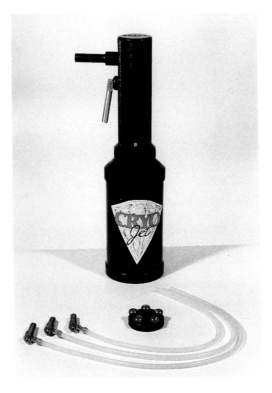

Fig. 12.17. Crojet unit (CryoTech Ltd, Ripley, UK) with a variety of probes. These are interchangeable with different sized spray attachments.

removal of surface tumours in all species, especially sarcoids in horses, the removal of some tumours of the oropharynx, the treatment of chronic infective lesions such as anal furunculosis, as a cryoneurectomy technique, for disbudding of goats, for the removal of anal sacs and for many other procedures.

Bibliography

Amstutz, H.E. (1980) *Bovine Medicine and Surgery*, Vols I and II. American Veterinary Publications, Santa Barbara, California.

Auer, J.A. (1992) *Equine Surgery*. W.B. Saunders, Philadelphia.

Barnett, K.C. (1989) *A Colour Atlas of Veterinary Ophthalmology*. Wolfe Medical Publications, London.

Blowey, R. & Weaver, A.D. (1991) *Colour Atlas of Diseases and Disorders of Cattle*. Wolfe Publishing, London.

Bojrab, M.J. (1990) *Current Techniques in Small Animal Surgery*, 3rd edn. Lea & Febiger, Philadelphia.

Brinker, W.O., Hohn, R.B. & Prieur, W.D. (1984) *Manual of Internal Fixation in Small Animals*. Springer-Verlag, Berlin.

Brinker, W.O., Piermattei, D.L. & Flo, G.L. (1990) *Handbook of Small Animal Orthopaedics and Fracture Treatment*, 2nd edn. W.B. Saunders, Philadelphia.

Colahan, P.T., Mayhew, I.G., Merritt, A.M. *et al.* (1991) *Equine Medicine and Surgery*, 4th edn. (2 vols). American Veterinary Publications, Santa Barbara, California.

Cox, J.E. (1987) *Surgery of the Reproductive Tract in Large Animals*, 3rd edn. Liverpool University Press, Liverpool.

Fackelman, G.E. & Nunamaker, D.M. (1982) *Manual of Internal Fixation in the Horse*. Springer-Verlag, Berlin.

Gelatt, K.N. (1991) *Veterinary Ophthalmology*. Lea & Febiger, Philadelphia.

Hall, L.W. & Clarke, K.W. (1991) *Veterinary Anaesthesia*, 9th edn. Baillière Tindall, London.

Helper, L.C. (1989) *Magrane's Canine Ophthalmology*. Lea & Febiger, Philadelphia.

Hickman, J. (1966) *Equine Surgery and Medicine*, Vols I and II. Academic Press, London.

Hickman, J. (1988) *Hickman's Farriery*, 2nd edn. J.A. Allen, London.

Houlton, J.E.F. & Collinson, R.W. (1994) *Manual of Small Animal Arthrology*. British Small Animal Veterinary Association, Cheltenham.

Jennings, P.B. (1984) *The Practice of Large Animal Surgery*, Vols 1 and 2. W.B. Saunders, Philadelphia.

McIlwraith, C.W. (1989) *Diagnostic and Surgical Arthroscopy in the Horse*, 2nd edn. Lea & Febiger, Philadelphia.

McIlwraith, C.W. & Turner, A.S. (1988) *Equine Surgery: Advanced Techniques*. Lea & Febiger, Philadelphia.

Mayhew, I.G. (1989) *Large Animal Neurology*. Lea & Febiger, Philadelphia.

Newton, C.D. & Nunamaker, D.M. (1985) *Textbook of Small Animal Orthopaedics*. Lippincott & Co., Philadelphia.

Oliver, J.E., Hoerlin, B.F. & Mayhew, I.G. (1987) *Veterinary Neurology*. W.B. Saunders, Philadelphia.

Piermattei, D.L. (1993) *An Atlas of Surgical Approaches to the Bones and Joints of the Dog and Cat*. W.B. Saunders, Philadelphia.

Short, C.E. (1987) *Principles and Practice of Veterinary Anaesthesia*. Williams & Wilkins, Baltimore.

Slatter, D.H. (1985) *Textbook of Small Animal Surgery*, Vols 1 and 2. W.B. Saunders, Philadelphia.

Stashak, T.S. (1987) *Adams' Lameness in Horses*. Lea & Febiger, Philadelphia.

Swaim, S.F. & Henderson, R.A. (1989) *Small Animal Wound Management*. Lea & Febiger, Philadelphia.

Walker, D.F. & Vaughan, J.T. (1980) *Bovine and Equine Urogenital Surgery*. Lea & Febiger, Philadelphia.

Wheeler, S.J. (ed.) (1989) *Manual of Small Animal Neurology*. British Small Animal Veterinary Association, Cheltenham.

White, N.A. (1989) *Equine Acute Abdomen*. Lea & Febiger, Philadelphia.

White, R.A.S. (ed.) (1991) *Manual of Small Animal Oncology*. British Small Animal Veterinary Association, Cheltenham.

Whittick, W.G. (1989) *Canine Orthopaedics*. Lea & Febiger, Philadelphia.

Wyn-Jones, G. (1988) *Equine Lameness*. Blackwell Scientific Publications, Oxford.

Index